The Duke Manual of Vitreoretinal Surgery

The Duke Manual of Vitreoretinal Surgery

Sharon Fekrat, MD, FACS
Professor, Ophthalmology
Associate Professor, Surgery
Duke University School of Medicine
Durham, North Carolina

Associate Editors

Avni Patel Finn, MD, MBA
Fellow, Vitreoretinal Surgery
Duke University School of Medicine
Durham, North Carolina

Akshay S. Thomas, MD, MS
Fellow, Vitreoretinal Surgery
Duke University School of Medicine
Durham, North Carolina

Illustrations by Xi Chen, MD, PhD
Assistant Professor, Ophthalmology
Duke University School of Medicine
Durham, North Carolina

Wolters Kluwer

Philadelphia • Baltimore • New York • London
Buenos Aires • Hong Kong • Sydney • Tokyo

DukeHealth

Acquisitions Editor: Chris Teja
Development Editor: Eric McDermott
Editorial Coordinator: John Larkin
Marketing Manager: Phyllis Hitner
Production Project Manager: Kim Cox
Design Coordinator: Teresa Mallon
Manufacturing Coordinator: Beth Welsh
Prepress Vendor: SPi Global

9 8 7 6 5 4 3 2 1

Printed in China

Cataloging-in-Publication Data available on request from the Publisher

ISBN: 978-1-9751-1790-0

Shop.lww.com

CCS0920

Contributors

Mohsin H. Ali, MD
Retina Group of Washington
Sterling, Virginia

Andrew N. Antoszyk, MD
Assistant Consulting Professor
Duke University Eye Center
Durham, North Carolina

Sruthi Arepalli, MD
Vitreoretinal Surgery Fellow
Cole Eye Institute
Cleveland Clinic
Cleveland, Ohio

Jorge Arroyo, MD, MPH
Associate Professor of Ophthalmology
Harvard Medical School
Director of the Retina Service
Division of Ophthalmology
Beth Israel Deaconess Medical Center
Boston, Massachusetts

Adam AufderHeide, MD, PhD
Retina Care Center
Medford, Oregon

Jaycob Avaylon, BS
Clinical Research Associate
Retina Macula Institute Research Center
Torrance, California

Claxton Baer, MD, PhD
Department of Surgery
Carolinas Medical Center–Northeast
Cabarrus Eye Center
Concord, North Carolina

Erica E. Ballard, MD
Vitreoretinal Surgery Fellow
Mercy Eye Clinic Specialists
Springfield, Missouri

Adam Berger, MD
Center for Retina and Macular Disease
Winter Haven, Florida

Durga S. Borkar, MD
Assistant Professor of Ophthalmology
Department of Ophthalmology
Duke University
Durham, North Carolina

Kevin Broderick, MD
Assistant Professor
Department of Surgery
Uniformed Services University of the Health Sciences
Bethesda, Maryland
Vitreoretinal Fellow
Department of Ophthalmology
The Retina Group of Washington
Chevy Chase, Maryland

Frank Brodie, MD, MBA
Vitreoretinal Fellow
Department of Ophthalmology
Duke University
Durham, North Carolina

Mark Cahill, MCh, MMedSci, FRCSI, FRCOphth, FEBO
Consultant Ophthalmologist
Royal Victoria Eye and Ear Hospital
Dublin, Republic of Ireland

Cindy X. Cai, MD
Vitreoretinal Surgery Fellow
Duke Eye Center
Duke University
Durham, North Carolina

Antonio Capone Jr, MD, FACS
Professor
Department of Ophthalmology
School of Medicine
Oakland University William Beaumont Hospital
Auburn Hills, Michigan

Sai H. Chavala, MD
Professor, Pharmacology and Neuroscience
Director, Translational Research
North Texas Eye Research Institute
University of North Texas Health Science Center
Fort Worth, Texas

Xi Chen, MD, PhD
Assistant Professor of Ophthalmology
Department of Ophthalmology
Duke University
Durham, North Carolina

Lawrence P. Chong, MD
Clinical Professor of Ophthalmology
Department of Ophthalmology
Keck School of Medicine
University of Southern California
Los Angeles, California

Mohammad Dahrouj, MD, PhD
Vitreoretinal Surgery Fellow
Retina Department
Massachusetts Eye and Ear/Harvard Medical School
Boston Massachusetts

Pouya N. Dayani, MD
Vitreoretinal Surgery and Ocular Inflammation
Retina-Vitreous Associates Medical Group
Los Angeles, California

Eugene de Juan Jr, MD
Clinical Professor
Department of Ophthalmology
University of California, San Francisco
San Francisco, California

Asad F. Durrani, MD
Resident Physician
Department of Ophthalmology and Visual Sciences
University of Michigan Kellogg Eye Center
Ann Arbor, Michigan

Justis P. Ehlers, MD
The Norman C. and Donna L. Harbert Endowed Chair for Ophthalmic Research
Cole Eye Institute
Cleveland Clinic
Cleveland, Ohio

Dean Eliott, MD
Stelios Evangelos Gragoudas Professor
Department of Ophthalmology
Harvard Medical School
Director, Retina Service
Department of Ophthalmology
Massachusetts Eye and Ear Infirmary
Boston, Massachusetts

Francisco A. Folgar, MD
Vitreoretinal Surgery Fellow
Carolina Eyecare Physicians
Charleston, South Carolina

Thomas R. Friberg, MD, MS
Professor
Department of Ophthalmology and Bioengineering
University of Pittsburgh
Chief
Retina Service
Department of Ophthalmology
University of Pittsburgh Medical Center
Pittsburgh, Pennsylvania

Ron P. Gallemore, MD, PhD
Assistant Professor
Department of Ophthalmology
School of Medicine
University of California, Los Angeles
Surgeon
Department of Ophthalmology
Good Samaritan Hospital
Los Angeles, California

Karen Gehrs, MD
Clinical Professor of Ophthalmology
Department of Ophthalmology and Visual Sciences
University of Iowa Hospitals and Clinics
Iowa City, Iowa

Shelley Day Ghafoori, MD
Clinical Assistant Professor
Department of Ophthalmology
Dell Medical School
University of Texas at Austin
Austin, Texas

Dilraj S. Grewal, MD
Associate Professor of Ophthalmology
Department of Ophthalmology
Duke University
Durham, North Carolina

Jóhann Ragnar Guðmundsson, MD
Adjunct Lecturer
School of Health Sciences
University of Iceland
Reykjavík, Iceland

Paul Hahn, MD
Partner
NJ Retina
Teaneck, New Jersey

Dean P. Hainsworth, MD
Professor
Department of Ophthalmology
University of Missouri
Columbia, Missouri

James T. Handa, MD
Robert Bond Welch Professor
Department of Ophthalmology
Johns Hopkins University
Chief
Retina Division
Wilmer Eye Institute
Johns Hopkins Medical Institutes
Baltimore, Maryland

Anne Hanneken, MD
Associate Professor
Department of Molecular Medicine
The Scripps Research Institute
Vitreoretinal Surgeon
Retina Consultants San Diego
Scripps Memorial Hospital
La Jolla, California

Thomas A. Hanscom, MD
Clinical Professor
Department of Ophthalmology
School of Medicine
University of California, Los Angeles
Los Angeles, California
The Retina Partners
Santa Monica, California

Christopher L. Haupert, MD
Adjunct Clinical Assistant Professor
Department of Ophthalmology
University of Iowa
Iowa City, Iowa

Glenn J. Jaffe, MD
Robert Machemer Professor of Ophthalmology
Chief, Vitreoretinal Division
Director, Duke Reading Center
Duke Eye Center
Durham, North Carolina

Alice C. Jiang, MD, MS
Resident Physician
Department of Ophthalmology
University of California, San Francisco
San Francisco, California

J. Michael Jumper, MD
West Coast Retina Medical Group
San Francisco, California

Joseph A. Khawly, MD, FACS
Assistant Professor of Clinical Ophthalmology
Institute for Academic Medicine
Houston Methodist/Weill Cornell Medical College
Clinical Instructor
Department of Ophthalmology
Baylor College of Medicine
Houston, Texas

James C. Lai, MD, MMM
Associate Clinical Professor
Department of Surgery
John A. Burns School of Medicine
University of Hawaii
Managing Partner
Retina Consultants of Hawaii
Honolulu, Hawaii

H. Michael Lambert, MD, FACS
Emeritus Professor
Department of Ophthalmology
Houston Methodist IAM/Weill Cornell/USUHS
Houston Methodist Hospital
Houston, Texas

Jeremy Lavine, MD, PhD
Assistant Professor
Department of Ophthalmology
Northwestern University
Chicago, Illinois

Phoebe Lin, MD, PhD
Associate Professor
Casey Eye Institute
Oregon Health & Science University
Portland, Oregon

Matthew W. MacCumber, MD, PhD
Professor and Associate Chair for Research
Department of Ophthalmology
Rush University Medical Center
Senior Physician
Illinois Retina Associates, SC
Chicago, Illinois

Tamer H. Mahmoud, MD, PhD
Professor
Department of Ophthalmology
School of Medicine
Oakland University William Beaumont
Royal Oak, Michigan

Joseph Martel, MD
Assistant Professor
Physician
Department of Ophthalmology
School of Medicine
University of Pittsburgh
Pittsburgh, Pennsylvania

Ankur Mehra, MD
Resident Physician
Department of Ophthalmology and Visual Sciences
University of Kentucky
Lexington, Kentucky

Alex Melamud, MD, MA
Retina Group of Washington
Sterling, Virginia

Lawrence S. Morse, MD, PhD
Professor of Ophthalmology
Department of Ophthalmology
University of California, Davis
Sacramento, California

Prithvi Mruthyunjaya, MD, MHS
Associate Professor of Ophthalmology
Ocular Oncology and Vitreoretinal Surgery
Director, Ocular Oncology Service
Director, Vitreoretinal Surgery Fellowship
Byers Eye Institute at Stanford University
Stanford, California

Roger L. Novack, MD, PhD, FACS
Retina Vitreous Associates Medical Group
Beverly Hills, California
Assistant Clinical Professor of Ophthalmology
Jules Stein Eye Institute
Geffen School of Medicine
University of California, Los Angeles
Los Angeles, California

Akousa Nti, MD
Vitreoretinal Fellow
The Wilmer Eye Institute
Department of Ophthalmology
Johns Hopkins School of Medicine
Baltimore, Maryland

Karl Olsen, MD
Clinical Assistant Professor
Department of Ophthalmology
University of Pittsburgh
Children's Hospital of Pittsburgh
Pittsburgh, Pennsylvania

Sally S. Ong, MD
Vitreoretinal Fellow
The Wilmer Eye Institute
Department of Ophthalmology
Johns Hopkins School of Medicine
Baltimore, Maryland

Carl H. Park, MD
Assistant Professor of Ophthalmology
Department of Ophthalmology
Thomas Jefferson University
Assistant Professor
Retina Service
Wills Eye Hospital
Philadelphia, Pennsylvania

Shriji Patel, MD
Assistant Professor of Ophthalmology
Co-Fellowship Director
Vitreoretinal Diseases and Surgery
Vanderbilt Eye Institute
Nashville, Tennessee

Andrew Pearson, MD
Professor and Chairman
Department of Ophthalmology and Visual Science
University of Kentucky
Lexington, Kentucky

Michelle Y. Peng, MD
West Coast Retina Medical Group
San Francisco, California

Eric Postel, MD
Professor
Duke University Eye Center
Chief, Ambulatory Surgery, Ophthalmology and Vice Chair, Ophthalmology
Department of Ophthalmology
Duke University Health System
Durham, North Carolina

Jawad Qureshi, MD, MBA
Founding Partner
Retina Center of Texas
Dallas, Texas

Jeffrey Rinkoff, MD
Staff
Department of Surgery
Ashland Asante Hospital
Ashland, Oregon

Nicholas Saba, BS
Medical Student
Department of Surgery
University of Connecticut School of Medicine
Farmington, Connecticut

Naryan Sabherwal, MD
Department of Ophthalmology
Rush University Medical Center
Illinois Retina Associates, SC
Chicago, Illinois

Christian J. Sanfilippo, MD
Associate Physician
The Retina Partners
Los Angeles, California

Ananth Sastry, MD
Vitreoretinal Surgery, PA
Minneapolis, Minnesota

Eric W. Schneider, MD
Tennessee Retina
Nashville, Tennessee

Adrienne Scott, MD
Associate Professor
Department of Ophthalmology
The Wilmer Eye Institute
Associate Professor
Department of Ophthalmology
Johns Hopkins School of Medicine
Baltimore, Maryland

Michael Seider, MD
Assistant Clinical Professor of Ophthalmology
Department of Ophthalmology
University of California–San Francisco
Codirector of Ocular Oncology and Vitreoretinal Surgeon
Department of Ophthalmology
The Permanente Medical Group
San Francisco, California

Harsha A. Sen, MD
Adjunct Instructor
Department of Ophthalmology
University of Alabama Birmingham
Birmingham, Alabama
Medical Director and Director of Retina Services
Eye Center South
Dothan, Alabama

Brendan Seto, BA
Clinical Research Assistant
Department of Ophthalmology
Beth Israel Deaconess Medical Center
Boston, Massachusetts

Sumit Sharma, MD
Assistant Professor of Ophthalmology
Cleveland Clinic–Cole Eye Institute
Cleveland Clinic Lerner College of Medicine
Cleveland, Ohio

Fadi Shaya, BSc
Clinical Research Coordinator
Dr Kent W. Small Macula and Retina Institute
Los Angeles, California

Belinda Shirkey, MD
Vitreoretinal Surgeon
Retina Associates of Kentucky
Lexington, Kentucky

R. Keith Shuler Jr, MD
Physician Partner
Southeastern Retina Associates
Clinical Assistant Professor
Department of Surgery
College of Medicine
The University of Tennessee Health Science Center
Knoxville, Tennessee

Jack O. Sipperley, MD
Director of Research
Retina Department
Barnet Dulaney Perkins Eye Center
Phoenix, Arizona

Kent Small, MD
President
Retina Department
Molecular Insight Research Foundation/Macula and Retina Institute
Glendale and Los Angeles, California

Einar Stefánsson, MD, PhD
Professor of Ophthalmology and Physiology
Editor-in-Chief
Acta Ophthalmologica University of Iceland
National University Hospital
Reykjavík, Iceland

Paul Sternberg Jr, MD
G.W. Hale Professor and Chair
Department of Ophthalmology and Visual Science
Chief Medical Officer
Vanderbilt Medical Group
Vanderbilt University Medical Center
Nashville, Tennessee

Eric Steuer, MD, PhD
Vitreoretinal Disease Specialist
Retina Associates, PC
Winchester, Virginia

Kenneth Taubenslag, MD
Second Year Fellow in Vitreoretinal Diseases and Surgery
Instructor in Ophthalmology and Visual Sciences
Department of Ophthalmology and Visual Sciences
Vanderbilt University Medical Center
Nashville, Tennessee

Daniel Ting, MD, PhD
Bay Area Retina Associates
Oakland, California

Cynthia A. Toth, MD
Joseph A.C. Wadsworth Professor of Ophthalmology
Professor of Biomedical Engineering
Department of Ophthalmology
Duke University Health System
Durham, North Carolina

Max Treacy, BA, BAI, MSc, FRCSI, FRCOphth, FEBO
Ophthalmologist and Managing Director
Medical Optics
Dublin, Ireland

Michael T. Trese, MD
Clinical Professor
Department of Ophthalmology
Oakland University William Beaumont
Rochester Michigan
Chief of Retina Service
Department of Ophthalmology
William Beaumont Hospital
Royal Oak, Michigan

Lejla Vajzovic, MD
Associate Professor of Ophthalmology
Department of Ophthalmology
Duke University Eye Center
Durham, North Carolina

Ryan N. Vogel, MD
Retina and Vitreous Consultants of Wisconsin
Milwaukee, Wisconsin

Scott D. Walter, MD, MSc
Assistant Clinical Professor
Department of Surgery
University of Connecticut School of Medicine
Farmington, Connecticut
Assistant Chief
Department of Ophthalmology
Hartford Hospital
Hartford, Connecticut

Johnathan Warminski, MD
Vitreoretinal Surgeon
Retina Center of Texas
Grapevine, Texas
Clinical Assistant Professor
Department of Ophthalmology
UT Southwestern Medical Center
Dallas, Texas

R. Joel Welch, MD
Vitreoretinal Surgery Fellow
Ophthalmology and Vision Science
UC Davis Eye Center
UC Davis Medical Center
Sacramento, California

Charles Wilson, MD
Retina Specialist
Department of Ophthalmology/Surgery
Cape Fear Valley Medical Center
Fayetteville, North Carolina

Glenn C. Yiu, MD, PhD
Associate Professor
Department of Ophthalmology & Vision Sciences
University of California, Davis
Davis, California
University of California, Davis Health
Sacramento, California

Wenlan Zhang, MD
Retina Northwest
Portland, Oregon

Xinxin Zhang, MD
Department of Ophthalmology
Duke University School of Medicine
Durham, North Carolina

John D. Zilis, MD
Clinical Associate Professor
Department of Ophthalmology
University of Colorado
Aurora, Colorado

Foreword

Vitreoretinal surgery at the Duke Eye Center has a rich tradition of surgical innovation. From the development of pars plana vitrectomy by Robert Machemer, MD, to the introduction of novel surgical instrumentation and techniques, to sharing it with others through the Advanced Vitreous Surgery (AVS) Course, many pioneers in our field can trace their inspiration to their time in the operating rooms in Durham, North Carolina. It is hard to believe that it has nearly been 30 years since I completed my vitreoretinal surgery fellowship training at Duke—a time when 20-gauge vitrectomy was the frontier of vitreoretinal surgery. As I peruse the 69 chapters in *The Duke Manual of Vitreoretinal Surgery*, it is a treat to delve into the surgical philosophies and practices of over 30 years of Duke vitreoretinal fellows and faculty summarized into this literary contribution.

Whether you are a casual home cook or a seasoned professional chef, having a tried and tested recipe at hand provides a framework that may be either improvised upon or followed step-by-step. Similarly, *The Duke Manual of Vitreoretinal Surgery* provides a roadmap for the simplest to the most complex vitreoretinal surgical scenarios and will prove to be invaluable, for both trainees at all levels as well as experienced vitreoretinal surgeons alike. The chapters have been configured to be essentially a cookbook for almost any surgical retina case. The chapters are concise yet comprehensive and ideal for a quick review the night before or the morning of a planned surgical procedure. Beyond a step-by-step description of surgical techniques, the Duke team shares the secret sauce for surgical success with the inclusion of a wide variety of topics including how and when to remove subretinal perfluorocarbon liquid, how to perform a direct perfluorocarbon silicone oil exchange, and tools to perform a chorioretinal biopsy, among many others. The illustrations, surgical photos, and online videos augment this impressive distillation of our current knowledge on vitreoretinal surgical techniques with tips and tricks from the Duke experience.

I congratulate the editors and all the chapter authors on this body of work that will have an enduring impact and domino effect on current and future vitreoretinal surgeons all over the world as they strive to save the vision of those patients who sit in their examination chair and enter their operating rooms.

Daniel F. Martin, MD
Chair, Cleveland Clinic Cole Eye Institute
Barbara and A. Malachi Mixon III Institute Chair in Ophthalmology
Professor of Ophthalmology
Cleveland Clinic Lerner College of Medicine of Case Western Reserve University
1990-91 Duke Vitreoretinal Surgery Fellow

Series Foreword

When you need to know how to approach a case that you may not be that familiar with, or when you want to review the many ways to drain subretinal fluid, or even when you need to know what to do next in the operating room when tackling a particularly challenging case, look no further. The answer lies here in the pages of *The Duke Manual of Vitreoretinal Surgery*. In one handy reference book such as this, you are able to explore reliable methods and techniques outlined by some of the most accomplished and competent vitreoretinal surgeons in order to achieve your surgical goals.

At the Duke Eye Center, we decided that we should not only share vitreoretinal surgical pearls in *The Duke Manual of Vitreoretinal Surgery* but also put in print some of the tips and tricks relied on in the operating room by some of the Duke Eye Center faculty in not only retina but also other ophthalmic subspecialties through *The Duke Manuals*. The intent of *The Duke Manuals* are not to circumvent traditional ophthalmic surgical training or create a substitute for the tried-and-true path to becoming a competent and skilled ophthalmic surgeon but instead to provide the student, resident, fellow, and practicing physician a review of the important factual and practical aspects of performing the different ophthalmic surgical procedures, step-by-step. *The Duke Manuals* are also an invaluable resource for the surgical assistant as well as the operating room nurse as they prepare for the surgical case and anticipate the surgeon's next move.

As Series Editor of *The Duke Manuals*, it has been especially rewarding to collaborate with many outstanding individuals in the profession of ophthalmology across the country who contributed to the series. All editors and authors have either trained at Duke or trained others as faculty at Duke. This series represents countless hours of involvement and work by so many busy surgeons; it could not have come together without their dedication to sharing their knowledge with all of you.

It is our hope that *The Duke Manuals* will serve as excellent resources and valuable references for students, residents, fellows, and practicing surgeons alike.

Sharon Fekrat, MD, FACS
Series Editor
Duke Vitreoretinal Surgery Faculty

Contents

Abbreviations

AC—anterior chamber
ACIOL—anterior chamber intraocular lens
AFX—air fluid exchange
AIDS—acquired immunodeficiency syndrome
AMD—age-related macular degeneration
AP—anterior-posterior
APD—afferent pupillary defect
BP—blood pressure
BRVO—branch retinal vein occlusion
BSS—balanced salt solution
CME—cystoid macular edema
CMV—cytomegalovirus
CNV—choroidal neovascularization
cpm—cuts per minute
CSF—cerebrospinal fluid
CT—computed tomography
D_5W—dextrose 5% in water
DD—disc diameter
DDX—differential diagnosis
EBV—Epstein-Barr virus
ERG—electroretinogram
ERM—epiretinal membrane
EUA—examination under anesthesia
FAX—fluid air exchange
FDA—Food and Drug Administration
FEVR—familial exudative vitreoretinopathy
FTMH—full-thickness macular hole
G—gauge
GA—geographic atrophy
GRT—giant retinal tear
HIV—human immunodeficiency virus
HOB—head of bed
HSV—herpes simplex virus
HZV—herpes zoster virus
ICG—indocyanine green
ILM—internal limiting membrane
IOFB—intraocular foreign body
IOL—intraocular lens
IOP—intraocular pressure
IRF—intraretinal fluid
IRH—intraretinal hemorrhage
IV—intravenous
LASIK—laser-assisted *in situ* keratomileusis
LP—light perception
mcg—microgram
MIVS—microincisional vitrectomy surgery
mL—milliliter
MRI—magnetic resonance imaging
ms—millisecond
MVR—microvitreoretinal
mW—milliwatt
NCVH—nonclearing vitreous hemorrhage
NLP—no light perception
nm—nanometer
NSAID—nonsteroidal anti-inflammatory drug
NV—neovascularization
NVD—neovascularization of the disc
NVI—neovascularization of the iris
OCT—optical coherence tomography
OR—operating room
PCIOL—posterior chamber intraocular lens
PCR—polymerase chain reaction
PCV—polypoidal choroidal vasculopathy
PFCL—perfluorocarbon liquid
PI—peripheral iridotomy
PPV—pars plana vitrectomy
PRH—preretinal hemorrhage
PRK—photorefractive keratectomy
PRP—panretinal laser photocoagulation
PVD—posterior vitreous detachment
PVR—proliferative vitreoretinopathy

RAM—retinal arterial macroaneurysms
RD—retinal detachment
ROP—retinopathy of prematurity
RP—retinitis pigmentosa
RPE—retinal pigment epithelium
RRD—rhegmatogenous retinal detachment
rtPA—recombinant tissue plasminogen activator
SB—scleral buckle
SRF—subretinal fluid
SRH—subretinal hemorrhage
TB—tuberculin
TRD—tractional retinal detachment
UGH—uveitis-glaucoma-hyphema
VA—visual acuity
VEGF—vascular endothelial growth factor
VH—vitreous hemorrhage
VMT—vitreomacular traction
VR—vitreoretinal
VZV—varicella-zoster virus

Section I

Just the Basics

CHAPTER 1

The Preoperative Discussion

Christian J. Sanfilippo, MD • Thomas A. Hanscom, MD

GOALS OF THE PREOP DISCUSSION

- Educate the cognitively competent patient or their appointed health care power of attorney to make an informed decision about whether to agree to or refuse the proposed surgical intervention.
- Educate about what to expect before, during, and after the intervention.
- Strengthen the trust and relationship between the doctor and patient.

INFORMED CONSENT DISCUSSION

Include the following about the proposed procedure:

- The diagnosis, if known
- An explanation of the purpose of and type of procedure
- An explanation of anticipated benefits, risks, and alternatives including what might be expected without intervention

Document this discussion in the medical record.

When multiple surgical options with different risk/benefit profiles are feasible options, as in the case of retinal detachment, discuss enough information during the informed consent process to allow an understanding as to why one particular surgical approach may be preferred over the other available options.

Include the following in the written informed consent document, at a minimum:

- The name of the surgical center or hospital where the surgery will take place
- The name of the procedure(s) to be performed
- The name of the surgeon(s) performing the procedure
- The indication(s), risks, benefits, and alternatives
- Specific risks and burdens of the surgery

Include other information in the consent form:

- Whether there will be videotaping of the surgical procedure
- Whether there will be observers present during the surgical procedure

- Whether there will be an M.D. assistant performing portions of the procedure
- Whether the surgeon will be running more than one room concurrently and available for critical portions of each procedure

The patient must have the ability to understand and cognitively process the information. If a patient lacks the ability to do so (cognitive capacity), obtain consent from their health care power of attorney. Specific state laws govern who may act as the health care power of attorney. When a language barrier exists, obtain an interpreter and provide a consent form written in the preferred language. Allow sufficient time for the patient or designee to read and understand the consent form, preferably in the clinic and not outside the OR room. Provide a signed copy of this document.

PLANNING FOR POSTOP CARE

Provide information about what to expect during the postop period.

Common Temporary Postop Changes: Pink (bloody) tears, eye redness, periorbital bruising/swelling, stinging during administration of postop eye drops, and expected vision impairment from tamponade agent use, among others.

Common Long-Term Postop Changes: Cataract progression in phakic individuals undergoing PPV, refractive changes in patients undergoing SB or lensectomy, recurrent RD, PVR, and need for silicone oil removal if used, among others.

Activity Restrictions: Temporary driving restrictions, positioning requirements, limited lifting/exercise, avoidance of exposure of the eye to water (bathing and swimming), avoidance of eye makeup, and altitude and flying restrictions. Estimate time off work and restrictions upon return to work.

Follow-Up Schedule: Give your patient an anticipated follow-up schedule. Tell them that they may need to be seen sooner if anything unexpected arises.

Specific Situations

Intraocular Gas

Vision is impaired while the gas bubble remains within the vitreous cavity, especially when it is in front of the macula. Explain this to the patient prior to surgery. Travel to altitudes higher than where the surgery was performed or travel by air must be restricted until the gas bubble has resolved. If an anesthetic agent is needed while the patient has gas in the eye, nitrous oxide should be avoided. Estimate the length of time that the gas is expected to remain within the eye prior to surgery. Consider having the patient wear a gas bubble bracelet or carry a card in their wallet notifying medical personnel that there is a gas bubble in the eye. See chapter titled *Gas Tamponade*.

Even a 10% intraocular gas bubble can cause a doubling of the IOP during changes in altitude, including the rapid ascent of air flight. Therefore, air travel should be completely restricted until the gas bubble has entirely resolved. In the event that a patient must travel by land to altitudes more than 1500 ft higher than where the surgery was performed, suggest a travel stop for 1 hour for each additional 1000 ft climbed before continuing on.

Silicone Oil

If used, the patient should be informed of the need for subsequent silicone oil removal. Silicone oil might be the tamponade of choice to avoid travel restrictions or to enhance a patient's visual function during the postop period. See chapter titled *Silicone Oil Tamponade*.

Positioning

When required, stress the importance of positioning to the ultimate success of the surgery to the patient. Give a complete explanation and demonstration of the exact position(s) that is needed for optimal gas tamponade. Enlisting the help and understanding of family members is important. In cases where prolonged facedown positioning is required, tell the patient about the option of renting a facedown massage chair or table for ergonomics and comfort. See chapter titled *Postop Positioning*.

Return Precautions

Educate the patient and family about which symptoms should prompt a call to the office or the on-call doctor, including severe or increasing ocular pain, headache, nausea, vomiting, or decreasing vision. Or, if they are unsure, tell them to contact the office or emergency contact numbers if any changes that do not seem right are noticed or if they want to talk about the symptoms so that the health care team can help decide when an examination is indicated.

CHAPTER 2

Vitrectomy Systems

Mohsin H. Ali, MD

See chapter titled *Vitrectomy Machine Settings*.

STELLARIS PC AND STELLARIS ELITE VISION ENHANCEMENT SYSTEMS (FIGS. 2.1 AND 2.2)

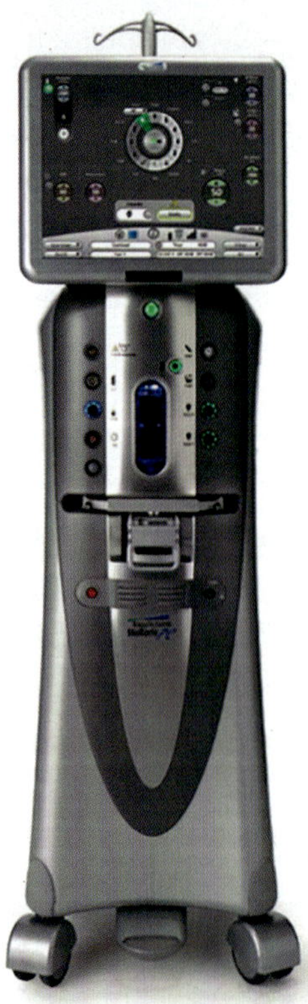

FIGURE 2.1. Stellaris PC (Bausch & Lomb, St. Louis, MO).

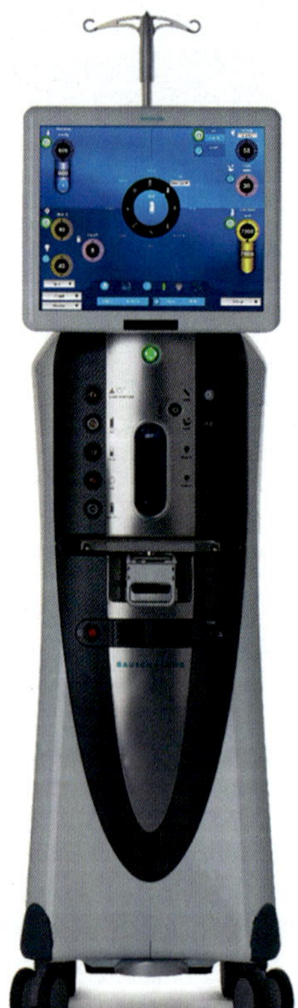

FIGURE 2.2. Stellaris Elite (Bausch & Lomb, St. Louis, MO).

Manufacturer: Bausch & Lomb (St. Louis, MO)

Pump Mechanism: Venturi (PC and Elite)

Phacoemulsification/Fragmatome Capability: Yes

Viscous Fluid Injection/Extraction Capability: Yes

Available Gauges: Stellaris PC: 20/23/25 gauge; Stellaris Elite: 20/23/25/27 gauge

Trocars/Cannulas/Valves: The translucent valves fit like caps over the cannulas. These can be easily removed (intentionally or inadvertently). Be careful handling the cannulas and passing them off the surgical field to ensure the translucent valves do not come off and become misplaced.

Maximum Cutter Speed

- Stellaris PC 5000 cpm
- Single-port cutter 7500 cpm (20/23/25 gauge, Stellaris Elite only)
- Bi-Blade cutter 15000 cpm (Fig. 2.3) (25/27 gauge, Stellaris Elite only)
- Vitesse cutter 1.7 million "virtual cuts per minute," hypersonic vitrector that causes hypersonic liquefaction of vitreous at the edge of the port (Stellaris Elite only) rather than traditional guillotine cutting.

Maximum Vacuum: 600 mm Hg (PC and Elite)

Color Filters: 3 color filters are available: amber, green tint, yellow tint. Try amber filter during FAX. Try green tint filter during membrane peeling.

Integrated Laser: Yes, 532 nm in both Stellaris PC and Elite. See chapter titled *Endolaser Types and Settings.*

Foot Pedal

- Stellaris Elite has a wireless, dual-linear foot pedal with integrated laser control.
- A separate laser pedal is not needed—the laser control is integrated into the base of the foot pedal (under the heel). A small cover over the heel area is raised to access the laser pedal.
- The dual-linear capability of the foot pedal allows independent control of 2 continuous functions simultaneously. This is most useful during fragmentation when the fragmatome vacuum control and fragmentation power can be controlled separately.

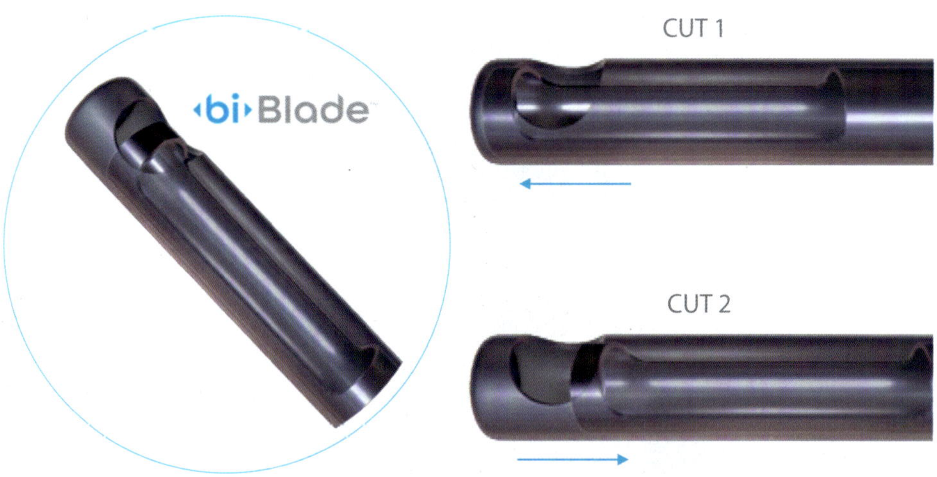

FIGURE 2.3. Bi-Blade cutter (Bausch & Lomb, St. Louis, MO) has a dual-port design that allows it to cut in two directions per cycle.

CONSTELLATION (FIG. 2.4)

Manufacturer: Alcon (Fort Worth, TX)

Pump Mechanism: Venturi

Phacoemulsification/Fragmatome Capability: Yes

Viscous Fluid Injection/Extraction Capability: Yes

Available Gauges: 20/23/25/27 gauge

Trocars/Cannulas/Valves: The valves are built into the cannula head (as opposed to caps that sit on the surface of the cannulas).

Maximum Cutter Speed

- Dual pneumatic cutter 7500-10 000 cpm. The 10k cutters have the additional advantage of a beveled end with a port closer to tip of the instrument shaft—helpful with the dissection of preretinal membranes (eg, diabetic TRD). The 7.5k cutters do not have beveled ends. Look for the "10k" label on the cutter handle to know which cutter you are using.
- The duty cycle open time can be varied between >50% (core mode—often used during the core vitrectomy), <50% (shave mode—often used when shaving the vitreous base or removing vitreous over detached, mobile retina), or 50% of the time (50/50 mode—rarely used).
- You can operate on proportional vacuum vitrectomy mode in which a high fixed cut rate is set (usually the maximum allowable, eg, 7500 or 10000 cpm) and vacuum is linearly varied with the foot pedal. Dual dynamic drive (3D) vitrectomy allows the cut rate and vacuum to be simultaneously linearly varied.

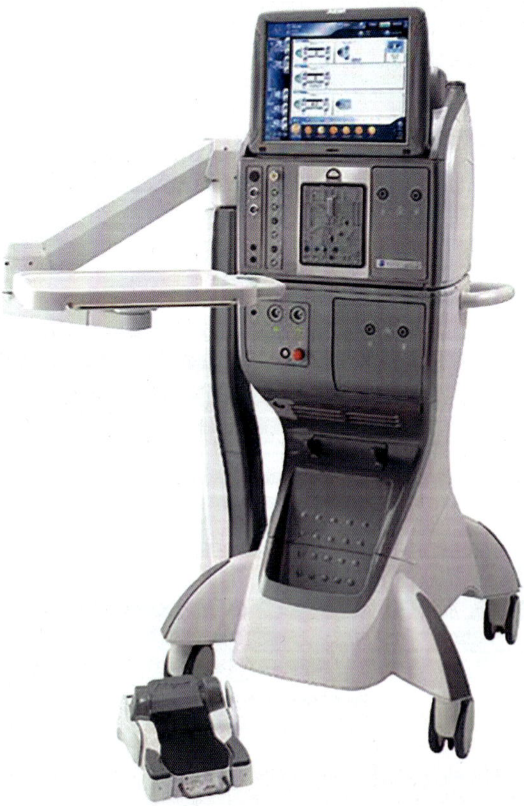

FIGURE 2.4. Constellation (Alcon, Fort Worth, TX).

Maximum Vacuum: 650 mm Hg

Chromovitrectomy: Built-in color filters are not available.

Integrated Laser: Yes, 532 nm. See chapter titled *Endolaser Types and Settings.*

Foot Pedal: Linear control and separate laser pedal

IOP Control

- Unlike other vitrectomy machines included here, the Constellation has an IOP compensation control that allows maintenance of particular IOP within approximately +/− 2 mm Hg of the value set on the machine. This feature can be toggled on or off. In general, the IOP compensation mode is activated during the entirety of most cases. You may elect to turn IOP compensation off during cannula placement.
- For IOP compensation to be properly calibrated, the patient's eye level must align with the lowest row of tubing connectors on the cassette. For example, if the patient's eye level is below the connectors, the actual IOP will be higher than that stated on the machine.

EVA (ENHANCING VISUAL ACUITY) (FIG. 2.5)

Manufacturer: Dutch Ophthalmic Research Corporation—DORC (Zuidland, The Netherlands)

Pump Mechanism

- Fluid control system combines a peristaltic pump system (in which vacuum is variable and flow is set) and Venturi pump system (in which vacuum is set and flow is variable).

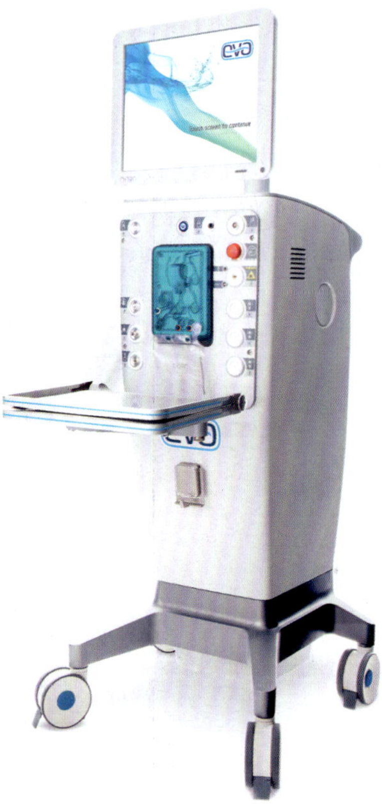

FIGURE 2.5. DORC EVA (Dutch Ophthalmic Research Corporation—DORC—Zuidland, The Netherlands).

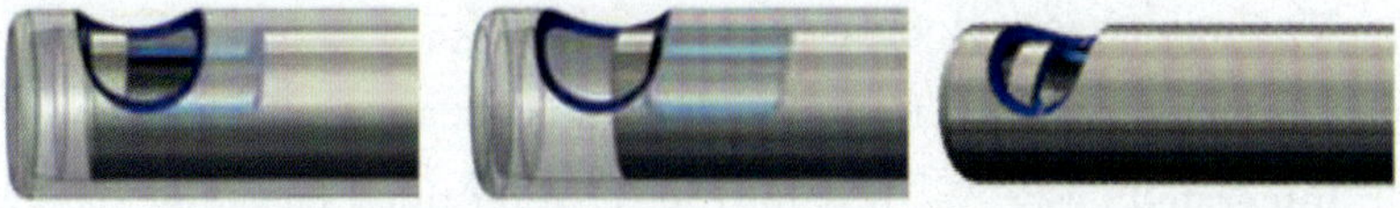

FIGURE 2.6. Similar to the Bi-Blade, the DORC TDC (two-dimensional cutting) cutter (Dutch Ophthalmic Research Corporation—DORC—Zuidland, The Netherlands) has a double opening in the internal guillotine blade to allow cutting during forward and backward movement of the blade.

- Vacuum mode is used for tasks in which efficiency is required (eg, core vitrectomy), and flow mode is used for shaving vitreous over detached, mobile retina. In contrast to operating with the Stellaris and Constellation machines, you may find that shaving with the flow mode on the EVA allows and requires bringing the cutter very close to the retina.

Phacoemulsification/Fragmatome Capability: Yes

Viscous Fluid Injection/Extraction Capability: Yes

Available Gauges: 20/23/25/27 gauge

Trocars/Cannulas/Valves: Silicone caps attached to the cannulas serve as valves and can be removed as needed. The valve should be removed prior to connecting the cannula to the high-flow infusion line.

Maximum Cutter Speed
- 8000 cpm with traditional, non-TDC cutter
- 16 000 cpm (constant open duty cycle of 92%) with two-dimensional cutting (TDC) (Fig. 2.6)
- TDC cutter achieves this high cut rate and duty cycle by having a double opening in the internal guillotine blade such that the vitreous is cut during both forward and backward movements of the blade.
- Prime the machine using a TDC cutting setting to benefit fully from the enhanced efficiency of the TDC cutter.

Maximum Vacuum: 680 mm Hg

Color Filters: LED illumination can be varied from white to yellow.

Integrated Laser: Yes, 532 nm. See chapter titled *Endolaser Types and Settings.*

Foot Pedal: Foot pedal is capable of dual linear control and integrated laser control.

VERSAVIT 2.0 (FIG. 2.7)

Manufacturer: Synergetics/Bausch & Lomb (St. Louis, MO)

Pump Mechanism: Micro-response diaphragm

Phacoemulsification/Fragmatome Capability: No

Viscous Fluid Injection/Extraction Capability: Yes

Available Gauges: 20/23/25/27 gauge

Trocars/Cannulas/Valves: Cannulas with removable valve caps available. Also available as a 3-in-1 cannula entry system in which all 3 cannulas are preloaded on a single blade.

Maximum Cutter Speed: 6000 cpm

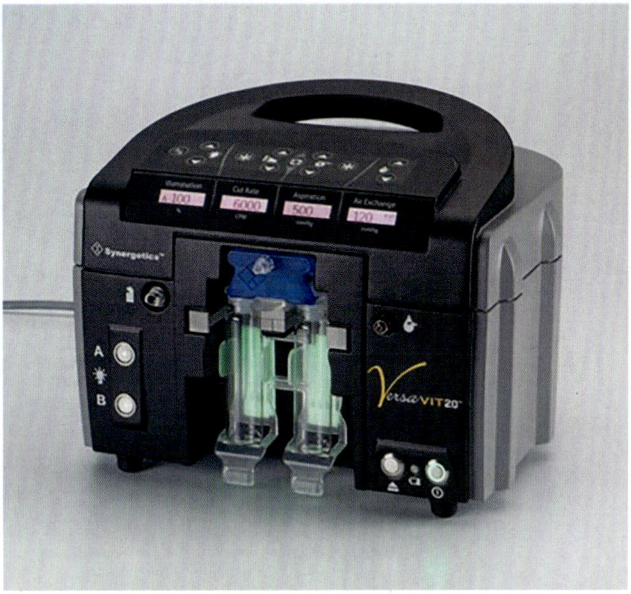

FIGURE 2.7. VersaVIT 2.0 (Synergetics/Bausch & Lomb, St. Louis, MO).

Maximum Vacuum: 500 mm Hg

Color Filters: Built-in color filters are not available.

Integrated Laser: No integrated laser. See chapter titled *Endolaser Types and Settings.*

Foot Pedal: Linear control

Other Considerations: Unlike other machines, this is small in size, lightweight, portable, low cost, and has a quick power-up time (30 seconds or less).

CHAPTER 3

Vitrectomy Machine Settings

Fadi Shaya, BSc ● Kent Small, MD

INFUSION AND INTRAOP IOP CONTROL

- Set the infusion IOP between 25 and 35 mm Hg.
  - Some machines may allow an "IOP compensation control" that allows you to maintain a particular IOP within ~+/– 2 mm Hg of the value set on the machine. See chapter titled *Vitrectomy Systems*.
- Utilizes flow sensors at the bottom of the cassette in the vitrectomy machine to automatically compensate to maintain a set IOP.
- IOP may be raised when there is bleeding to achieve hemostasis.
- Closely monitor increases in intraop infusion pressure and IOP in eyes with glaucoma.
- If performing PPV with high aspiration, be careful not to outrun the infusion as this can result in hypotony and consequences such as choroidal hemorrhage.
- Monitor perfusion of the central retinal artery.
  - In patients with retinal vascular disease or who are hypotensive, perfusion of the central retinal artery may require a lower infusion pressure.

Infusion fluids. BSS has a pH of 7.5 and osmolality of 300 mOsm/kg, 155.7 micromol/L sodium, 10.1 micromol/L potassium, 3.3 micromol/L calcium, 1.5 micromol/L magnesium, 128.9 micromol/L chloride, 5.8 micromol/L citrate, and 28.6 micromol/L acetate. BSS PLUS has pH of 7.4 and osmolality of 305 mOsm/kg, 160 micromol/L sodium, 5.0 micromol/L potassium, 1.0 micromol/L calcium, 1.0 micromol/L magnesium, 130 micromol/L chloride, 25 micromol/L bicarbonate, 3 phosphorus, 5 micromol/L glucose, and 0.3 micromol/L glutathione. The addition of glucose, glutathione, and bicarbonate to BSS PLUS decreases the likelihood of lens and corneal decompensation. 0.3 mL of 50% dextrose micromol/L can be added to the bottle in diabetics to prevent crystalline lens opacification. 0.3 mL of 1:1000 preservative-free epinephrine can be added to the bottle to maintain hemostasis and pupillary dilation. Do not use epinephrine in infusion fluid for sickle cell patients.

Cutter size: Smaller vitrectomy probes have allowed transition to the MIVS

- 23G, 25G, and 27G systems are currently used.
- The smaller gauge may decrease vitreous flow rate and reduce efficiency, particularly for the 27G system, though this is partially overcome by higher cutting speeds.

- One challenge of the 27G system when more manipulation is required is the increased flexibility of the instruments.

Cut rate: Measured as the number of cuts per minute (cpm).

- Increased cut rates result in smaller bites of vitreous and less traction on the retina, potentially decreasing the risk of iatrogenic retinal breaks.
- Currently available cut rates may vary from 5000 up to 16 000 cpm for bi-blade cutters or even 1.7 million virtual cuts per minute with hypersonic "cutters." See chapter titled *Vitrectomy Systems*.
- A higher cut rate may decrease traction on the vitreous and improve efficiency.
- The cut rate is lower on "dense mode" which is typically employed during lensectomy or the cutting of denser tissues.

CONSTELLATION SETTINGS

	20 gauge	**CPM**	**Vacuum**	**Infusion**	**FAX**	**Duty cycle**
Core Vit	Proportional/Core Vitrectomy	5000	0→300	25-30	25-30	Core
Retina Shave	Proportional/Shave Mode	3000	0→300	25-30	25-30	Shave
Vit Scissors	Proportional/Shave Mode	250	0→150	25-30	25-30	Shave
Vit Frag	Proportional/Core Vitrectomy	3500	0→300	25-30	25-30	Core
	Momentary	300	650	25-30	25-30	Core
	Extrusion		150→200	25-30	25-30	
	Diathermy Extra Ocular	40				
	Diathermy Intra Ocular	20				
	Proportional Diathermy	40				
	Micro Reflux	50→75				
	Proportional Reflux	0→120			Pulse	
	Frag All Modes		120	35	100 pps	

	23 gauge	**CPM**	**Vacuum**	**Infusion**	**FAX**	**Duty cycle**
Core Vit	Proportional/Core Vitrectomy	10 000	0→450	25-30	25-30	Core
Retina Shave	Proportional/Shave Mode	10 000	0→300	25-30	25-30	Shave
Vit Scissors	Proportional/Shave Mode	250	0→300	25-30	25-30	Shave
Vit Frag	Proportional/Core Vitrectomy	4000	0→650	25-30	25-30	Core
	Momentary	300	650	25-30	25-30	Core
	Extrusion		475			
	Diathermy Extraocular	40				
	Diathermy Intraocular	20				
	Proportional Diathermy	40				
	Micro Reflux	75→100				
	Proportional Reflux	0→120			Pulse	
	Frag All Modes		120	35	100 pps	

	25 gauge	**CPM**	**Vacuum**	**Infusion**	**FAX**	**Duty cycle**
Core Vit	Proportional/Core Vitrectomy	10 000	0→650	25-30	25-30	Core
Retina Shave	Proportional/Shave Mode	10 000	0→450	25-30	25-30	Shave
Vit Scissors	Proportional/Shave Mode	250	0→425	25-30	25-30	Shave
Vit Frag	Proportional/Core Vitrectomy	4000	0→650	25-30	25-30	Core
	Momentary	300	650	25-30	25-30	Core
	Extrusion		475			
	Diathermy Extra Ocular	40				
	Diathermy Intra Ocular	20				
	Proportional Diathermy	40				
	Micro Reflux	100				
	Proportional Reflux	0→120			Pulse	
	Frag All Modes		120	35	100 pps	

(Continued)

CONSTELLATION SETTINGS (*Continued*)

	27 gauge	CPM	Vacuum	Infusion	FAX	Duty Cycle
Core Vit	Proportional/Core Vitrectomy	10 000	0→650	25-30	25-30	Core
Retina Shave	Proportional/Shave Mode	10 000	0→650	25-30	25-30	Shave
Vit Scissors	Proportional/Shave Mode	250	0→425	25-30	25-30	Shave
Vit Frag	Proportional/Core Vitrectomy	4000	0→650	25-30	25-30	Core
	Momentary	300	650	25-30	25-30	Core
	Extrusion		475			
	Diathermy Extraocular	40				
	Diathermy Intraocular	20				
	Proportional Diathermy	40				
	Micro Reflux	100				
	Proportional Reflux	0→120				

Vacuum, Infusion, and FAX expressed in mm Hg.
PPS = pulses per second.

STANDARD ELITE AND STELLARIS PC SETTINGS

Elite	CPM	Vacuum	Infusion	Stellaris PC	CPM	Vacuum	Infusion
20G Proportional Core	5000	300-450	25-30		3000-5000	300-450	25-30
20G Proportional Shave	7500	150-200	25-30		5000	150-200	25-30
20G Extrusion		300-600	25-30			300-600	25-30
23G Proportional Core	5000	450	25-30		3000-5000	450-600	25-30
23G Shave	7500	150-200	25-30		5000	150-200	25-30
23G Extrusion		450-600	25-30			450-600	25-30
23G Bi-Blade Proportional Core	7500	300-450	25-40	N/A			
23G Bi-Blade Proportional Shave	7500	150	25-35	N/A			
25G Proportional Core	5000	450-600	25-30		3000-5000	450-600	25-30
25G Proportional Shave	7500	150-200	25-30		5000	150-200	25-30
25G Extrusion		600	25-30			600	25/30
25G Bi-Blade Proportional Core	7500	450-600	25-35	N/A			
25G Bi-Blade Proportional Shave	7500	150-200	25-35	N/A			
27G Extrusion		600	25-30			600	25-30
27G Bi-Blade Proportional Core	7500	600	25-30	N/A			
27G Bi-Blade Proportional Shave	7500	150-200	25-30	N/A			
FRAG (both systems)	U/S	PPS	Duty Cycle	Vacuum			
20G needle	10	80	40	450			
23G needle	10	80	40	450-600			

Vacuum, Infusion, and FAX expressed in mm Hg.
PPS = pulses per second.

23G EVA SETTINGS

Step 1: Core Vitrectomy	23G Standard	23G TDC	
VACUUM			
Cut Rate—Position 1	7000 CPM 3D	8000 CPM 3D or Linear	
Cut Rate—Position 2	3000 CPM 3D	8000 CPM 3D or Linear	
Vacuum—Normal	Vacuum Linear 0 Start	Vacuum Linear 0 start	
Vacuum—Normal	Vacuum Linear 400 mm Hg max	Vacuum Linear 350 mm Hg max	
AIC Vacuum	Tamponade 60/Start Point = 30 Air & Fluid Alt. Pressure AIC = 30-75, 30-40 if High Flow	Tamponade 60/Start Point = 30 Air & Fluid Alt. Pressure AIC = 30-75, 30-40 if High Flow	Consider static start at 20 mm Hg with same AIC Max
FLOW			
Cut Rate—Position 1	7000 CPM 3D	8000 CPM 3D or Linear	
Cut Rate—Position 2	3000 CPM 3D	8000 CPM 3D or Linear	
Flow—Position 1	Flow Linear Start 0 mL/min with 400 vac	Flow Linear Start 0 mL/min with 350 vac	
Flow—Position 2	Flow Linear Max 30 mL/min with 400 vac	Flow Linear Max 30 mL/min with 350 vac	
AIC Flow	Tamponade 60/Start Point = 30 Air & Fluid Alt. Pressure Flow AIC = 30-75, 30-40 if High Flow	Tamponade 60/Start Point = 30 Air & Fluid Alt. Pressure Flow AIC = 30-75, 30-40 if High Flow	Consider static start at 20 mm Hg with same AIC Max
Diathermy	20%		
Light	70% with 0 yellow		
Viscous Fluid Injection	Off		
Step 2: Shave	**23G Standard**	**23G TDC**	
VACUUM			
Cut Rate—Position 1	7000	8000	
Cut Rate—Position 2	3000	8000	
Vacuum—fastest	Shave can be achieved by using core settings and easing off the pedal	Shave can be achieved by using core settings and easing off the pedal	
AIC Vacuum	30-50, 30-30 if High Flow	30-50, 30-30 if High Flow	
FLOW			
Cut Rate—Position 1	7000 CPM 3D or Linear	8000 CPM with 3D or Linear	
Cut Rate—Position 2	7000 CPM 3D or Linear	8000 CPM with 3D or Linear	
Flow—Position 1	Flow Linear Start 0 mL/min with 400 vac	Flow Linear Start 0 mL/min with 300 vac	
Flow—Position 2	Flow Linear Max 2.8 mL/min with 400 vac	Flow Linear Max 02.8 mL/min with 300 vac	
AIC Flow	Tamponade 60/Start Point = 30 Air & Fluid Alt. Pressure Flow AIC = 30-50, 30-30 if High Flow	Tamponade 60/Start Point = 30 Air & Fluid Alt. Pressure Flow AIC = 30-50, 30-30 if High Flow	Consider static start at 20 mm Hg with same AIC Max
Diathermy	20%		
Light	70% with 0 yellow		
Viscous Fluid Injection	Off		
Step 3: Extrusion	**23G Soft Tip**		
VACUUM			
Cut Rate—Position 1	NA		
Cut Rate—Position 2	NA		
Vacuum—fastest	Vacuum—Linear Start—0 mm Hg		
Vacuum—fastest	Vacuum—Linear Max—500 mm Hg		
AIC Vacuum	Tamponade 60/Start Point = 30 Air & Fluid Alt. Pressure Same as core		Consider static start at 20 mm Hg with same AIC Max

(Continued)

23G EVA SETTINGS (*Continued*)		
FLOW		
Cut Rate—Position 1	NA	
Cut Rate—Position 2	NA	
Flow—Position 1	Flow—Linear Flow Start = 0 mL/min with 500 mm Hg	
Flow—Position 2	Flow—Linear Flow Max = 28 mL/min with 500 mm Hg	
AIC Flow	Same as core	
Diathermy	20%	
Light	70%	
Viscous Fluid Injection	Off	
Step 4: Viscous Fluid Control (Silicone Oil Removal)	**Use 1363DD Kit for both VFI and VFE**	
Vacuum		
Vacuum—Position 1	0 mm Hg	
Vacuum—Position 2	660 mm Hg	
Diathermy	20%	
Light	70%	
AIC Venturi	NA	Consider static start at 20 mm Hg with same AIC Max
Viscous Fluid Injection	Off	
Step 5: Viscous Fluid Control (Viscous Fluid Injection)	**1363DD Kit and 1272BFI06 (23G Needle)**	
Viscous Fluid Injection	0-3.5 Bar	
Diathermy	20%	
Light	70%	
Air	Tamponade 60/Start Point = 30 Air & Fluid Alt. Pressure	
AIC	NA	
Step 6: PHACO/FRAG	**20G/23G Frag Needle**	
Top Left Box	Select Frag Icon Select Linear Mode Select Continuous at 30%	
Aspiration Threshold 20G/23G	120 mm Hg/170 mm Hg	
Aspiration Preset Max 20G/23G	220 mm Hg/270 mm Hg	
Diathermy	20%	
Light	70%	
Air	Tamponade 60/Start Point = 30 Air & Fluid Alt. Pressure	
AIC	NA	
Foot Pedal	15/60/100	
Viscous Fluid Injection	N/A	

25G EVA SETTINGS		
Step 1: Core Vitrectomy	**25G Standard**	**25G TDC**
VACUUM		
Cut Rate—Position 1	7000 CPM 3D	8000 CPM 3D or Linear
Cut Rate—Position 2	3000 CPM 3D	8000 CPM 3D or Linear
Vacuum—fastest	Vacuum Linear 0 Start	Vacuum Linear 0 Start
Vacuum—fastest	Vacuum Linear 500 mm Hg Max	Vacuum Linear 450 mm Hg Max
AIC Vacuum	Tamponade 60/Start Point = 30 Air & Fluid Alt. Pressure AIC = 30-80, 30-50 if High Flow	Tamponade 60/Start Point= 30 Air & Fluid Alt. Pressure AIC = 30-80, 30-50 if High Flow

25G EVA SETTINGS (*Continued*)

FLOW			
Cut Rate—Position 1 Peristaltic	7000 CPM 3D	8000 CPM 3D or Linear	
Cut Rate—Position 2 Peristaltic	3000 CPM 3D	8000 CPM 3D or Linear	
Vacuum—Position 1 Peristaltic	Flow Linear Start 0 mL/min with 500 mm Hg	Flow Linear Start 0 mL/min with 400 mm Hg	
Vacuum—Position 2 Peristaltic	Flow Linear Max 20 mL/min with 500 mm Hg	Flow Linear Max 20 mL/min with 400 mm Hg	
AIC Flow	Tamponade 60/Start Point = 30 Air & Fluid Alt. Pressure	Tamponade 60/Start Point = 30 Air & Fluid Alt. Pressure	
	Flow AIC = 30-80, 30-50 if High Flow	Flow AIC = 30-80, 30-50 if High Flow	Consider static start at 20 mm Hg with same AIC Max
Diathermy	20%		
Light	80%		
Viscous Fluid Injection	Off		
Step 2: Shave	**25G Standard**	**25G TDC**	
VACUUM			
Cut Rate—Position 1	Not recommended	Not recommended	
Cut Rate—Position 2			
Vacuum—fastest	Shave can be achieved by using core settings and easing off the pedal	Shave can be achieved by using core settings and easing off the pedal	
AIC Vacuum			
FLOW			
Cut Rate—Position 1	7000 CPM 3D or Linear	8000 CPM with 3D or Linear	
Cut Rate—Position 2	7000 CPM 3D or Linear	8000 CPM with 3D or Linear	
Flow	Flow Linear Start 0 mL/min with 500 vac	Flow Linear Start 0 mL/min with 500 vac	
Flow	Flow Linear Max 5 mL/min with 500 vac	Flow Linear Max 5 mL/min with 500 vac	
AIC Flow	Tamponade 60/Start Point = 30 Air & Fluid Alt. Pressure	Tamponade 60/Start Point = 30 Air & Fluid Alt. Pressure	
	Flow AIC = 30-55, 30-35 if High Flow	Flow AIC = 30-55, 30-35 if High Flow	Consider static start at 20 mm Hg with same AIC Max
Diathermy	20%		
Light	80%		
Viscous Fluid Injection	Off		
Step 3: Extrusion	**25G Soft Tip**		
VACUUM			
Cut Rate—Position 1	NA		
Cut Rate—Position 2	NA		
Vacuum—fastest	Vacuum—Linear Start—0 mm Hg		
Vacuum—fastest	Vacuum—Linear—600 mm Hg		
AIC Vacuum	Tamponade 60/Start Point = 30 Air & Fluid Alt. Pressure		
	Vacuum AIC = 30-80		Consider static start at 20 mm Hg with same AIC Max
FLOW			
Cut Rate—Position 1	NA		
Cut Rate—Position 2	NA		
Flow—Position 1	Flow—Linear Flow Start = 0 mL/min with 600 mm Hg		
Flow—Position 2	Flow—Linear Flow Max = 20 mL/min with 600 mm Hg		
AIC Flow	Flow AIC = 30-80		Consider static start at 20 mm Hg with same AIC Max
Diathermy	20%		
Light	80%		
Viscous Fluid Injection	Off		

(*Continued*)

25G EVA SETTINGS (*Continued*)		
Step 4: Viscous Fluid Control (Silicone Oil Removal)	**Use 1363DD kit for both VFI and VFE**	
VACUUM		
Vacuum—Position 1	0 mm Hg	
Vacuum—Position 2	660 mm Hg	
Diathermy	20%	
Light	80%	
Air	Tamponade 60/Start Point = 30 Air & Fluid Alt. Pressure	
AIC	NA	Consider static start at 20 mm Hg with same AIC Max
Viscous Fluid Injection	Off	
Step 5: Viscous Fluid Injection	**1363DD Kit and 1272BFI05 (25G Needle)**	
Viscous Fluid Injection	0-5 Bar	
Diathermy	20%	
Light	80%	
Air	Tamponade 60/Start Point = 30 Air & Fluid Alt. Pressure	
AIC	Off	
Step 6: PHACO/FRAG	**20G/23G Frag Needle**	
Top Left Box	Select Frag Icon Select Linear Mode Select Continuous at 30%	
Aspiration Threshold 20G/23G	120 mm Hg/170 mm Hg	
Aspiration Preset Max 20G/23G	220 mm Hg/270 mm Hg	
Diathermy	20%	
Light	80%	
Air	Tamponade 60/Start Point = 30 Air & Fluid Alt. Pressure	
AIC	NA	
Foot Pedal	15/60/100	
Viscous Fluid Injection	N/A	

27G EVA SETTINGS			
Step 1: Core Vitrectomy	**27G Standard**	**27G TDC**	
VACUUM			
Cut Rate—Position 1	6000 CPM 3D	8000 CPM 3D or Linear	
Cut Rate—Position 2	2000 CPM 3D	8000 CPM 3D or Linear	
Vacuum—Fastest	Vacuum Linear 0 Start	Vacuum Linear 0 Start	
Vacuum—Fastest	Vacuum Linear 680 mm Hg Max	Vacuum Linear 500 mm Hg Max	
AIC Vacuum	Tamponade 60/Start Point = 30 Air & Fluid Alt. Pressure AIC = 30-50, 30-30 if High Flow	Tamponade 60/Start Point = 30 Air & Fluid Alt. Pressure AIC = 30-50, 30-30 if High Flow	Consider static start at 20 mm Hg with same AIC Max
FLOW			
Cut Rate—Position 1	6000 CPM 3D	8000 CPM 3D or Linear	
Cut Rate—Position 2	2000 CPM 3D	8000 CPM 3D or Linear	
Flow	Flow Linear Start 0 mL/min with 680 mm Hg	Flow Linear Start 0 mL/min with 500 mm Hg	
Flow	Flow Linear Max 10 mL/min with 680 mm Hg	Flow Linear Max 10 mL/min with 500 mm Hg	
AIC Flow	Tamponade 60/Start Point = 30 Air & Fluid Alt. Pressure AIC = 30-50, 30-30 if High Flow	Tamponade 60/Start Point = 30 Air & Fluid Alt. Pressure AIC = 30-50, 30-30 if High Flow	Consider static start at 20 mm Hg with same AIC Max

27G EVA SETTINGS (*Continued*)			
Diathermy	20%		
Light	100%		
Viscous Fluid Injection	Off		
Step 2: Shave	**27G Standard**	**27G TDC**	
VACUUM			
Cut Rate—Position 1	Not recommended	Not recommended	
Cut Rate—Position 2			
Vacuum—fastest	Shave can be achieved by using core settings and easing off the pedal	Shave can be achieved by using core settings and easing off the pedal	
AIC Vacuum			Consider static start at 20 mm Hg with same AIC Max
FLOW			
Cut Rate—Position 1	7000 CPM 3D or Linear	8000 CPM 3D or Linear	
Cut Rate—Position 2	7000 CPM 3D or Linear	8000 CPM 3D or Linear	
Flow	Flow Linear Start 0 mL/min with 680 vac	Flow Linear Start 0 mL/min with 680 vac	
Flow	Flow Linear Max 2 mL/min with 680 vac	Flow Linear Max 2 mL/min with 680 vac	
AIC Flow	Tamponade 60/Start Point = 30 Air & Fluid Alt. Pressure Flow AIC = 30-40, 30-30 if High Flow	Tamponade 60/Start Point = 30 Air & Fluid Alt. Pressure Flow AIC 30-40, 30-30 if High Flow	Consider static start at 20 mm Hg with same AIC Max
Diathermy	20%		
Light	100%		
Viscous Fluid Injection	Off		
Step 3: Extrusion	**27G Soft Tip**		
VACUUM			
Cut Rate—Position 1	NA		
Cut Rate—Position 2	NA		
Vacuum—fastest	Vacuum—Linear Start 0 mm Hg		
Vacuum—fastest	Vacuum—Linear Max 680 mm Hg		
AIC Vacuum	Tamponade 60/Start Point = 30 Air & Fluid Alt. Pressure Vacuum AIC = 30-50		Consider static start at 20 mm Hg with same AIC Max
FLOW			
Cut Rate—Position 1	NA		
Cut Rate—Position 2	NA		
Flow—Position 1	Flow—Linear Start = 0 mL/min with 680 mm Hg		
Flow— Position 2	Flow—Linear Max = 10 mL/min with 680 mm Hg		
AIC Flow	Flow AIC = 30-50		Consider static start at 20 mm Hg with same AIC Max
Diathermy	20%		
Light	100%		
Viscous Fluid Injection	Off		
Step 4: Viscous Fluid Control (Silicone Oil Removal)	**Use 1363DD Kit for both VFI and VFE**		
VACUUM			
Vacuum—Venturi Position 1	0 mm Hg		
Vacuum—Venturi Position 2	660 mm Hg		
Diathermy	20%		
Light	100%		
Air	Tamponade 60/Start Point = 30 Air & Fluid Alt. Pressure		
AIC	NA		Consider static start at 20 mm Hg with same AIC Max
Viscous Fluid Injection	Off		

(*Continued*)

27G EVA SETTINGS (*Continued*)	
Step 5: Viscous Fluid Control (Viscous Fluid Injection)	**1363DD Kit and 1272BFI04 (27G Needle)**
Viscous Fluid Injection	0-6 Bar
Diathermy	20%
Light	100%
Air	Tamponade 60/Start Point = 30 Air & Fluid Alt. Pressure
AIC	Off
Step 6: PHACO/FRAG	**20G/23G Frag Needle**
Top Left Box	Select Frag Icon Select Linear Mode Select Continuous at 30%
Aspiration Threshold 20G/23G	120 mm Hg/170 mm Hg
Aspiration Preset Max 20G/23G	220 mmHg/270 mm Hg
Diathermy	20%
Light	100%
Air	Tamponade 60/Start Point = 30 Air & Fluid Alt. Pressure
AIC	NA
Foot Pedal	15/60/100
Viscous Fluid Injection	N/A

The EVA utilizes either "vacuum mode," where the surgeon controls the vacuum or "flow mode," where the surgeon controls the flow. The individual settings for each mode are expressed above.
AIC, automatic infusion compensation.

Duty cycle: The amount of time the port is open during the cutting cycle (open port time/time of complete *cut* cycle).

- Increasing the duty cycle will increase the flow.
- You can control this, independent of the aspiration and cut rate.
- Three possible settings are usually available.
  - Open-bias duty cycle: Port primarily open, increases flow rate, and used for core PPV
  - 50/50
  - Closed-bias duty cycle: Port primarily closed, decreases flow rate, and is used for shaving vitreous in areas of RD

Core vitrectomy: Utilizes a higher cut rate along with higher vacuum

Shave vitrectomy: Utilizes a lower vacuum setting with higher cut rate

- Used over detached or peripheral retina to allow cutting vitreous with little retinal movement

Dense tissue vitrectomy: Utilizes a lower cut rate along with higher vacuum

- Used for denser material and tissues such as retained lens fragments

Fluidics and vacuum

Two main pump systems are available on vitrectomy machines.

- Flow-controlled peristaltic pump
  - Keeps fluid turnover in an eye exactly at the rate controlled by the pedal, while the vacuum adjusts to the lowest required level.
  - Drawbacks include pulsatile vacuum and potential flow fluctuations.

- Vacuum-controlled venturi pump
  - Directly controls vacuum to generate flow
  - Keeps suction vacuum exactly at the level controlled by the foot pedal, while the fluid turnover depends on the vacuum, gauge, cut rate, and material being aspirated

Vacuum: Can be increased from 0 to 650 mm Hg on current systems

Newer systems allow for a dual dynamic drive (3D) or proportional vitrectomy mode.

- 3D vitrectomy
  - Allows for simultaneous linear control of the cut rate and vacuum pressures
  - Depress the foot pedal to change the settings linearly from a preset start point for cutting and vacuum to a preset endpoint
- Proportional vitrectomy
  - High fixed cut rates and vacuum are varied linearly, reducing pulsatile traction.

OTHER SETTINGS

- Internal diathermy: Used for intraop bleeding such as in a diabetic TRD or to mark a retinal break during RD repair.
- Lighting: See chapter titled *Illumination During Vitreous Surgery* for detailed information on endoillumination.

CHAPTER 4

Lenses and Viewing Systems

R. Joel Welch, MD • Lawrence S. Morse, MD, PhD

- **Non–Wide-Angle Viewing—Direct Image Contact Surgical Lenses**
  - Several lenses are available for on-axis or off-axis (offset) viewing.
  - These surgical lenses create a direct image that does not need inversion.
  - Many are available as disposable or reusable lenses.
  - Most lenses require a viscous coupling agent, while some use an irrigating system.
  - The lens can be held by an assistant, or a lens ring can be sutured to the limbal sclera and the contact lens positioned within the lens ring for hands-free stabilization. Newer hands-free contact lenses have skirts around the rim of the base of the lens to stabilize it.
  - Smaller field of view but with greater resolution for ILM and ERM peeling.
    - On-axis lenses (often termed "flat" lenses) are used for macular surgery.
      - Field of view: 20-50 degrees, depending on the lens
      - Magnification: 0.5×-1.4×, depending on the lens
    - Off-axis or prism lenses are used for more peripheral surgery, outside the macula.
      - Degree of offset: 15-45 degrees, depending on the lens
      - Field of view: 30-40 degrees, depending on the lens
      - Magnification: 0.5×-1.0×, depending on the lens
- **Wide-Angle Viewing Systems**
  - Used in conjunction with the operating microscope to provide a wide-angle or magnified intraop view of the ocular fundus or macula.
  - Several systems are available; the more popular options are listed below (Table 4.1).
    - **Noncontact Wide-Angle Systems**
      - Advantages: No assistant required to manipulate the lens, easy adaptability with both peripheral and macular work.
      - Disadvantages: Corneal drying requires application of viscous solution such as cornea coat, irrigating fluid, viscoelastic, and others.
        - Hoya lens (Hoya Corporation, Tokyo, Japan) is a single-use, contact lens with zero refractive power that prevents corneal drying and improves visualization in eyes with poor corneal status. Used in conjunction with noncontact wide-angle viewing systems.

TABLE 4.1. Wide-angle viewing during vitreoretinal surgery

System or lens	Manufacturer	Field of view (degrees)
Noncontact wide-angle viewing		
BIOM	Oculus Surgical	130
RESIGHT	Carl Zeiss Meditec	130[a]
OFFISS	Topcon Medical Systems	130
PWL[b]	Ocular Instruments	130
Merlin	Volk Optical	120
EIBOS	Haag-Streit	124
NGENUITY	Alcon Laboratories	N/A[c]
Beyeonics One	Beyeonics	N/A
Contact wide-angle viewing		
AVI	Advanced Visual Instruments	130
MiniQuad	Volk Optical	127[d]
MiniQuad XL	Volk Optical	134[d]
HRX	Volk Optical	150[d]
Landers	Ocular Instruments	146[d]
Single-use SMT 037	Sensor Medical Technology	155[d]

[a]*With disposable Super View lens (Oculus).*
[b]*PWL 132D lens used as part of the Ocular Landers Wide-Angle Surgical Viewing System.*
[c]*Not currently available as stand-alone system, field of view varies depending on the wide-angle viewing system.*
[d]*Dynamic field of view.*
BIOM, binocular indirect ophthalmoscopy microscope; OFFISS, optic fiber–free intravitreal surgery system; PWL, Peyman-Wessels-Landers; AVI, Advanced Visual Instruments.

- BIOM (Oculus Surgical, Inc., Port St. Lucie, FL) (Fig. 4.1).
  - Elements: SDI (stereoscopic diagonal invertor), noncontact lens (reusable or disposable)
  - Field of view: 60-130 degrees, depending on lens
- RESIGHT (Carl Zeiss Meditec, Inc., Dublin, CA) (Fig. 4.2).
  - Elements: Focusing/inverting unit, noncontact lens (reusable)
  - Field of view: 60D lens for posterior pole, 120D lens for wide-angle viewing
  - The disposable Super View lens (Oculus, Lucie, FL) can be exchanged for the 120D lens, which increases 130 degrees for improved peripheral viewing in tractional or retinal detachment repair.
- 3D "Heads up" Wide-Angle System: NGENUITY (Alcon Laboratories, Inc., Fort Worth, TX).
  - Elements: 3D HDR Camera, 3D 4K OLED 55-in monitor, viewing glasses (3D, polarized)
  - Field of view: Currently available as complement to other viewing systems; therefore, field of view depends on the system.

- **Other Noncontact Wide-Angle Viewing Systems**
  - OFFISS (Topcon Medical Systems, Oakland, NJ): Illumination incorporated into the microscope, no light pipe needed.
  - Ocular Landers Wide-Angle Surgical Viewing System (Ocular Instruments, Inc., Bellevue, WA): Mounted to wrist rest or surgical bed
  - Merlin (Volk Optical, Inc., Mentor, OH)
  - EIBOS (Haag-Streit Surgical, Wedel, Germany)

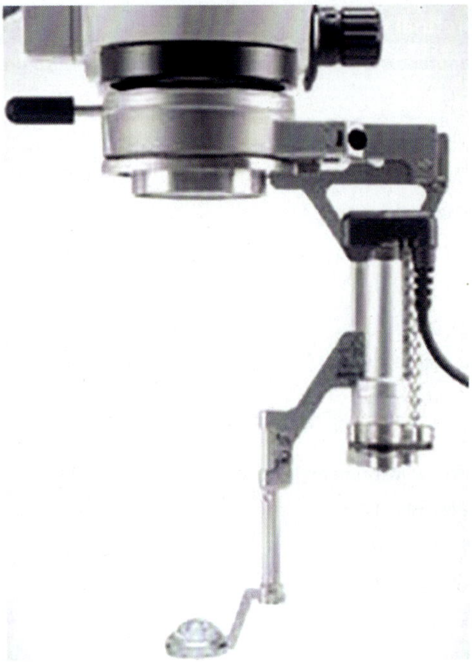

FIGURE 4.1. BIOM wide-angle viewing system lens attached to Leica scope. Each lens system allows retraction of lens so standard viewing for anterior segment can be facilitated. Other lens for retina work can be attached, that is, Oculus Surgical Super View lens for RESIGHT system which adds 10 degrees more of peripheral view.

- **Contact Wide-Angle Systems or Lenses**
  Coupled to the cornea with a coupling agent and often handheld by an assistant. A lens ring can be sutured to the limbal sclera and the contact lens positioned within the lens ring for hands-free stabilization. Newer hands-free contact lenses have skirts around the rim of the base of the lens to stabilize it.
  - Advantages: Better image resolution and stereo viewing than noncontact systems
  - Disadvantages: May contribute to intraop corneal epithelial edema, may require an assistant to manipulate lens
  - AVI Panoramic Viewing System (Advanced Visual Instruments, Inc., New York, NY)
    - Elements: Stereo image inverter, contact lens (reusable)
    - Field of view: 68 or 130 degrees, depending on lens

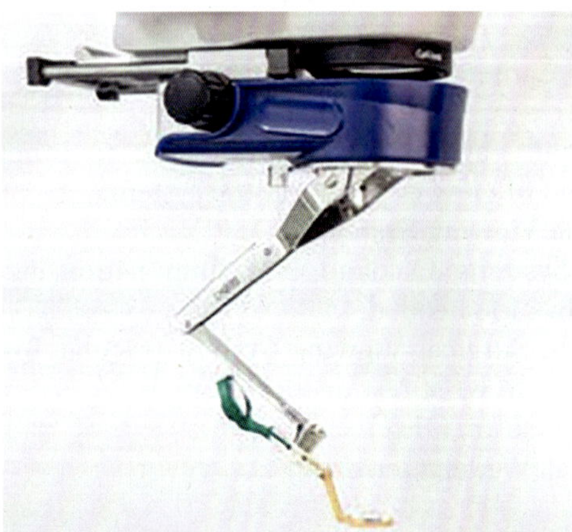

FIGURE 4.2. Zeiss RESIGHT wide-angle viewing system with 128D (*yellow*) peripheral lens and 60D (*green*) macular lens.

- Indirect contact surgical lenses from various vendors
  These lenses create an inverted image and are most often coupled with an inverter device on the microscope.
  - Field of view: 57-150 degrees
  - Magnification: 0.38×-1.030×

SUMMARY

Several advances in wide-angle viewing systems and magnifying lenses for vitreoretinal surgery have been developed. Preferences for the various systems depend on the surgical microscope in use and surgeon choice. Newer imaging systems have been developed (NGENUITY and Beyeonics, Haifa, Israel) which provide similar field of view but utilize digital enhancement to improve peripheral and macular retinal imaging.

CHAPTER 5

Setting Up for Vitreoretinal Surgery

Jack O. Sipperley, MD

After written informed consent is obtained and a surgery date chosen, the patient is brought to the OR. See chapter titled *The Preoperative Discussion*.

- Choice of anesthesia
  - Consider the patient's age, medical comorbidities, and expected length of the surgical procedure when choosing monitored anesthesia sedation (MAC) or general anesthesia.
  - Local anesthetic (retrobulbar or peribulbar block) with MAC is often the preferred method.

The block usually consists of a 50:50 mixture of 5 mL of 4% lidocaine and 5 mL of 0.75% bupivacaine and with 150 units of hyaluronidase (Wydase) and is prepared in a 10-mL syringe and then capped with a 25G Atkinson retrobulbar needle or a sharp 25G needle. No epinephrine is used. About 4-6 mL of block is often administered.

After cleaning the lower lid about 2/3 temporally along the inferior orbital rim with an alcohol wipe, place your gloved index finger between the infraorbital rim and globe, pushing the globe away from the needle path. Insert the needle tip perpendicular to the skin in this location (Fig. 5.1). You will feel two "pops": one as your pass through the orbital septum and a second pop when you enter the muscle cone. Administer the block. Remove the needle and apply on-off alternating pressure to the globe with gauze for about 1-2 minutes. This same technique can be used with a transconjunctival approach through the inferotemporal conjunctival cul-de-sac instead of a trans-lid approach.

  - Your anesthesia team may administer the blocks—make sure you are comfortable with their technique. If you have any concerns, do the block yourself.

For patients who must remain on oral anticoagulation or who have a bleeding disorder, consider performing a cut down block, also known as a sub-Tenon peribulbar block, instead of a needle retrobulbar or needle peribulbar block. After the patient has been prepped and draped, open conjunctiva and Tenon in the inferonasal quadrant as posteriorly as possible using Westcott scissors and 0.12 forceps. Insert the blunt cannula that is attached to the syringe containing the block (Fig. 5.2) into the open conjunctival buttonhole and guide it posteriorly through sub-Tenon space into the peribulbar space.

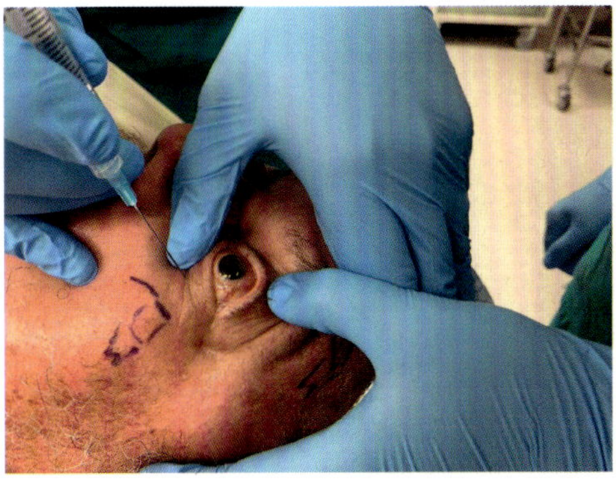

FIGURE 5.1. After cleaning the lower lid about 2/3 temporally along the inferior orbital rim with an alcohol wipe, place your gloved index finger between the infraorbital rim and globe, pushing the globe away from the needle path. Insert the needle tip perpendicular to the skin in this location. This same technique can be used with a transconjunctival approach through the inferotemporal conjunctival cul-de-sac instead of a trans-lid approach.

If a significant retrobulbar hemorrhage occurs, perform an immediate lateral canthotomy and cantholysis. A swab of Betadine can be placed on the skin of the lateral canthus. Clamp a hemostat along the lateral canthus toward the temporal rim of the orbit for 20 seconds. Remove the hemostat. Compressing the tissue decreases bleeding after the canthotomy and allows visualization of the line to cut. Use straight scissors to cut along this line down to the temporal orbital rim. Use cautery for hemostasis of this incision.

  - Discuss the level of anesthesia during the procedure with the anesthesiologist. Goal is to keep the patient sedated and not agitated so that they remain still for the procedure.
  - General anesthesia may be beneficial for younger patients, anyone who is not able to reliably cooperate while under monitored sedation including some of those with cognitive challenges, Parkinson disease, head tremor, claustrophobia, psychiatric conditions, or a significant language barrier preventing comprehension with intraop instructions.
- Patient positioning
  - Position your patient comfortably on stretcher with a pillow under the knees.
  - Adjust the head so it is at the edge of the head support with the zygoma and maxilla in the same flat plane and with the head turned 15 degrees away from the operative eye.
    - Consider placing tape across the forehead so that the head is secured to the stretcher's head support to facilitate intraop stability.
  - Consider using a wrist rest.
    - Keep the rest at patient's ear level.
      - A high wrist rest may inhibit your ability to angle the surgical instruments toward the anterior vitreous and AC.
  - Use a drape retractor to keep the drape elevated around the patient's nose and mouth, which improves patient comfort.

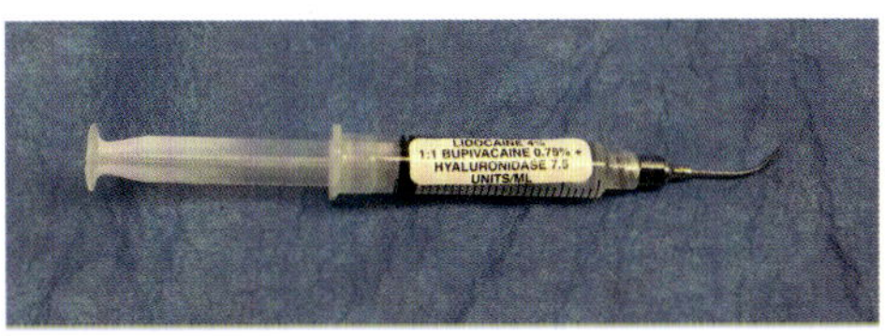

FIGURE 5.2. Cut down block. Place a blunt cannula on the syringe containing the block in preparation for the sub-Tenon peribulbar or retrobulbar block.

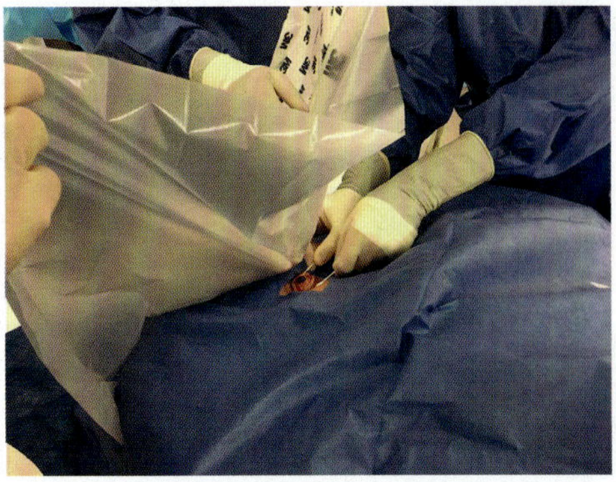

FIGURE 5.3. Evert the eyelids with sterile cotton-tipped applicators while placing the drape over the operative eye.

- Prepping
  - Place a drop of 5% Betadine in the fornix.
  - Starting at the lashes and moving outward to the eyelids and periorbital area, prep the lids and surrounding skin with 5% Betadine.
    - Use cotton-tipped applicators to apply the Betadine to the eyelash area and then use Betadine-soaked sponges to clean the lids and periorbital area.
    - Repeat three times, working from the eyelids outward to the periorbital area.
    - Dry the eyelids with a sterile gauze or towel.
- Draping
  - Various drapes may be used.
  - Evert the eyelids with sterile cotton-tipped applicators while placing the drape over the operative eye (Fig. 5.3).
  - Make sure the drape is adherent to the skin on the nasal side to prevent air leakage from under the drape into the surgical field and fluids from escaping from the field over the nasal bridge toward the fellow eye.
  - Position a towel between the wrist rest and head to keep the field dry intraop.
- Speculum
  - Use a speculum to retract the lids and keep the lashes covered with the drape without interfering with surgical instrument manipulation. Eighty-five percent of postop endophthalmitis infections come from organisms on the eyelids and eyelashes.
  - Most commonly, a wire lid speculum or Lieberman lid speculum is used. A Rappazzo speculum is also a good option.
- Microscope position
  - Maintain proper posture to protect yourself against neck, shoulder, and back problems in the future. Avoid unnatural flexion and extension of your neck.
  - Keep your back straight and the oculars positioned so that there is no severe flexion or extension of your neck during surgery.
- Foot pedal position
  - Place the microscope control, vitrectomy control, and laser pedal in the same position for each case, so they are easily accessible to you.
- Music
  - If you want, play music in the OR since it can decrease any associated stress.

Section II

Pars Plana Vitrectomy

CHAPTER 6

Gauge Selection and Cannula Placement

Ryan N. Vogel, MD • Sally S. Ong, MD • James T. Handa, MD

Transconjunctival MIVS has essentially replaced the 20G vitrectomy system. MIVS sizes include the 23G, 25G, and 27G vitrectomy systems (Fig. 6.1). See chapter titled *Vitrectomy Machine Settings*.

ADVANTAGES AND DISADVANTAGES OF CANNULAS VS SCLEROTOMIES WITHOUT CANNULAS

Advantages

- Easier insertion and removal of instruments and reduced trauma to the edges of the sclerotomy, which increases the chance of a self-sealing wound at the end of the case.
- The location of the infusion line can be quickly interchanged between any of the cannulas to overcome challenges related to visualization, ease of access, and untoward events.

Disadvantages

- Fixed internal diameter limits both the size and curvature of instruments, such as scissors. This size limitation precludes the use of most multifunctional instruments that were available with 20G systems.

Valved cannulas are more commonly used than nonvalved cannulas. Valved cannulas allow better fluid control and thus IOP control and, in turn, less turbulence and reduced chance of incarcerating retina in the cannula. It can be challenging to insert certain instruments through valved cannulas, especially the softtip cannula.

Trocar Insertion and Cannula Placement

- Sclerotomy sites are chosen so that the trocars, cannulas, and instruments pass through the pars plana, thereby avoiding puncture of the retina or vascular pars plicata.
  - For adults and children over age 3, trocars are generally placed between 3 and 3.5 mm posterior to the limbus in aphakic and pseudophakic eyes.

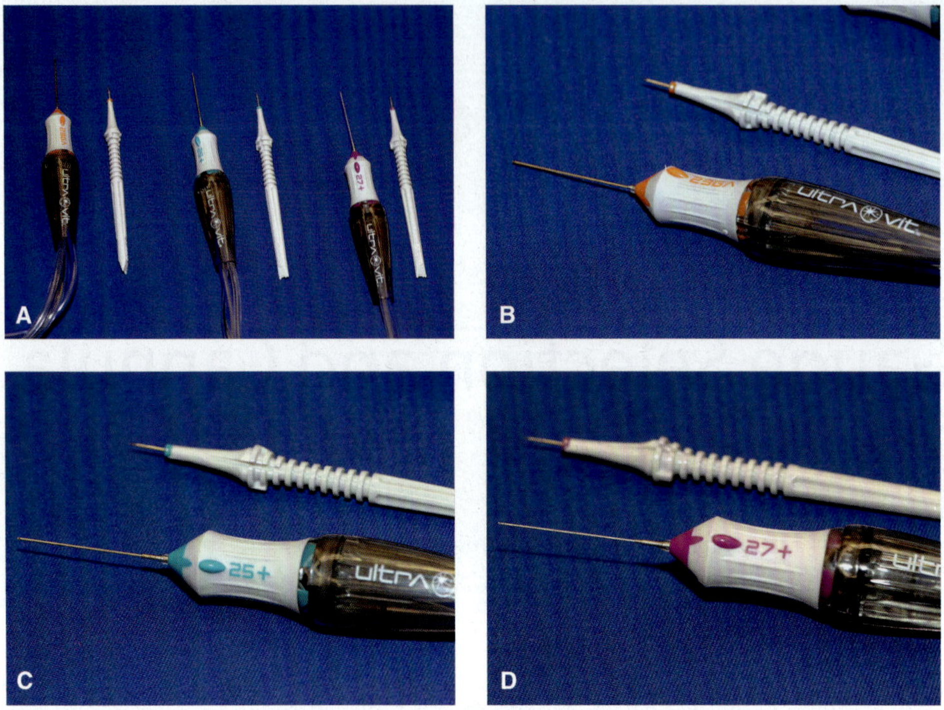

FIGURE 6.1. The range of cannula gauge sizes (Alcon is used as an example). **A.** Some of the 23G (orange), 25G (blue), and 27G (purple) vitrector and trocar cannulas. **B.** Higher magnification view of 23G vitrectomy handpiece and trocar cannula. **C.** Higher magnification view of 25G vitrectomy handpiece and trocar cannula. **D.** Higher magnification view of 27G vitrectomy handpiece and trocar cannula.

- In phakic eyes, the risk of lens injury can be reduced during trocar insertion and instrument manipulation if trocars and cannulas are inserted 4 mm posterior to the limbus.
- Consider adjusting the entry distance based on the axial length, since eyes with shorter axial lengths may be more prone to inadvertent retinal penetration when standard entry distances are used.
- In young children, use indirect ophthalmoscopy or transillumination to assess the location of the pars plana prior to placing the ports.

> **Children may have particularly tough sclera. Twisting the trocar while inserting can facilitate entry. See chapter titled *Pediatric RRD* for trocar cannula insertion tips in neonate and infant eyes.**

- Oblique and biplanar insertion techniques promote better wound apposition compared to straight perpendicular entry techniques.
  - Oblique insertion of the trocar cannula most commonly involves inserting the trocar in a direction parallel to the limbus, while the wide dimension of the blade is oriented perpendicular to the limbus.
  - Based on the radial direction of the scleral fibers, this technique may displace the scleral fibers rather than cut them.
  - Insert the trocar parallel to the limbus to avoid inadvertently contacting the retina or lens.
- Displace the conjunctiva prior to inserting the trocar so that the entry site at the conjunctiva is not aligned with the sclerotomy upon cannula removal (Video 6.1).

> **If the eye is hypotonous, check all preexisting wounds for a leak and suture if there is a leak, and pump up the AC or vitreous cavity with infusion fluid on a 30G needle.**

> **If the eye is hypotonous and no preexisting wounds are leaking, use counter traction with toothed forceps to facilitate trocar insertion or pump up the AC or vitreous cavity with infusion fluid on a 30G needle prior to inserting a trocar.**

Cannula Removal

- Sclerotomies close by a combination of scleral edema and plugging of residual vitreous into the wound. Upon removing the cannula at the end of the case, gently compress the sclerotomy with a cotton tip and wait for scleral edema to develop, which closes the unsutured sclerotomy.
- Raising the infusion pressure while compressing the wound allows the walls of the wound to better appose.
- Partial FAX may increase the surface tension at the sclerotomy and reduce the chance of wound leak.

> **Longer 6-mm cannulas may be useful in eyes where there has been prolonged preop hypotony or a RD with a thicker choroid. In cases in which there is no view to the posterior segment, consider placing the infusion cannula and vitreous cutter in the AC through the limbus to clear anterior segment opacities, such as fibrotic pupillary membranes. Once you clear the view, use standard PPV techniques to complete the surgery.**

Advantages of Smaller Gauge Vitrectomy

- Decreased inflammation, improved patient comfort, and reduced conjunctival scarring which may better preserve the conjunctiva if future glaucoma surgery is indicated.
- Sclerotomies with smaller gauge cannulas are less likely to require sutures to close, which can decrease postop pain, corneal astigmatism, and operating time.
- Smaller gauge vitreous cutters can access tighter spaces, and the mouth of the probe can be safely brought closer to the retinal surface. The vitreous cutter can also function as a pick, forceps, and scissors for tissue dissection.
- Smaller gauge vitreous cutters, with decreased flow rates, can reduce post-occlusion surge, which reduces the risk of inadvertently aspirating mobile areas of the detached retina.
- Smaller vitrectomy ports have a reduced "sphere of influence," limiting tractional disturbance on surrounding tissues and possibly reducing the risk of iatrogenic retinal breaks.

> **Smaller gauge sclerotomies should be sutured if the sclerotomy is leaking especially if silicone oil is used.**

Disadvantages of Smaller Gauge Vitrectomy

Disadvantages are related to the smaller diameter. This reduced diameter translates into decreased efficiency of aspiration, weaker vacuum hold, smaller grasping platforms on forceps, shorter scissor blades, unwanted flexibility of instrument shafts, especially when operating in the anterior vitreous cavity, and limitations in designing multifunctional instruments. These factors should all be considered when selecting a gauge size for vitrectomy. Most cases can be successfully completed with either large or small gauges.

INTRAOPERATIVE CONSIDERATIONS (VIDEO 7.1)

- **Microscope**
  - Fogging can occur in the surgeon oculars or on the BIOM/RESIGHT lens. Both are caused by respirations from either the surgeon (oculars) or patient (BIOM/RESIGHT lens) in some cases. This can be managed by taping of mask or drape to the nose bridge to prevent exhaled air from entering the surgical field. See chapter titled *Setting Up For Vitreoretinal Surgery*. Sometimes if the BIOM/RESIGHT lens is too close to the eye, the patient's body temperature can also contribute to fogging. Putting anti-fog solution on the surgeon oculars or onto the posterior surface of the BIOM/RESIGHT lens and then drying it can help prevent fogging.
- **Cornea**
  - Corneal epithelium

Corneal Epithelial Edema and Scraping

- **This can initially be managed conservatively by placing glycerin on the epithelium or "squeegeeing" the epithelium by rolling a cotton tip over the cornea.**
- **If these maneuvers fail, the epithelium can be removed using either a cotton tip or broad (Beaver) blade. The epithelium should be removed first centrally and then expanded, ideally leaving 2 mm of corneal epithelium around the limbus intact. Remove the debrided epithelium with a Weck-Cel sponge, and then rinse any remaining epithelium away. Maintain defined edges and remove any redundant epithelium to ensure good and rapid healing postop. Remember to alert the patient to possible surface discomfort after the anesthesia wears off.**
- **The surface will dry more rapidly after epithelial scraping. Use either viscoelastic or an alternative ocular surface coating gel to maintain even and persistent surface lubrication.**
- **Place a bandage contact lens on the cornea at the end of the case to promote corneal epithelial healing.**

    - Edema is common during vitreous surgery and can be exacerbated by prolonged surgery times, preexisting epitheliopathy from conditions like diabetes, and preop povidone-iodine prep.
      - In diabetics as well as in Stickler syndrome, epithelial scraping should be avoided unless absolutely necessary as healing may be prolonged.
      - Methylcellulose, viscoelastic, and hypromellose are options to keep cornea moist during surgery.
  - Corneal stroma/endothelium
    - The stroma can become edematous intraop and develop Descemet's folds due to long case time or elevated IOP causing endothelial dysfunction and edema. Preexisting conditions as well as combined phacoemulsification increase the risk for corneal edema.
    - Normalize the IOP when possible.
    - Use glycerin to help deturgess the cornea.
    - Coating the posterior cornea with dispersive viscoelastic will prevent additional aqueous from entering the cornea and help smooth out any Descemet's folds.
- **Anterior chamber**
  - Hyphema
    - Find the source.
      - Blood may egress from the trabecular meshwork during hypotony.

        - Vitreous hemorrhage can enter AC.
        - Active bleeding can occur after iridectomy or clearing of vascularized pupillary membrane in eyes with NVI.
    - If neovascular etiology, consider intraop anti-VEGF, if not given preop, at the end of the case to prevent postop bleeding.
    - Displace hyphema by filling AC with viscoelastic (remove viscoelastic at end of the case to prevent postop IOP spikes).
  - Gas
    - Vitreous air or gas may enter the AC, either around the IOL or through a zonular defect, and impair the view.
    - Remove air or gas in the AC via needle aspiration. Alternatively, displace gas by filling AC with viscoelastic (remove viscoelastic at end of the case to prevent postop IOP spike).
  - Fibrin
    - Remove clots and fibrin with forceps as cohesive sheet; sometimes the vitreous cutter is needed.
- **Pupil**
  - Determine if posterior synechiae or pupillary membrane is preventing dilation.
    - Lyse synechiae or excise pupillary membrane.
  - Pharmacologic approaches.

Pharmacologic Pupil Management

Preop
- Use higher concentration of phenylephrine, cardiac considerations permitting.
- Pledgets soaked in dilating drops can enhance intraocular penetration.
- Use topical NSAID preop to maintain intraop mydriasis.
- If there is history of alpha-agonist use (ie, risk for floppy iris), consider preop topical atropine 1%.
- Avoid clonidine for periop BP management as it can cause miosis.

Intraop
- Add intracameral lidocaine (1%) or ketorolac (0.3%), if available, to augment.

  - Fill AC with viscoelastic for mechanical mydriasis.
    - If pupillary dilation still inadequate for viewing, use iris hooks.

Iris Hook Tips

a. Create four entry sites into AC at limbus at 10, 2, 4, and 8 o'clock (Fig. 7.1) using a Ziegler knife or equivalent. Recommend placing all incisions into AC prior to inserting hooks. Slant the incision slightly posteriorly which will help when trying to engage the iris with the hook. It is okay to have trace bleeding from small conjunctival vessels at the limbus, as this will help identify incisions.
b. Place all iris hooks on the field.
c. Small amounts of viscoelastic can be placed under the pupillary iris border to elevate the iris margin so easier to hook.
d. Be careful not to engage anterior capsule in pseudophakic eyes.
e. Secure the hook in place by advancing the silicone sleeve on the hook shaft up to the limbus.
f. Disengage the hooks from the iris prior to removal to prevent any iris trauma or bleeding.

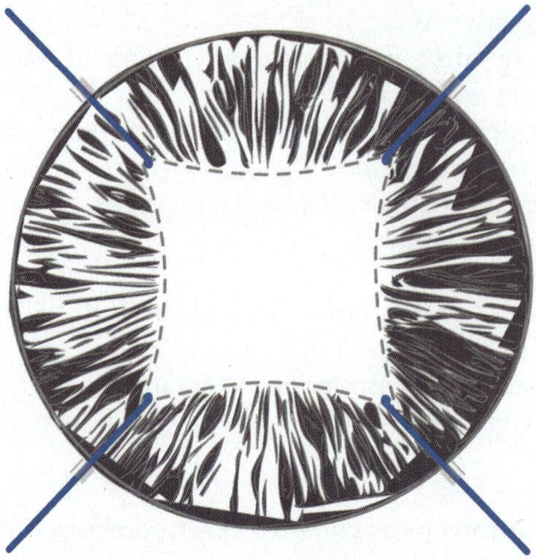

FIGURE 7.1. Properly placed iris hooks can enlarge a small pupil and improve the view during vitreous surgery.

- **Lens**
  - Phakic
    - Underestimation of preexisting lens opacity can require concurrent phacoemulsification or lensectomy at time of surgery.
    - Slight lens feathering that occurs during FAX is rarely visually significant for the surgeon and can be observed unless loss of view precludes additional surgical maneuvers.
    - In diabetics, using supplemental glucose (ie, BSS PLUS) in the irrigating fluid has been suggested to minimize intraop lens clouding. Can also add dextrose to non-BSS PLUS infusion fluid to create a 0.5% dextrose solution.
  - Pseudophakic
    - Posterior capsule opacification can be limiting and is managed by using the vitreous cutter to remove the central posterior capsule. If the IOL is silicone or hydrophobic acrylic and tamponade (either gas or oil) is planned, the posterior capsule should be preserved if at all possible to prevent later formation of IOL condensations or opacities.
    - After posterior capsulotomy, intraop condensation can occur on the posterior surface of the IOL. This can be temporarily wiped away with the soft-tip cannula or resolved with a small amount of viscoelastic placed on the posterior IOL surface.

CHAPTER 8

Vitrectomy Surgery Steps

Naryan Sabherwal, MD • Mathew W. MacCumber, MD, PhD

PREOPERATIVE CONSIDERATIONS

- Know the lens status. This may change the planning and approach to surgery.
  - Cannula location varies depending on lens status. See chapter titled *Gauge Selection and Cannula Placement*.
  - For phakic patients with diabetes, add dextrose to the infusion fluid to make a 0.5% dextrose solution in order to decrease intraop lens feathering. See chapter titled *Getting and Maintaining Your View*.
  - For eyes with a visually significant cataract that may interfere with intraop visualization, consider a pars plana lensectomy or simultaneous phacoemulsification with IOL placement to improve the view. See chapter titled *Pars Plana Lensectomy*. If the PPV is elective, consider phacoemulsification with IOL placement separately at an earlier date.

SURGICAL STEPS (VIDEO 8.1)

- Cannula insertion
  - Place the cannulas at 8, 10, and 2 o'clock in the right eye (Fig. 8.1) and 10, 2, and 4 o'clock in the left eye. Clock-hour location of cannula placement may vary to accommodate patient factors such as a small orbit, a deep orbit, a prominent nasal bridge, or the presence of a functioning trabeculectomy or tube shunt(s).
  - Insert the trocar cannula 4.0 mm posterior to the limbus in phakic eyes, 3.5 mm posterior to the limbus in pseudophakic eyes, and 3.0 mm posterior to the limbus in aphakic eyes.
    - Measure this distance using the opposite end of the trocar, which has built-in scleral markers measuring 3.0 and 4.0 mm.
  - Displace the conjunctiva with a cotton tip and then insert the trocar at a beveled angle. If the angle of entry is too shallow, the infusion may end up in the suprachoroidal space. If the angle of entry is too steep, there is a higher chance of sclerotomy leakage. Insert the trocar smoothly starting at 10-30 degrees and gradually pointing the tip of the trocar more perpendicularly toward the center of the eye just before the cannula is fully inserted.

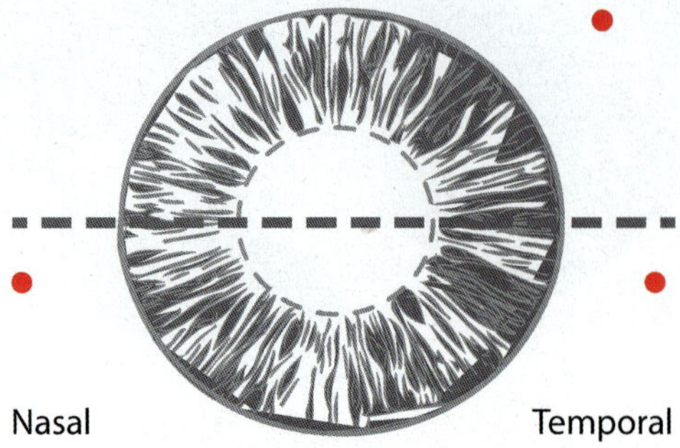

FIGURE 8.1. Surgeon's view of the right eye. The *red dots* mark the ideal placement of the three cannulas inferotemporally, superotemporally, and superonasally. The superonasal and superotemporal cannulas are typically placed at about 10 and 2 o'clock.

- Prior to inserting the infusion line into the inferotemporal cannula, turn the infusion on to clear any air bubbles in the line, and then turn off the infusion. Then, insert infusion line firmly into the inferotemporal cannula.
- Visualize the tip of the infusion line in the vitreous cavity prior to turning on the infusion. You can visualize the infusion line tip by turning off the microscope and room lights and shining the light pipe through the cornea and pupil (Fig. 8.2). The shiny metallic tip of the infusion line should not have any tissue overlying it.

Sometimes, the tip of the infusion line may be covered by nonpigmented ciliary epithelium or even retina, or there may be media opacity that prevents visualization. In these situations, infusion fluid will flow into the suprachoroidal space or subretinal space. If this should occur, immediately turn off the infusion. Remove the infusion line and place it in one of the other two cannulas. Make sure you can visualize the tip of the infusion line before turning on the infusion. If you still cannot see the tip, consider using a 6-mm cannula instead; when inserting the 6-mm cannula, do not shelve the entry, but instead enter the vitreous cavity directly and more perpendicular to the sclera. Another option particularly for aphakic and pseudophakic eyes is the placement of the cannula and infusion line at the limbus.

- When the infusion is turned on, continue to visualize the infusion tip in the same manner to confirm that the fluid is flowing into the vitreous cavity.
- Tape the infusion line to the drape near the eye to prevent inadvertent removal of the infusion line during surgery. Angle the infusion line so the infusion is pointed toward the midvitreous cavity.
- Place the remaining trocars. If the infusion line is placed first and turned on, then you can increase the IOP to ensure smooth placement of the other trocars.

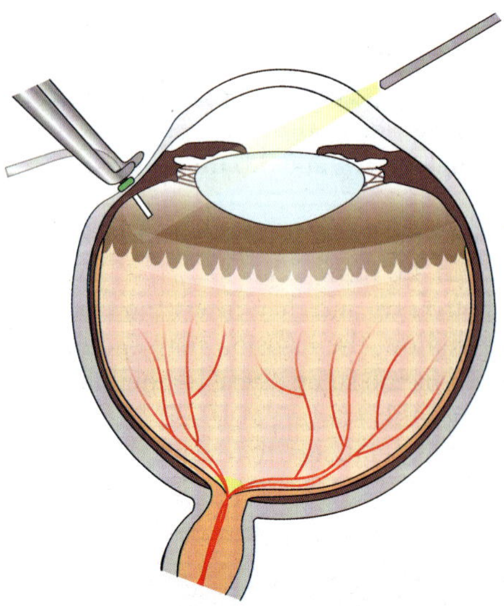

FIGURE 8.2. The infusion line should be directly visualized in the vitreous cavity prior to running the infusion by turning off the microscope and room lights and shining the light pipe through the cornea and pupil.

- Core vitrectomy
  - Coat the cornea with methylcellulose, hypromellose, or viscoelastic for lubrication.
  - Noncontact widefield viewing systems such as the BIOM or ReSight or contact widefield viewing systems such as the AVI "short fat" lens are used. See chapter titled *Lenses and Viewing Systems*.
  - Insert the light pipe and vitrector handpiece each through one of the two superior sclerotomies so that you can visualize the instruments in the midvitreous cavity through the pupil. Avoid the phakic lens.
  - Perform core vitrectomy in the midvitreous cavity to debulk the central vitreous.
  - Use higher flow (achieved using higher aspiration rates) for the core vitrectomy, and use lower flow for peripheral vitrectomy.
  - See chapter titled *Vitrectomy Machine Settings*.

Foot-pedal position varies among surgeons, with some preferring to manipulate the microscope pedal with the dominant foot, while others prefer using the dominant foot for the vitrectomy pedal. Program the pedal and microscope buttons to your preference. Proportional vitrectomy allows for higher cut rates and variable flow, with flow increasing with increased aspiration as you depress the pedal. During core and peripheral vitrectomy, use a high flow and high cut rate for maximum efficiency in vitreous removal. While shaving or vitrectomizing over a detached retina, use lower flow and higher cut rates. Set IOP pressure control between 25 and 35 mm Hg, and only use higher pressures (up to 60 mm Hg) intermittently to avoid corneal edema and retinal vascular effects.

- PVD induction. See chapter titled *PVD Induction*.
  - If there is a preexisting PVD, vitrectomize the peripheral vitreous. If there is no PVD, induce a PVD.
  - Turn the cutter off. Position the vitreous cutter close to the optic nerve head, engage vitreous, and aspirate at the maximum vacuum. Fill the port with vitreous.
  - While aspirating maximally, slowly lift the hyaloid as the vitrector is moved into the midvitreous while remaining aligned with the optic nerve head below. To avoid the formation of a retinal break, detach the hyaloid no farther than the midperiphery.
  - Once the posterior hyaloid has been lifted, turn the cutter back on and continue with PPV.
  - If the first attempt at PVD induction fails,
    - Highlight the vitreous with triamcinolone (Triesence suspension, Alcon Laboratories Inc., Fort Worth, TX). May need to stain it more than once. See chapter titled *Intraoperative Visualization Agents*.

Off-label use of triamcinolone (Kenalog, Bristol-Myers Squibb, Peapack, NJ) can be used instead of Triesence to highlight the vitreous, but contains benzyl alcohol as a preservative.

    - Briefly increase the vacuum on the machine. It may also be necessary to increase the IOP setting on the machine. See chapter titled *Vitrectomy Machine Settings*.
    - Use a lighted pick, if available, to engage the Weiss ring while aspirating with the cutter.
    - Engage peripapillary vitreous overlying the peripapillary retina. Lift while moving slightly toward the periphery. Do this around the optic nerve.
- Peripheral vitrectomy
  - Trim the vitreous from the core out to the periphery. Start at either 12 or 6 o'clock, and move in a clockwise or counterclockwise fashion, cutting at the edge of visible vitreous skirt.

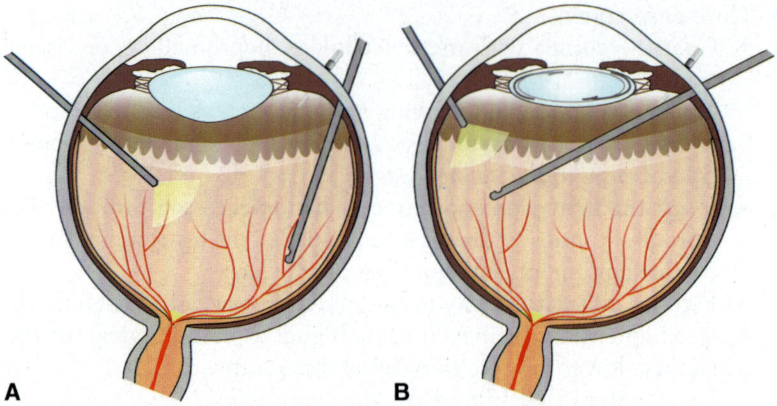

FIGURE 8.3. **A.** In a phakic eye, do not reach across the vitreous cavity with the surgical instruments so as to avoid damaging to the native lens. **B.** In a pseudophakic or aphakic eye, you can safely reach across the vitreous cavity with the surgical instruments without risk of damage to the IOL.

  - If the vitreous skirt edge is not visible, there may not be a PVD.
  - Stay engaged with the vitreous.
  - Adequate visualization is key during peripheral vitrectomy. Illuminate the retina under and ahead of the vitrector port. This allows avoidance of the retina particularly if it is mobile.
  - In phakic eyes, do not reach over to the other side of the vitreous cavity in order to avoid touching the lens with the instruments during surgery. You can reach from temporal to nasal or vice versa but only up to the equator (Fig. 8.3A).
  - In pseudophakic or aphakic eyes, you can safely reach across the eye with surgical instruments (Fig. 8.3B).
- Shaving with scleral depression
  - Ensure a more complete vitrectomy by shaving the peripheral vitreous while scleral depressing.
  - Without an assistant, use the microscope light in pseudophakic eyes or a chandelier light in phakic eyes to facilitate scleral depression.
  - With an assistant, clear communication is key so that you know when there will actually be some depression. This will avoid inadvertent vitrector tip–retina touch.
  - When depressing around the infusion cannula, pay attention to the infusion line so that the depressor does not get caught in the infusion tubing. If this happens, the cannula may be partly pulled out of the eye and can cause infusion fluid to flow into the suprachoroidal space. See chapter titled *Choroidals*.
  - Lower flow rates achieved using lower aspiration are used in the periphery and over detached retina to decrease the risk of creating an iatrogenic retinal tear.

If there is a RD present, keep the vitreous cutter port pointed away from the detached retina during PPV to prevent iatrogenic retinal breaks. Lower vacuum settings and higher cut rates will also minimize retinal mobility when removing the vitreous cutter closer to the detached retinal surface.

Consider these subconjunctival injections at the end of the case: 0.5 mL of cefazolin (Ancef) at a concentration of 200 mg/mL and 0.5 mL of dexamethasone (Decadron) at a concentration of 10 mg/mL. For children, decrease the volume to 0.25 mL.

CHAPTER 9

PVD Induction

Shriji Patel, MD ● Paul Sternberg Jr, MD

PREOPERATIVE CONSIDERATIONS

- Assess the status of the posterior hyaloid during dilated fundus examination.
- Examine the peripheral retina to identify lattice degeneration, retinal breaks, areas of retinal thinning, or other peripheral pathology.
- Get an OCT to identify VMT and areas of vitreous adhesion (Fig. 9.1) and to assess whether the hyaloid is still attached to the nerve.
- If the view is limited, perform a B-scan ultrasound to determine if a PVD is present.

SURGICAL PROCEDURE (VIDEO 9.1)

- Insert each trocar and cannula in the typical beveled fashion. Ensure appropriate infusion line placement and position. See chapter titled *Gauge Selection and Cannula Placement*.
- Remove vitreous near trocar insertion sites to decrease vitreous traction and iatrogenic breaks with instrument manipulation.
- Vitrectomize any vitreous obstructing the infusion tip to improve fluidics.
- Perform core vitrectomy to clear the central vitreous gel. Spare the vitreous directly over the optic nerve to allow for subsequent hyaloid elevation.
- If using a chromovitrectomy agent to improve visualization, inject this over the optic nerve and posterior pole. See chapter titled *Intraoperative Visualization Agents*.

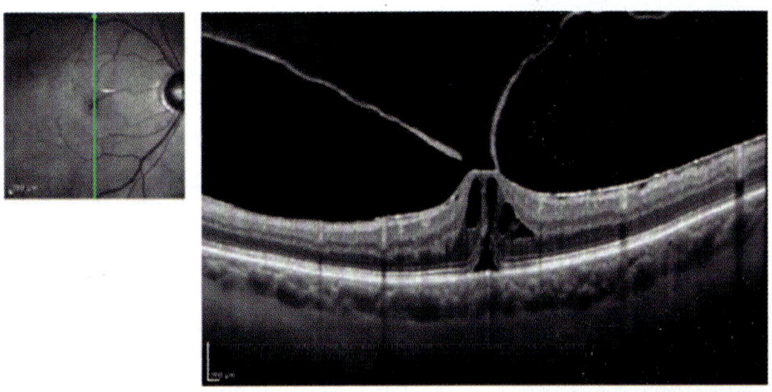

FIGURE 9.1. Preop and intraop OCT can help identify if the posterior hyaloid is already separated from the macula and optic nerve. In this preop image, the posterior hyaloid remains attached to the fovea.

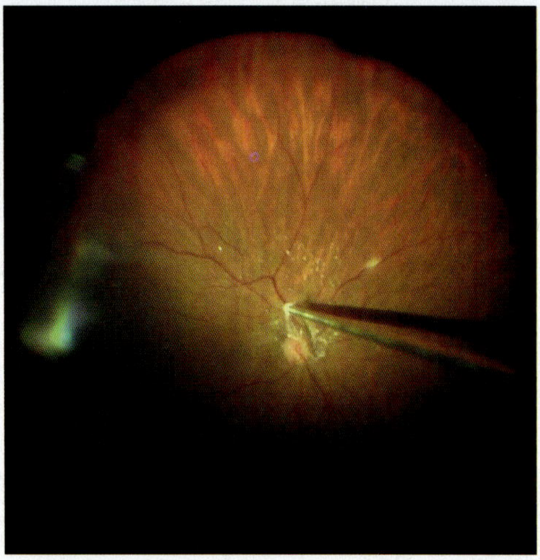

FIGURE 9.2. Using the vitrector (aspiration only), start directly above or at the edge of the optic nerve with the vitrector mouth faceup. Triamcinolone highlights the posterior hyaloid.

  - Use preservative-free triamcinolone acetonide (Triesence, Alcon Laboratories, Inc., Fort Worth, TX), which is FDA approved for use in visualization during PPV.
    - Dilute the triamcinolone with BSS to a 1:30 to 1:10 dilution.
  - Off-label use of triamcinolone (Kenalog, Bristol-Myers Squibb, New York City, NY) can be administered similarly, but contains benzyl alcohol as a preservative.
- Using the vitrector (set on aspiration only), place the vitrector tip directly above or at the edge of the optic nerve with the vitrector mouth faceup (Fig. 9.2).
- Gradually increase aspiration, allowing the vitreous to fully occlude the cutter mouth, and move the vitrector tip toward the optic nerve rim to engage the Weiss ring.
- Once the vitreous and hyaloid edge are engaged, gently pull the vitrector upward toward the midvitreous cavity, staying in line with the optic nerve axis and closely observing the peripherally advancing edge of the vitreous (Fig. 9.3).
  - Alternatively, move the cutter radially out from the optic nerve, taking care to initially stay parallel to the retinal surface and then slowly elevating upward.
  - Prior to repeating this maneuver, turn the cutter on to remove any vitreous in the cutter mouth to prevent unnecessary VR traction.
- Ideally, separate the vitreous from the retinal surface as peripherally as possible without retinal break formation or lens damage.

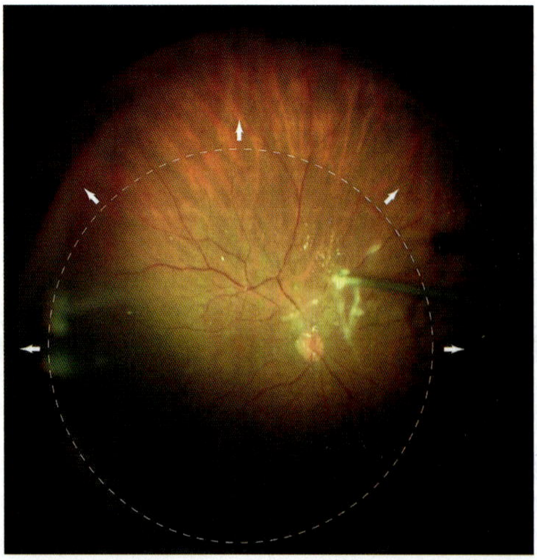

FIGURE 9.3. Once the vitreous and hyaloid edge are engaged, gently pull the vitrector upward toward the midvitreous cavity, staying in line with the optic nerve axis and closely observing the peripherally advancing edge of the vitreous (*dotted circle*).

- At a minimum, separate the posterior hyaloid from the optic nerve and macula.
- Position the vitrector opening away from detached retina to prevent inadvertent retinal incarceration and iatrogenic breaks.
- Once the PVD has been induced, perform a peripheral vitrectomy and shave the vitreous base.
    - Put the vitrectomy machine setting on shave mode will increase the cut rate (5000 cpm or greater) and lower the maximum vacuum (300 mm Hg) to minimize retinal movement as the vitreous gel is removed. See chapter titled *Vitrectomy Machine Settings*.
- Prior to case completion, perform 360-degree scleral depression using widefield viewing or indirect ophthalmoscopy to look for any iatrogenic peripheral retinal breaks that would require retinopexy and tamponade.

MANAGING A TIGHTLY ADHERENT POSTERIOR HYALOID

- Use a pick (either a 25G needle or MVR blade with a bent tip) to engage the Weiss ring and manually elevate the hyaloid.
- Use a soft-tipped cannula on aspiration or forceps to elevate the Weiss ring and posterior hyaloid.
- Use PFCL to dissect the hyaloid from the retina and stabilize detached retina.
- Bimanual PVD induction: use the vitrector handpiece or soft-tip aspiration cannula in combination with a lighted pick (Fig. 9.4).

Tips for PVD induction in pediatric eyes

- **Consider using forceps, a pick, or Finesse Flex Loop (Grieshaber/Alcon) under a magnifying contact lens to engage the hyaloid edge.**
- **Consider multiple rounds of staining with triamcinolone to ensure that the hyaloid is adequately separated.**
- **Avoid creation of a retinal break during hyaloid elevation.**

POSTOPERATIVE CONSIDERATIONS

The reported rates of intraop and postop retinal break formation following small gauge surgery can be as high as 16%. The rate in the setting of PVD induction increases significantly. In the postvitrectomy eye, peripheral retinal breaks can rapidly evolve into a RRD due to the absence of vitreous tamponade. Perform a thorough peripheral exam postop and counsel patients on symptoms of RD.

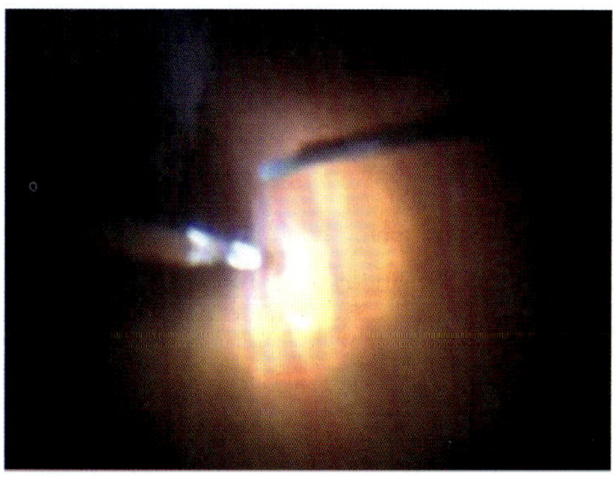

FIGURE 9.4. Bimanual PVD induction: the vitrector handpiece or soft-tip aspiration cannula in combination with a lighted pick can initiate hyaloid elevation.

CHAPTER 10

Illumination During Vitreous Surgery

Jaycob Avaylon, BS • Ron P. Gallemore, MD, PhD

Adequate intraop illumination is a critical aspect of VR surgery. In some cases, such as a non-clearing VH, the method of illumination is not as important. In other cases, such as ILM peeling, the illumination technique and tools can make or break the case, particularly if there are other compounding variables such as lenticular or other media opacities. Some illumination sources are highlighted here (Table 10.1); there are others that are in use but are not included herein.

TABLE 10.1. Select light sources. There are others that are not depicted

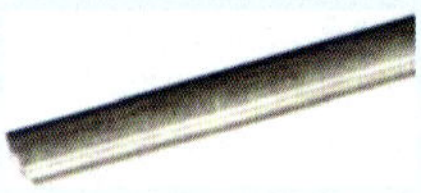	Name: Vivid Focal Endoilluminator Manufacturer: Synergetics Inc. Light cone angle: 65° Purported use: higher intensity light
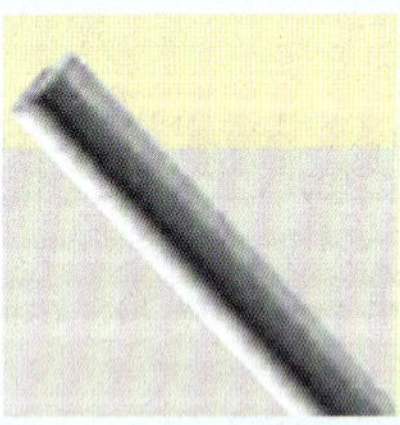	Name: Straight Endoilluminator Manufacturer: Alcon Constellation System Light cone angle: 85° Purported use: higher intensity light
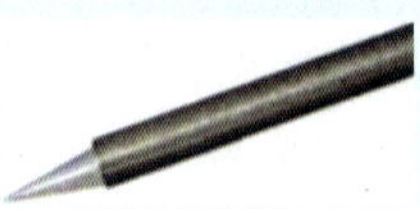	Name: Widefield Endoilluminator Manufacturer: Synergetics Inc. Light cone angle: 135° Purported use: standard widefield lighting
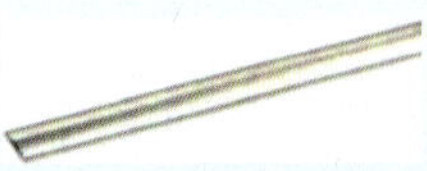	Name: Widefield Diffusion Endoilluminator Manufacturer: Synergetics Inc. Light cone angle: 135° Purported use: widefield light with focal bright spot
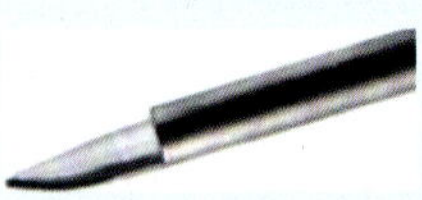	Name: Shielded Corona Widefield Endoilluminator Manufacturer: Synergetics Inc. Light cone angle: 135° Purported use: widefield light with shield to decrease glare

(*Continued*)

TABLE 10.1. Select light sources (*Continued*). There are others that are not depicted

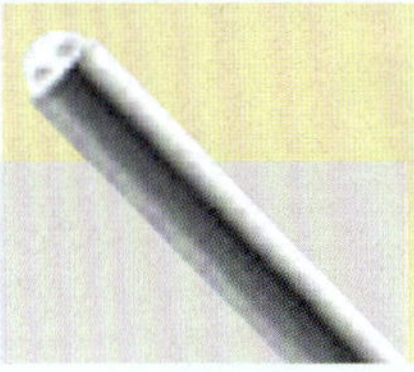	Name: Sapphire Widefield Endoilluminator (Video 10.1) Manufacturer: Alcon Constellation System Light cone angle: 106° Purported use: widefield lighting
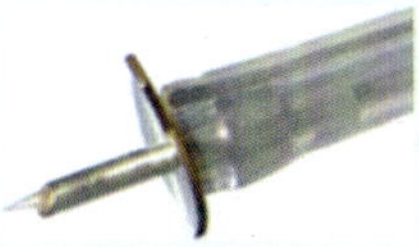	Name: Illuminated Infusion Chandelier Manufacturer: Synergetics Inc. Light cone angle: panoramic Purported use: bimanual surgery without extra sclerotomy
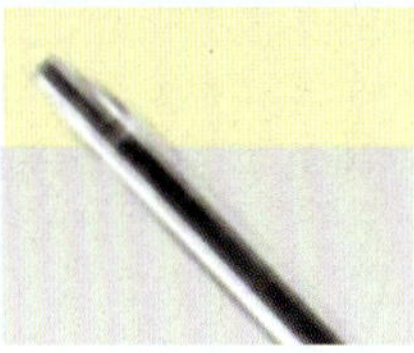	Name: Chandelier Lighting System Manufacturer: Alcon Constellation System Light cone angle: panoramic Purported use: bimanual surgery

FOCAL ILLUMINATION (FIG. 10.1)

- Advantages: Increased focal light intensity. Improves contrast and resolution. Particularly useful for membrane peeling of ERM, ILM, PVR membranes, etc.
- Disadvantages: May not be able to observe peripheral pathology, such as retinal breaks, evolving choroidal detachment, or suprachoroidal infusion placement

DIFFUSE ILLUMINATION (FIG. 10.2)

- Advantages: Allows widefield retinal visualization. May be better for NCVH, removal of IOFB, and primary RDs since all retinal breaks and areas of SRF can be visualized.
- Disadvantages: Lower illumination in any given area, with less contrast and resolution. Not optimal for detailed work such as ILM peeling, etc.

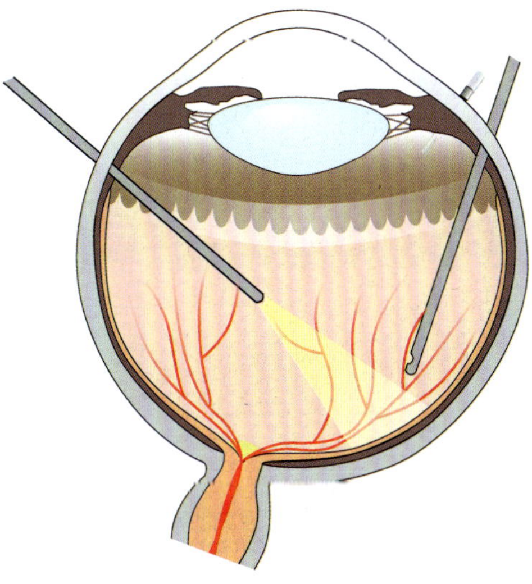

FIGURE 10.1. Focal illumination allows increased focal light intensity.

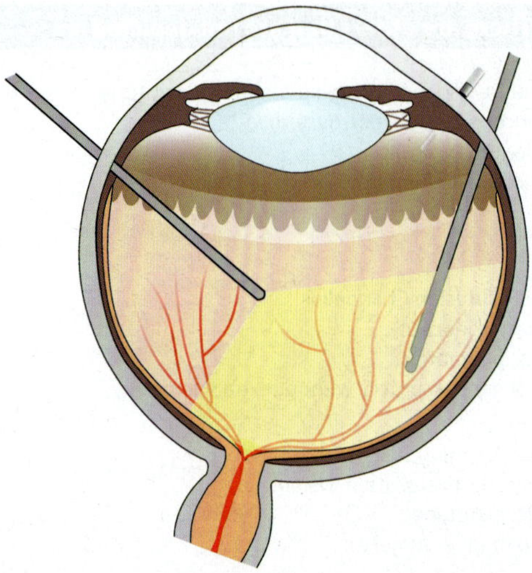

FIGURE 10.2. Diffuse illumination allows widefield retinal illumination.

CHANDELIER ILLUMINATION (FIG. 10.3)

- Advantages: Provides broad diffuse illumination for the entire fundus and great for bimanual surgery. Can be used with both 23G and 25G. Comes with an additional trocar and can be inserted like an infusion line cannula but as a fourth port typically placed inferiorly near 6 o'clock.
- Disadvantages: Additional cost and additional sclerotomy

ILLUMINATED INSTRUMENTS

- Types of illuminated instruments: Illuminated forceps, scissors, membrane peelers (picks), laser probes, and light pipes are all available.
- Specific applications of specific instruments:
  - Illuminated forceps: Useful when trying to peel fine membranes and in complex RD cases with PVR or PDR. Adjusting the tip location of the fiber optic light relative to the working portion of the forceps can impact visualization of the membranes.

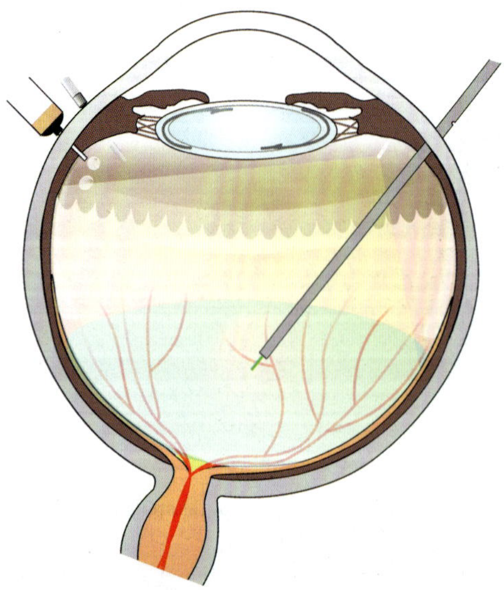

FIGURE 10.3. Chandelier illumination provides broad diffuse illumination for the entire fundus and helpful for bimanual surgery. Direct PFCL silicone oil exchange using chandelier illumination depicted herein.

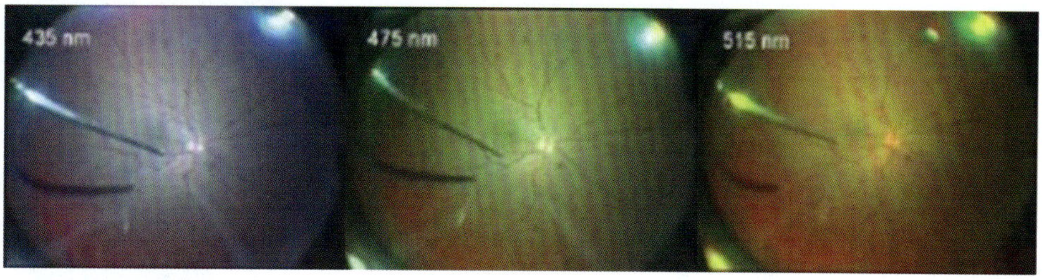

FIGURE 10.4. Three light filters improve visualization. Demonstrated on the Stellaris PC (Bausch + Lomb):
435 nm: Filters out harmful blue and UV light.
475 nm: Yellowish/green light highlights tissues.
515 nm: Amber tint helps reduce glare when under air. Safest.
(Reprinted with permission from Bausch & Lomb.)

  - Illuminated pick: Aids in bimanual techniques in complex RD cases. Available in 23G and 25G.
  - Illuminated scissors: Aids in bimanual techniques and reduces the need for chandelier lighting.
  - Illuminated laser probes: Particularly useful in lasering retinal breaks on posterior slope of SB and allows self-scleral depression. See chapter titled *Endolaser Types and Settings*.
  - Infusion light pipe: Available in 20G. Great option for straightforward NCVH and silicone oil removal cases. This may eliminate the need for a third port.

Light filters

- Improves visualization (Fig. 10.4).
  - 435 nm: Filters out harmful blue and UV light
  - 475 nm: Yellowish/green light highlights tissues in the eye
  - 515 nm: Amber tint reduces glare when under air. Safest

SOME LIGHT SOURCES

- Standard
  - Xenon: Intense light with optimal visualization for currently available standard light sources. Often utilized with filters to protect the retina from phototoxicity. Present in Bausch & Lomb Stellaris Elite machine.
  - Halogen: Warmer color with more yellow wavelength but not as powerful, so contrast may be less but is safer.
- Constellation System by Alcon
  - Utilizes RFID (radio-frequency identification technology) so when you plug in a particular light pipe into the system, the light pipe is recognized, and the appropriate amount of light is used to keep it within the FDA standards for phototoxicity limits. Only functions with Alcon instruments.
- NGENUITY System
  - 3D heads-up visualization, as opposed to binocular microscopy, allows surgery with less light and improves and enhances resolution and contrast. As little as 5% illumination may be adequate compared to the usual 40%-50% for coaxial microscopic visualization.

and variation in underlying pigmentation. Keep the laser probe moving if using continuous.

- Under PFCL, air, gas, and silicone oil
  - Endolaser
    - Spot intensity increases under PFCL, air, or gas due to insulating effect on the retina and diminished heat dissipation.
  - Indirect laser
    - Spot size increases under silicone oil or scleral depression.
    - Spot size decreases under air or gas.
    - Spot intensity increases under PFCL, air, or gas due to insulating effect on the retina and diminished heat dissipation.
- If not getting desired spot intensity,
  - Increase power, decrease spot size, and increase duration
  - Remove SRF, blood, silicone oil, or PFCL if present

WORKFLOW

- Preplace laser pedal between vitrectomy pedal and microscope pedal or on the side opposite the assistant. Some systems such as the Bausch and Lomb Stellaris Elite have an integrated laser pedal in the vitrectomy foot pedal with a hinged cover. The cover is lifted to access the laser pedal.
- Choose the probe type depending on where you need to apply laser.
- Connect the probe to laser console.
- Use protective eyewear for staff per facility protocol.
- Insert the laser probe into the vitreous cavity, and avoid phakic lens if using nonflexible, fixed curved probe.
- Only turn the laser from "standby" to "ready" once in the eye.
- For initial settings, see above.
- See Video 11.1.

Tips

- Panretinal laser photocoagulation: Wall off and demarcate the temporal arcades to avoid inadvertently lasering the macula by placing the posteriormost row anterior to temporal arcades and disc (Fig. 11.3). Work anteriorly from that posterior row. Place laser burns about one to two burn widths apart.
- Retinal breaks: Apply three rows of confluent laser spots to tightly surround the retinal breaks with spots just touching. You can use single pulse, repeated pulse, or continuous paint.

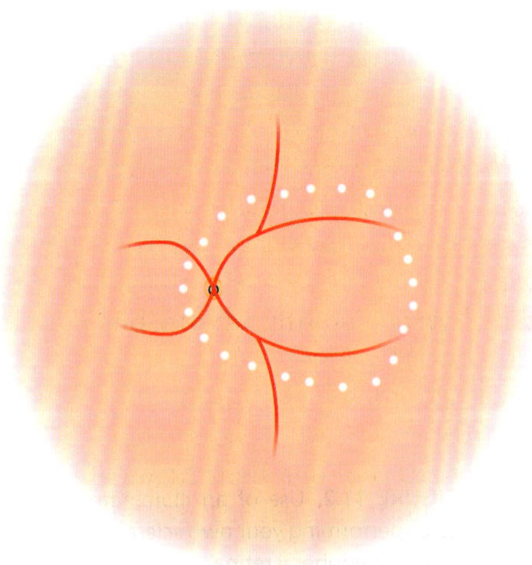

FIGURE 11.3. Panretinal laser photocoagulation. Wall off and demarcate the temporal arcades since you want to avoid the macula by placing the posteriormost row anterior to temporal arcades and disc.

- Retinal arteriolar macroaneurysm and capillary hemangioma: Larger spot, lower power, and longer duration.
- Avulsed and segmented retinal vessel: Diathermy works better than laser.
- Increase the distance between the tip of the laser probe and the retina as you move more anteriorly since the eye wall curves. This way, you will avoid hitting the retina with your laser tip. Also, since the anterior retina is thinner, this will prevent hot burns.

Indirect Laser

- Used primarily to treat pathology in the fellow eye
- Integrated into vitrectomy console or separate laser unit
- Less efficient than endolaser for operative eye since you may need to clear condensation on posterior surface of IOL, drain reaccumulated SRH, or remove PRH, SRH, or VH in order to continue lasering.

Laser Risks

Here are some complications and precautions.

- Retinal necrosis/vaporization from a hot laser burn can lead to retinal hole formation. What to do if this occurs: Encircle laser-induced hole with three rows of laser, +/− tamponade. See chapters titled *Fluid Air Exchange* and *Air Gas Exchange* and *Gas Tamponade*.
- Choroidal bleeding can occur with intense laser. What to do: Temporarily increase the infusion pressure, and consider diathermy if a retinal break is present. If the macula is detached, keep SRH out of the fovea by the rotating eye, and consider using PFCL to flatten the macula. Drain the subretinal subfoveal blood, particularly if thick and accessible from a posterior retinotomy.
- Inadvertent laser to the macula. Avoid by orienting and reorienting yourself throughout application of the laser. Ask yourself, "Where is the macula?"
- More retinal necrosis occurs with higher power, longer duration, and smaller spot size. Be careful when moving the probe tip closer to the retina since that creates a smaller spot size. At shorter durations, the power has to be increased to the point that it becomes more difficult to reproducibly create burns without inadvertently rupturing the retina, Bruch membrane, and choroid.
- Avoid lasering through PRH, IRH, and SRH.
- Choroidal effusions may occur, usually postop, especially when extensive amount of laser is applied. Use topical atropine 1% to help prevent the lens iris diaphragm from moving anteriorly.
- CNV can occur following rupture to Bruch membrane as a result of intense, hot laser burns.

Section III

Vitreoretinal Surgical Adjuncts

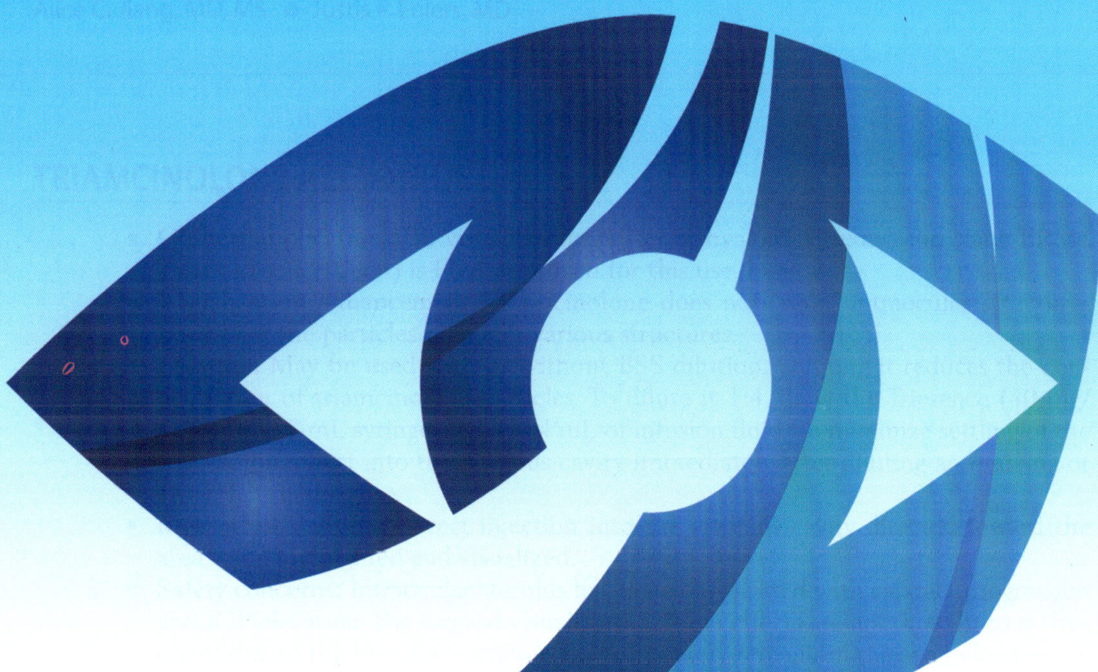

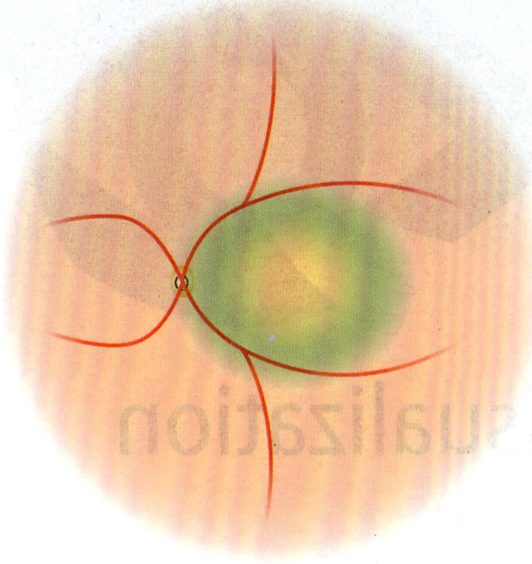

FIGURE 12.1. ICG stains ILM. "Negative staining" of ERM may be noted by the unstained central area occupied by an ERM.

  - *D5W*: The 25 mg ICG powder may be reconstituted with 20-mL D5W. Swirl. This will create a 1.25 mg/mL solution of ICG, which decreases the risk of RPE toxicity. Withdraw 2 mL from the ICG vial in a 3-mL syringe. Attach two green 0.22-µm filters to the 3-mL syringe. Attach a 22G needle to the filters. Inject 1 mL through both filters into TB syringe for the final product. Use promptly.
    - Using D5W provides a "heavy solution" (heavier than infusion fluid) that results in sinking of the ICG to the posterior pole without needing to be particularly close to the retinal surface during injection. Leave the ICG on the macular surface for the shortest time possible (< 30 seconds) and then remove. Aim to use the minimum concentration that achieves the required staining effect.
- **Method of delivery:** Direct injection into the vitreous cavity. Use soon after preparation.
- **Safety concerns:** Reports regarding the potential toxic effects of ICG to the retina and RPE have been cited. No randomized trials exist defining safety. When using ICG, the lowest concentration (<0.5 mg/mL) should be used for the shortest time possible to minimize potential risk. Allow staining with ICG for 30 seconds or less prior to its removal. Reduce the light pipe setting to about 25% of normal illumination to minimize the risk of phototoxicity.

> **Consider placing a small blob of viscoelastic over the macular hole prior to the use of ICG to decrease the likelihood of ICG coming into direct contact with the RPE.**

TRYPAN BLUE

- **Clinical applications:** Enhancing ERM visualization during membrane peeling procedures for PVR and/or ERM.
- **Stains:** ERM and ILM
- **Dilution:** Commercially available as a 0.15% concentration. "Heavy" trypan blue can be made by mixing it 1:1 with D5W. A heavy solution will allow for staining of the ERM/ILM without needing a FAX or injection close to the retinal surface.
- **Method of delivery:** Direct injection into the vitreous cavity.
- **Safety concerns:** Fewer safety concerns compared to ICG.

BRILLIANT BLUE

- **Clinical applications:** Selective staining of the ILM, a good alternative for ICG and trypan blue.
- **Stains:** ILM
- **Dilution:** Commercially available as a 0.025% concentration outside the United States and was recently FDA approved for use in the United States as well. It can be made heavy by diluting it with D5W.
- **Method of delivery:** Direct injection into the vitreous cavity.
- **Safety concerns:** Fewer safety concerns compared to ICG.

When injecting any of these substitutes close to the retinal surface, rapid and forceful injection could potentially result in an iatrogenic retinal break. Avoid direct injection into a FTMH.

Sometimes restaining is necessary.

CHAPTER 13

Perfluorocarbon Liquid

Eric Steuer, MD, PhD

PREOPERATIVE CONSIDERATIONS

- Alert OR team at the beginning of the case that you may be using PFCL.
- It is a very costly item, so ask the team not to open it until you are sure you need it.
- In very large or myopic eyes, be prepared to use two vials of PFCL.
- If your scrub or circulator is inexperienced, have your assistant help draw up the PFCL.

INDICATIONS

- Almost all cases of GRTs
- Frequently helpful in extensive PVR cases facilitating posterior to anterior peeling
- Helpful in stabilizing a detached retina while shaving the vitreous base
- Stabilizes the posterior retina during retinectomy
- Flattens a detached macula to facilitate ERM peel
- Some cases of complicated trauma:
  - To displace SRH
  - To stabilize the posterior retina during progressively anterior maneuvers
  - To protect the macula from posterior migration of SRH
  - To help with partial removal of an incarcerated retina
  - To help protect the macula during IOFB or dislocated IOL removal during repeated retrieval attempts

TECHNIQUES AND PEARLS (VIDEO 13.1)

- Consider reducing infusion pressure just prior to PFCL placement.
- Inject PFCL using a soft-tip cannula or dual-bore cannula. The dual-bore cannula allows for more control of the IOP by allowing fluid to egress from cannula shaft while PFCL is injected. See chapter titled *Posterior SRF During Vitrectomy for RRD*.

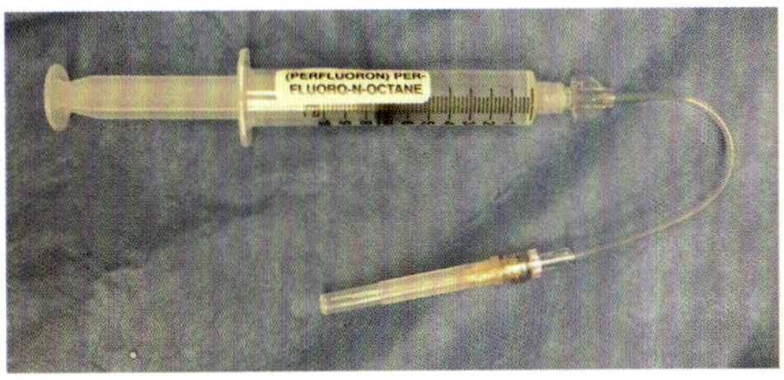

FIGURE 13.1. If bothered by an assistant's tendency to introduce tremor, separate the cannula and syringe with a short piece of small-bore tubing.

- Always inject slowly and under direct visualization with a widefield viewing system using an experienced assistant.
  - If bothered by an assistant's tendency to introduce tremor, separate the cannula and syringe with a short piece of small-bore tubing (Fig. 13.1).
  - If you favor injecting without an assistant, practice stabilizing your injecting hand with your thumb on the plunger.
- Begin by forming a bubble of PFCL over the nerve.
  - A high-speed stream of PFCL can penetrate the retina and cause a subretinal bleb or retinal hole.
  - Avoid beginning the initial stream of PFCL over the central macula to avoid creating a FTMH from the force of the PFCL stream.
- Immerse the tip of the cannula in the collection of PFCL to reduce the formation of smaller PFCL bubbles (Fig. 13.2). Avoiding bubbles lessens the chance of subretinal migration of PFCL through retinal breaks.
- If your view is disrupted by an infusion stream creating bubbles at the PFCL surface, try adjusting the infusion fluid pressure or redirecting and retaping the infusion line. This is less likely to happen with use of valved cannulas.

SPECIAL SCENARIOS

- Giant retinal tear. See chapter titled *Giant Retinal Tear*.
  - When performing PFCL air exchange, remove any remaining fluid above PFCL first (there almost always will be some, especially at the peripheral edge of the PFCL bubble). Patiently aspirate along the edge of the GRT, without touching the retina itself or RPE, making sure there is no residual infusion fluid before aspirating the PFCL posterior to the posterior edge of the GRT, as this will lessen the chance of the posterior edge of the GRT slipping. If it slips posteriorly, your

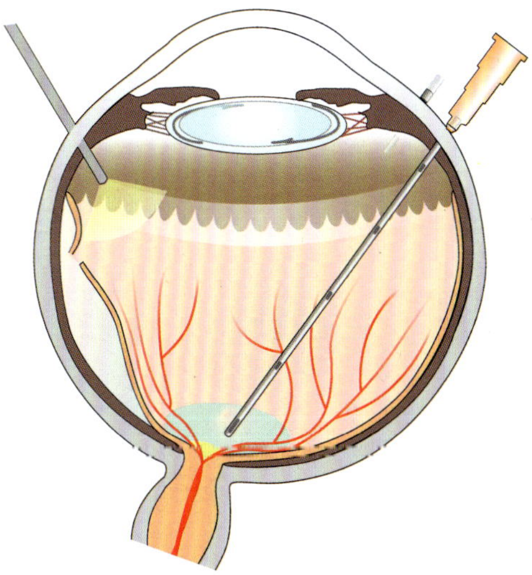

FIGURE 13.2. Immerse the tip of the cannula in the collection of PFCL to reduce the formation of smaller bubbles during injection.

choices are to repeat PFCL with a new vial, attempt a direct PFCL to silicone oil exchange, or try to position the patient postop hoping the slipped edge will smooth out (not likely). See chapters titled *Fluid Air Exchange* and *Perfluorocarbon Liquid Silicone Oil Exchange*.

- Floating a dislocated IOL
  - If using PFCL for floating up a dislocated IOL, remember that the refractive index of silicone plate haptic IOLs and PFCL is similar causing these IOLs to sometimes "disappear" in PFCL.
- Subretinal migration of PFCL
  - If PFCL migrates into the subretinal space via a break (typically a break under unrecognized traction), it should be removed.
  - Try to remove via the retinal break by tilting the eye toward the break, but you may need to create a posterior retinotomy directly over the subretinal PFCL.
  - Any remaining subretinal PFCL will inevitably migrate posteriorly and usually end up directly under the fovea where it will likely require a second PPV to remove it and may result in a permanent scotoma. See chapter titled *Subretinal Perfluorocarbon Liquid*.
- PFCL in AC
  - If you discover droplets of PFCL in the AC postop, these can be cautiously removed at the slit lamp with a 25G needle through a limbal paracentesis. Consider using povidone-iodine and postprocedure topical antibiotics.

CHAPTER 14

Gas Tamponade

Belinda Shirkey, MD

Intravitreal gas tamponade has multiple indications including pneumatic retinopexy, pneumatic vitreolysis, pneumatic displacement, SB for RRD, PPV for RRD, FTMH, and RRD prophylaxis in some eyes with retinal breaks, among others.

ADVANTAGES OF GAS AS AN INTRAVITREAL TAMPONADE

- Reportedly higher FTMH closure rates with gas than with air or silicone oil.
- Gas conforms to the undulations or divots of the retina and eye wall and provides more uniform tamponade, whereas silicone oil has an inherent surface tension that results in a smooth meniscus at its interface with the retina and thus does not conform to the contours of an irregular surface (Fig. 14.1).
- Gas reabsorbs over time, whereas silicone oil requires surgical removal.

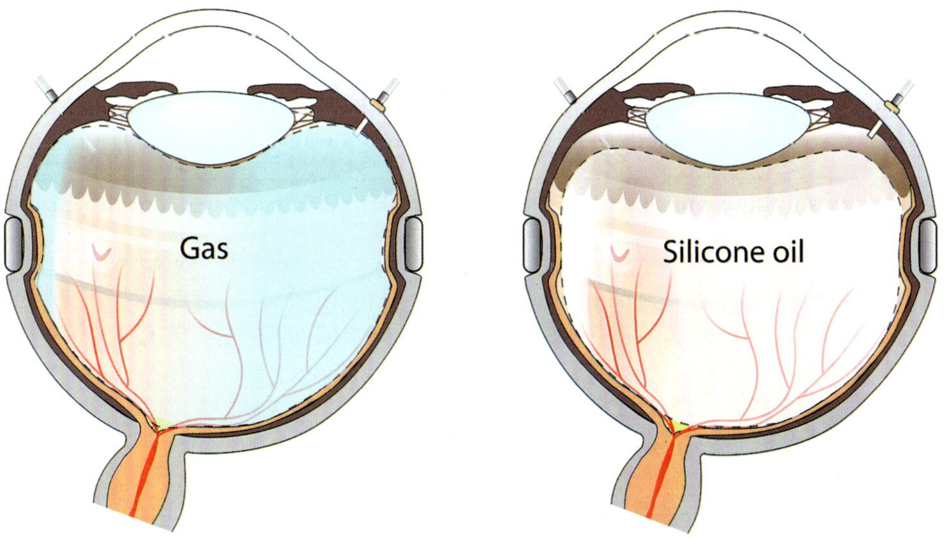

FIGURE 14.1. Gas conforms to the undulations or divots of the retina and eye wall and provides more uniform tamponade, whereas silicone oil has an inherent surface tension that causes a smooth meniscus at the interface with the retina and thus does not conform to the contours of irregular surfaces.

TABLE 14.1. Expansion and duration of common gas tamponade agents

	Expansion	Time to max expansion	Duration	Nonexpansile concentration
Air	0	None	5-7 d	0%-100%
SF_6	2×	1-2 d	2-4 wk	20%
C_3F_8	4×	3-4 d	6-8 wk	14%

- Gases can be used for intravitreal tamponade in either nonvitrectomized or vitrectomized eyes (Table 14.1).

CHOICES FOR GAS TAMPONADE

- Sterile air
  - Inert and nonexpansile
  - Drawn up from room air through a Millipore filter into a syringe (Fig. 14.2)
  - Administered either as an intravitreal injection, manually through a cannula after FAX, or from a vitrectomy machine
- Sulfur hexafluoride (SF_6)
  - Expansile medical grade gas
  - 100% SF_6 will expand twice its volume within 1-2 days.
  - 0.6 mL of 100% SF_6 is injected intravitreally in nonvitrectomized eyes. An AC paracentesis prior to gas injection may be performed to allow the administration of the 0.6 mL volume.
  - Nonexpansile concentration is 20% and is used in vitrectomized eyes.
  - Reabsorption occurs typically within 2-4 weeks, but it may last longer.
- Perfluoropropane (C_3F_8)
  - Expansile medical grade gas
  - 100% C_3F_8 gas will expand four times its volume within 3-4 days.
  - 0.3 mL of 100% C_3F_8 is injected intravitreally in nonvitrectomized eyes. An AC paracentesis prior to gas injection may be performed to allow the administration of the 0.3 mL volume.

Some prefer C_3F_8 in nonvitrectomized eyes to take advantage of the larger expansion and less initial volume.

  - Nonexpansile concentration is 14% and is used in vitrectomized eyes.
  - Reabsorption occurs typically within 6-8 weeks, but it may last longer.

If you are putting nonexpansile C_3F_8 in a vitrectomized aphakic eye, consider making an inferior PI.

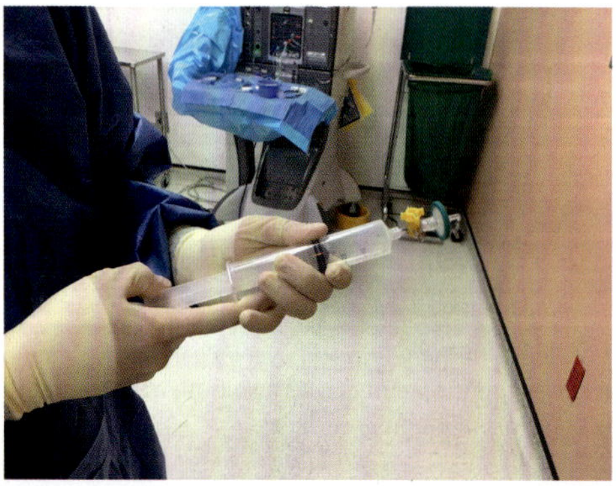

FIGURE 14.2. Sterile air can be drawn up from room air into a syringe through a Millipore filter. A 30-mL syringe is pictured here.

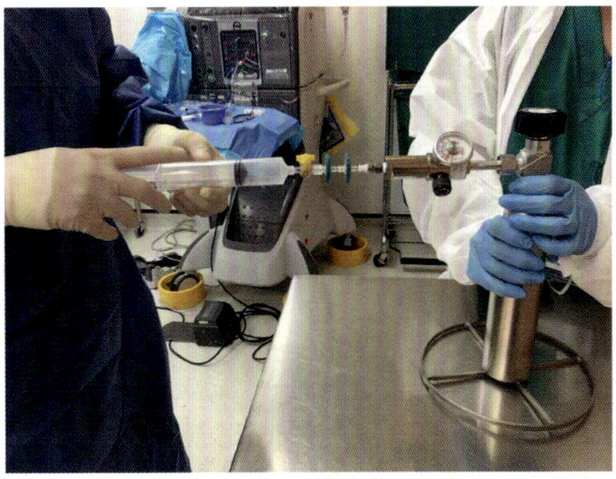

FIGURE 14.3. 100% (undiluted) gas is being drawn up into a 30-mL syringe through two Millipore filters.

HOW TO DRAW UP 100% (UNDILUTED) EXPANSILE GAS (FIG. 14.3, VIDEO 14.1):

VIDEO

- Check the gas name and expiration date.
- Connect two Millipore filters to gas tank canister.
- Connect a 1-mL TB syringe to the filter.
- Make sure both the gas tank valve and pressure chamber valve are closed (Fig. 14.4).
  - There is a valve from the gas tank canister to the pressure chamber and a valve from pressure chamber to outside.
  - The pressure chamber, sold separately, prevents the inadvertent emptying of all of the gas from the gas tank canister.
- Open the gas tank valve to fill the pressure chamber.
- Close the gas tank valve.
- Open the pressure chamber valve slowly to fill the attached syringe with the gas. Do not let the plunger fly off!
- Close the pressure chamber valve.
- Empty the gas in the syringe into room air in order to flush the line of any air pockets.
- Repeat steps 4-8.
- Promptly place a 30G needle on the syringe.
- The 100% gas is now ready for use. See above for quantities.
- How to draw up and dilute gas
- Check the gas name and expiration date.
- Connect a Millipore filter to gas tank.
- Connect a 30-mL syringe to the filter.

Some prefer a 60-mL syringe instead of a 30-mL syringe.

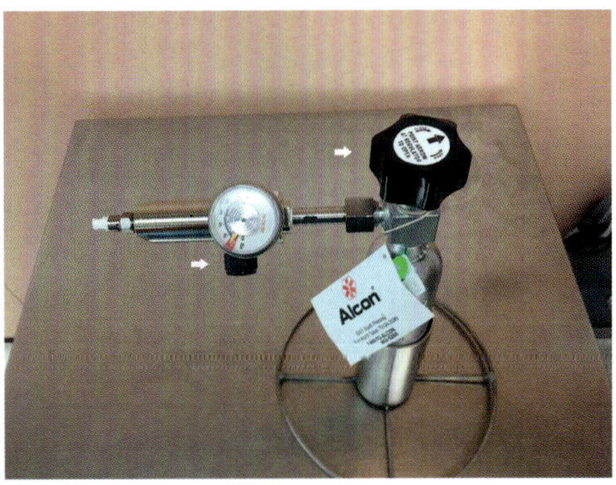

FIGURE 14.4. Make sure both gas tank valve (*arrow*) and pressure chamber valve (*arrow*) are closed.

- Make sure both the gas tank valve and pressure chamber valve are closed (Fig. 14.4).
  - There is a valve from the gas tank to the pressure chamber and a valve from pressure chamber to outside.
  - The pressure chamber, sold separately, prevents the inadvertent emptying of all of the gas from the canister.
- Open the gas take valve to fill the pressure chamber.
- Close the gas tank valve.
- Open the pressure chamber valve slowly to fill the attached syringe with the gas. Do not let the plunger fly off!
- Close the pressure chamber valve.
- Empty the gas in the syringe into room air in order to flush the line of any air pockets.
- Repeat steps 4-8.
- The 100% gas is now ready for dilution in the 30-mL syringe to a nonexpansile concentration.

You should either dilute the gas yourself or directly supervise the dilution.

- Promptly place a new Millipore filter on the gas-containing 30-mL syringe.
  - To obtain 20% SF_6: 6 mL of 100% gas is diluted with 24 mL of sterile air, for a total of 30 mL.
  - To obtain 14% C_3F_8: 4.5 mL of 100% gas is diluted with 25.5 mL of sterile air, for a total of 30 mL.

If using a 60-mL syringe, the following dilutions will result in nonexpansile concentrations.
- **To obtain 20% SF6: 12 mL of 100% gas is diluted with 48 mL of sterile air, for a total of 60 mL.**
- **To obtain 14% C3F8: 9 mL of 100% gas is diluted with 51 mL of sterile air, for a total of 60 mL.**
- **Promptly place a 30G needle on the syringe.**
- **The gas is now ready to use.**
- **When using a 60-mL syringe, flush 50 mL of the diluted nonexpansile gas through the vitreous cavity. See chapter titled Air Gas Exchange.**

- Promptly place a new Millipore filter on the gas-containing 30-mL syringe.
- To obtain 20% SF6: 6 mL of 100% gas is diluted with 24 mL of sterile air, for a total of 30 mL.
- To obtain 14% C3F8: 4.5 mL of 100% gas is diluted with 25.5 mL of sterile air, for a total of 30 mL.
- Promptly place a 30G needle on the syringe.
- The gas is now ready to use.
- When using a 30-mL syringe, flush 25 mL of the diluted nonexpansile gas through the vitreous cavity. See chapter titled Air Gas Exchange.

The Alcon Constellation machine can link the gas tanks to the machine so that the sterile scrubbed assistant can use the automated mechanism to fill a 30-mL syringe with 100% gas. Note that both the SF_6 and C_3F_8 tanks may be connected to the back of the machine. Care should be taken to identify that the gas that you plan to use is linked properly prior to surgery. This 100% gas will then need to be diluted to nonexpansile concentrations as outlined herein.

Be careful not to misidentify the gases and use the wrong concentration.

A complete fill of 100% undiluted gas can lead to a dangerously high IOP and irreversible visual loss.

TIPS

- Provide gas tamponade warnings to your patient and their family. A gas warning wristband and a gas warning wallet card are available reminder options.
- Flying in an airplane and other altitude changes are contraindicated for a patient with gas tamponade since changes in altitude lead to significant changes in bubble size. See chapter titled *The Preoperative Discussion*.
- Gas tamponade contributes to cataract formation and progression and may also lead to secondary elevation of IOP.
- VA through an intravitreal gas bubble is often at the hand motion level.
- Use of nitrous oxide is contraindicated in patients with an intravitreal gas bubble.

CHAPTER 15

Silicone Oil Tamponade

Erica E. Ballard, MD • Dean P. Hainsworth, MD

PREOPERATIVE CONSIDERATIONS

Consider silicone oil tamponade in the following cases:

- Complex or recurrent RRD
- PVR
- FTMH
- Retinal necrosis-related RD/viral retinitis RD
- When performing a retinectomy
- When postop positioning is not possible or feasible
- When air travel is necessary in the immediate postop period
- Inferior VR pathology
- Monocular status

TYPES OF SILICONE OIL

Two viscosities are available with similar endotamponade effects.

- Higher viscosity (5000 centistoke): more difficult to inject, slower to remove, and less likely to emulsify
- Lower viscosity (1000 centistoke): easier to inject, faster to remove, and more likely to emulsify

POTENTIAL COMPLICATIONS OF SILICONE OIL

Short Term

- Silicone oil in the AC
  - Causes include overfill, aphakia, poor zonular support, occluded inferior PI, open posterior capsule, and choroidal detachment.
- Signs include shimmering iris crypts, posterior bulging iris, or absent aqueous flare.
- Subconjunctival silicone oil
  - Suture all sclerotomies when using silicone oil.
  - Subconjunctival silicone oil can cause chronic irritation and is challenging to remove once it seeps into the tissues.

- High IOP due to silicone oil
  - Two causes
    - Pupillary block in aphakic and ACIOL eyes, without a patent PI.
    - Overfill (shallow AC) with secondary angle closure. Fluid is incompressible and the sclera is relatively inelastic; therefore, a slight overfill can lead to an exponential rise in IOP.

Long Term

- High IOP
  - Causes include emulsified oil droplets clogging the trabecular meshwork or causing trabeculitis.
- Chronic hypotony (IOP ≤ 5)
  - In the Silicone Oil Study, 18% of eyes at 36 months were hypotonous.
- Cataract
  - Progression may be faster in eyes with silicone oil.
- Recurrent RD
  - Rates similar to C_3F_8 gas use in the Silicone Oil Study. If the retina stays attached 3-5 months after silicone oil removal, redetachment is unlikely.
- Silicone oil emulsification
  - Can contribute to elevated IOP, inflammation, and PVR formation
- Bullous or band keratopathy
  - Usually due to silicone oil in the AC resulting in endothelial toxicity and cell loss or uveitis
- Unexplained visual loss
  - Refractive shifts secondary to silicone oil are well known; however, unexplained vision loss as demonstrated by multifocal ERG has shown only foveal involvement. The mechanism is unclear.

SILICONE OIL REMOVAL

Preoperative Considerations

- Remove silicone oil when it has served its purpose and when further retention may increase the risk of complications (the sweet spot).
- Silicone Oil Study: remove silicone oil after a minimum of 8 weeks.
- Remove silicone oil within 6 months, unless opt to retain silicone oil longer.
- Complications that may prompt earlier silicone oil removal include corneal touch, high IOP not controlled with medical management, and emulsification.

SURGICAL PROCEDURE (VIDEO 15.1)

- Set up a two-port vitrectomy system. Place the infusion line in the inferotemporal cannula. Place the second cannula for either the passive egress or active aspiration of silicone oil either superonasal or superotemporal. Passive egress works efficiently with 20G nonvalved cannula and is much less efficient with smaller gauges, even if the valve is removed.
- Allow infusion fluid to replace globe volume as silicone oil is either actively aspirated or allowed to passively egress.
- Keep the cannula or the aspiration tip within the silicone oil bubble to avoid aspiration of infusion fluid.

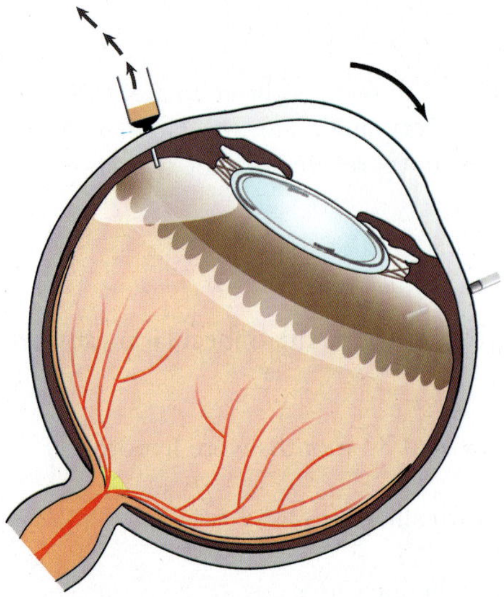

FIGURE 15.1. Near the end of silicone oil removal, a silicone oil-infusion fluid meniscus will be seen. Keep the cannula or the aspiration tip within the silicone oil bubble to avoid aspiration of infusion fluid. Tilting the eye may better position the remaining silicone oil bubble for removal.

VIDEO If silicone oil is being actively aspirated, typically a 23G automated viscous extraction device is used (Video 15.1).

- **The vitrectomy machine is set to "viscous fluid extraction."**
- **Before starting, make sure the rubber piece within the extraction syringe is at the end of the syringe closest to the tip. If not, you can switch the vitrectomy machine to "viscous fluid inject" and press down on the pedal to get the rubber stopper to the end of the syringe closest to the tip.**
- **Place the tip of the extraction device into the cannula while actively aspirating.**
- **Keep the tip of the extraction syringe in silicone oil at all times.**
- **As the silicone oil is removed, maneuver the eye so that silicone oil remains most elevated to ensure the tip of the extraction syringe remains in silicone oil at all times.**
- **If the syringe begins extracting infusion fluid instead, the eye will quickly soften. Stop aspirating.**

- Near the end of silicone oil removal, a silicone oil-infusion fluid meniscus will be seen. Tilting the eye may better position the remaining silicone oil bubble for removal (Fig. 15.1).
- In machine-assisted active suction of the silicone oil, slow aspiration once the silicone oil bubble appears nearly aspirated to avoid hypotony.
- After all visible silicone oil has been removed, perform scleral depression to search for any remaining silicone oil droplets.
- Remove the silicone oil as completely as possible, although complete removal is impossible. Consider multiple FAX to aspirate residual "oil slick." Silicone oil adheres to ciliary processes, zonules, and posterior iris.

Multiple FAX can help remove residual silicone oil.

- **Use a backflush cannula.**
- **Inject air that pushes any anteriorly remaining silicone oil toward the posterior pole so that a layer of oil is present between the air and infusion fluid.**
- **Use the tip of the backflush cannula to aspirate the thin film of silicone oil.**
- **Once the FAX is complete, partially refill the eye with infusion fluid.**
- **Any residual silicone oil on the retinal surface then reaccumulates at the surface of the fluid. Repeat the FAX to skim off any silicone oil on the surface.**
- **Repeat the FAX until any visible residual silicone oil is removed.**

- Aspirate any emulsified silicone oil droplets from the corneal endothelial surface using a TB syringe on a short 25G needle. Be careful not to touch the corneal endothelium.

POSTOPERATIVE CONSIDERATIONS

- Sometimes, silicone oil stays in the eye indefinitely when there is a poor visual prognosis or in patients unable to return to OR.
- Low IOP (<10 mm Hg) deters removal.
- Try a handheld corrective lens to determine visual potential in the silicone oil-filled eye such as +5.0D, whether the patient is phakic, aphakic, or pseudophakic.

Section IV

Exchanges

CHAPTER 16

Fluid Air Exchange

Joseph A. Khawly, MD, FACS

CONSIDERATIONS PRIOR TO FAX

- Remove all vitreous around the retinal break(s), and perform a thorough vitrectomy with shaving of the vitreous base. See chapter titled *Vitrectomy Surgery Steps*.
- Mark all retinal breaks, iatrogenic or preexisting, with endodiathermy so you can easily identify them under air. Often, the view under air is less than ideal, and having this high contrast of white diathermy against the orange color of the fundus will help you visualize the breaks to drain SRF through them if needed and laser them. See chapter titled *Endolaser Types and Settings*.
- Extremely small retinal breaks (smaller than the area of the tip of the soft-tip cannula) may be enlarged slightly with the vitreous cutter to avoid aspiration of the retina itself during FAX. Aspirating the retina can exert inadvertent traction on the retina and lead to bleeding or allow for subretinal migration of PFCL.
  - Consider doing a fluid-fluid exchange initially so that the turbid "schlieren" or SRF containing cellular and growth factor components that may contribute to PVR does not access the preretinal surface.

> **Fluid-fluid exchange. While infusion fluid remains on, place the soft-tip cannula or vitreous cutter in front of the retinal break, and aspirate SRF (Fig. 16.1).**

  - After a fluid-fluid exchange, there will be some reaccumulation of SRF, but this will be from infusion fluid that dilutes the remaining SRF and the components that promote PVR.
- Consider using humidified air during FAX.
  - Moisten the humidifying chamber (MoistAir, Iridex) by adding several mL of infusion fluid to it. Then, connect this between the air tubing coming from the vitrectomy machine and the infusion tubing that attaches to the cannula entering the eye (Fig. 16.2). You may have to cut the tubing to insert the chamber.
  - Humidified air may be beneficial if the eye is under air infusion for a prolonged period of time since it will delay posterior lens opacification in a phakic eye and decrease the risk of a visual field defect from a dehydration injury that may result

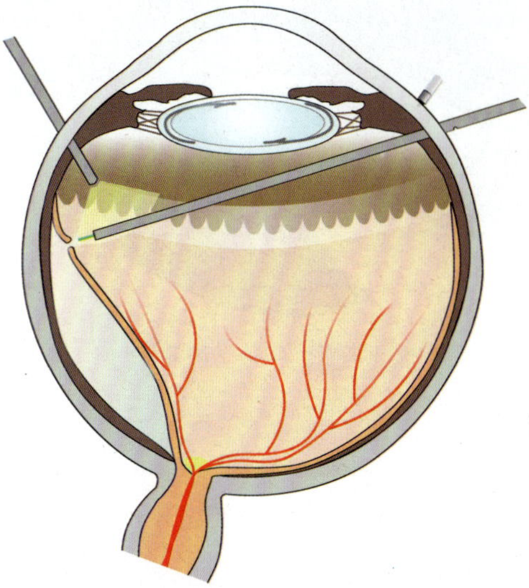

FIGURE 16.1. Fluid-fluid exchange. While infusion fluid remains on, place the soft-tip cannula or vitreous cutter in front of the retinal break, and aspirate SRF.

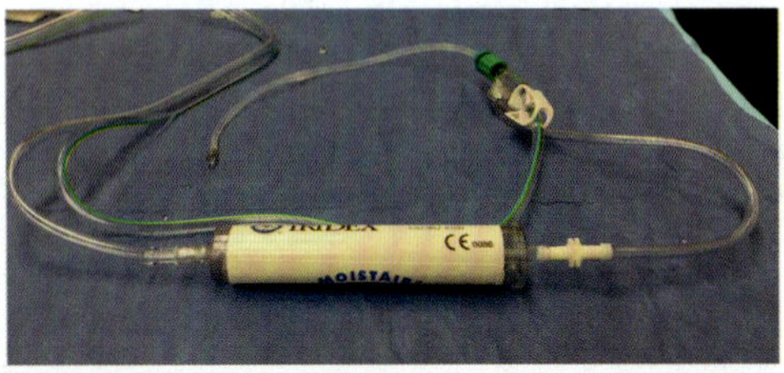

FIGURE 16.2. Connect the humidifying chamber (MoistAir, Iridex) between the air tubing coming from the vitrectomy machine and the infusion tubing that attaches to the cannula entering the eye. Moisten the humidifying chamber by adding several mL of infusion fluid.

when airflow is directed perpendicular to the retinal surface. These sequelae are less likely to occur nowadays with smaller-gauge vitrectomy and the use of valved cannulas as well as during FAX of relatively short duration.
- The main disadvantage of using a humidified chamber is the added cost to the procedure.

> **Ensure the infusion cannula is in the vitreous cavity during the FAX. If the infusion cannula tip slips into the choroidal space, air may inadvertently be infused into the choroidal circulation, which could lead to an air embolism.**

FAX WITHOUT THE USE OF PFCL (VIDEO 16.1)

- **Use a posterior drainage retinotomy to drain SRF.**
  - In the era of PFCL, creating a posterior drainage retinotomy is less commonly performed since it can contribute to PVR, ERM, RD, or CNV.
  - If PFCL is not available or if you are not as familiar with the intraop management of PFCL, then a posterior drainage retinotomy may be needed.
    - It should be considered only if there is adequate posterior SRF to create one, as in eyes with a total or subtotal RD.
    - In cases where only a more peripheral RD is present, then drain directly through the preexisting peripheral retinal break instead.
  - If possible, create your posterior drainage retinotomy adjacent to the optic nerve superonasally, ~1-2 DD from the edge of the nerve.
    - This superonasal and posterior location ensures maximal SRF drainage, yet its relative distance from the fovea helps minimize consequences related to ERM formation around the retinotomy.
    - Drainage retinotomies anywhere inferior to the nerve are often avoided because an inferior location may not be well tamponaded with air or gas. See chapter titled *Gas Tamponade*.

- A drainage retinotomy superotemporal to the nerve is often too close to the macula and increases the likelihood of visual sequelae from ERM formation.
- Mark the drainage retinotomy site with diathermy. Use a soft-tip cannula to punch through this spot from which you can then drain SRF. See chapter titled *Posterior SRF During Vitrectomy for RRD*.

- **Use an existing peripheral break to drain SRF.**
  - In cases where RD is confined to a few clock hours of peripheral retina, a FAX may be performed using the causative peripheral break to drain SRF.
  - Rotate the eye so the quadrant with the SRF is in as dependent a position as possible to maximize SRF drainage.
  - This technique almost never results in complete SRF drainage, but as long as enough SRF is drained to create chorioretinal apposition for laser retinopexy around the retinal break(s), it is not critical to drain all of the SRF.
  - If not all the posterior SRF is drained in eyes with a macula-involving rhegmatogenous RD, postop positioning to maximize the use of intraocular tamponade is key to assure macular re-attachment and to avoid formation of a retinal fold. See chapters titled *Postop Positioning* and *Postop Retinal Fold*.

FAX WITH THE USE OF PFCL

- No need for posterior drainage retinotomy. Instead, PFCL allows you to drain through a preexisting peripheral retinal break or a peripheral retinotomy.
- Ensure all traction on and adjacent to the retinal break is relieved before injecting PFCL into the eye. If not, PFCL may migrate into the subretinal space before FAX or shortly after FAX begins.
  - This is uncommon in eyes without PVR.
  - This can happen while attempting to use PFCL to unfold a GRT. Slow injection of PFCL is key to avoid "trapping" a folded flap of the retina under the PFCL.
- Inject PFCL slowly in all cases to allow simultaneous egress of infusion fluid in the vitreous cavity out of the eye. Injecting slowly into the established bubble of PFCL may avoid the creation of smaller PFCL bubbles at the peripheral fluid interface that could then migrate into the subretinal space through a break.
- Inject PFCL no higher than the posterior edge of the most peripheral retinal break (Fig. 16.3).

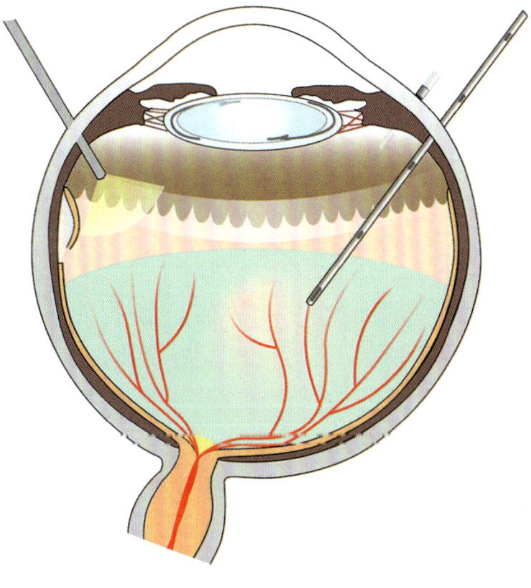

FIGURE 16.3. PFCL should be injected no higher than the posterior edge of the most peripheral retinal break.

- If that retinal break is covered with PFCL, then further PFCL injection will not allow SRF to exit the subretinal space.
- Laser is performed at this point or after FAX. See chapter titled *Endolaser Types and Settings*.

- Turn air infusion on, position the soft-tip cannula close to the retinal break, and aspirate slowly and continuously. As the fluid-air interface migrates past your view of the soft-tip cannula, there is a short period of compromised visualization. Once the interface passes over, a slight refocusing of the microscope and wide-angle viewing system is required to reestablish good focus.
- Once as much SRF has been removed as possible through the break, use the soft-tip cannula to aspirate the remaining PFCL by aspirating over the optic disc. Avoid aspirating the optic nerve tissue itself!
- Dry once more over the disc after waiting a few minutes to ensure all of the fluid has been removed.
- Continue aspirating as you remove the soft-tip cannula from the eye to prevent PFCL from dribbling back out of the soft-tip cannula into the vitreous cavity.

Consider a PFCL "washout" after removing the PFCL by injecting a small amount of infusion fluid while under air and then reaspirating that fluid with the soft tip over the optic disc to ensure no small droplets of PFCL remain (Fig. 16.4).

Because PFCL has a low boiling point, it is volatile and evaporates in an air-filled eye over time.

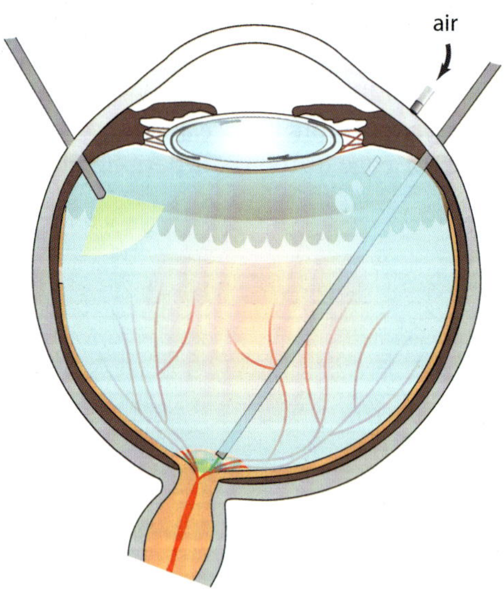

FIGURE 16.4. Consider a PFCL "washout" after removing the PFCL by injecting a small amount of infusion fluid while under air and then reaspirating that fluid with the soft tip over the optic disc to ensure no small droplets of PFCL remain.

CHAPTER 17

Air Gas Exchange

Adam Berger, MD

- The infusion line is clamped proximal to the Luer lock junction using a hemostat (Fig. 17.1). This ensures an airtight globe during subsequent maneuvers.
- The infusion line is separated from the air tubing at the Luer lock.
- The syringe of diluted gas is attached to the infusion line at the Luer lock. See chapter titled *Gas Tamponade*.
- While applying very light pressure to the plunger of the syringe, the hemostat is removed (Fig. 17.2).
- A vent or "chimney" is inserted into the opposite cannula (Fig. 17.3), simultaneously depressing the plunger on the syringe slowly to start the infusion of gas into the vitreous cavity as the air escapes and, thus, the air gas exchange. Air is allowed to escape from the chimney vent. Slow, steady continuous pressure is applied to the plunger to avoid elevating the IOP or allowing the eye to soften.

VIDEO

Alternate methods of venting the air from the vitreous cavity include removing the valve on the cannula, inserting a soft-tip cannula on a backflush handle, using a 25G needle attached to a small syringe with the plunger removed, or holding open the valve on the cannula with a toothed forceps (Video 17.1).

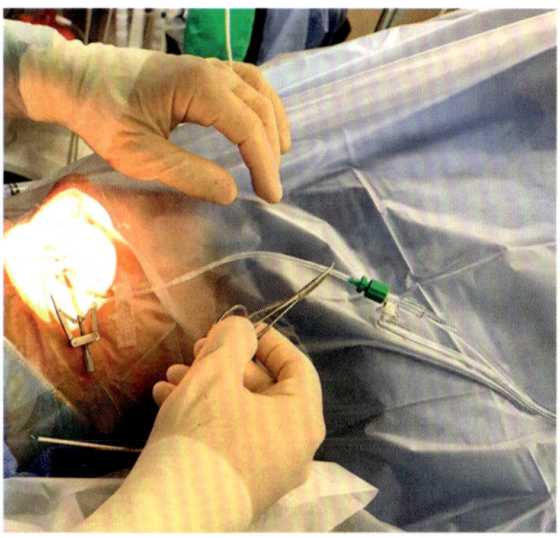

FIGURE 17.1 The infusion line is clamped proximal to the Luer lock so that the infusion line can be disconnected from the vitrectomy machine without depressurizing the eye.

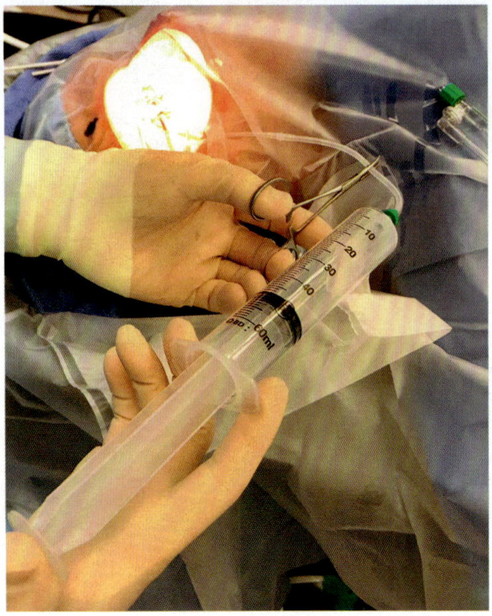

FIGURE 17.2. With light pressure on the plunger, the hemostat is removed. A 60-mL syringe containing a nonexpansile concentration of gas is being used.

- If there is any resistance to the flow of gas, check the vented cannula to make sure it is not obstructed with vitreous.
- When there is ~5 mL of gas left in the syringe if you are using a 30-mL syringe or 10 mL of gas left if you are using a 60-mL syringe, the pressure on the plunger is released and the venting device removed. See chapter titled *Gas Tamponade*.
- IOP may be adjusted at this time using tactile approximation. The infusion line is then again clamped with a hemostat.

Leave the residual gas in the syringe, and cap it with a 30G needle in case additional gas is needed at the end of the case.

- The transscleral cannulas are removed.
- If the eye is soft due to some gas escaping during removal of the cannulas, the residual gas capped with a 30G needle may be used to inject gas through the pars plana to "top off" the eye.

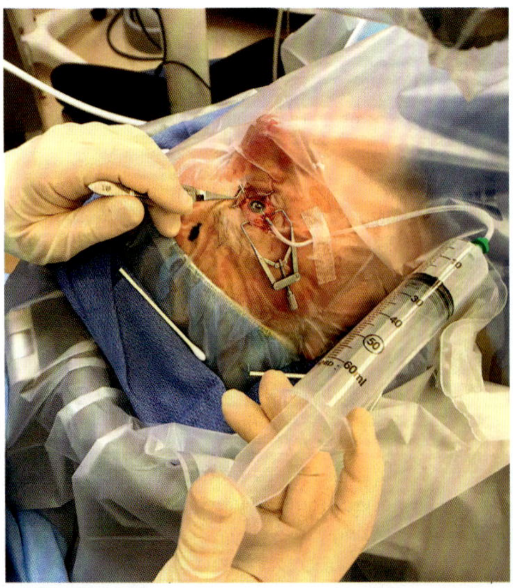

FIGURE 17.3. About 50 mL of gas is injected if using a 60-mL syringe as shown while simultaneously venting air out of the vitreous cavity through another port.

CHAPTER 18

Air Silicone Oil Exchange

John D. Zilis, MD

PREOPERATIVE CONSIDERATIONS

The indications for silicone oil in vitrectomy are many and include complex or recurrent RD, PVR, viral retinitis, as well as other situations like air travel, monocular status, and positioning challenges in children or those with limited mobility. It is often used when there is inferior VR pathology or need for long-term tamponade. See chapter titled *Silicone Oil Tamponade*.

Air silicone oil exchange is the most common approach to silicone oil placement in the eye and is performed at the conclusion of the case. A thorough vitrectomy and complete removal of retinal traction with flattening of the retina under air should be accomplished before silicone oil is introduced. Residual fluid inside the vitreous cavity should be removed as completely as possible. Due to surface tension differences, if the retina is not flat under air, silicone oil will not flatten it. Residual traction may also, occasionally, lead to subretinal silicone oil.

SURGICAL PROCEDURE

- Leave all three cannulas in place initially with the air infusion on.
- Attach a short, thin walled blunt needle to the silicone oil-filled syringe to allow the silicone oil to flow faster, with less required force.
    - If such a blunt needle is not available, shorten and use an angiocath needle of appropriate gauge instead.
- First, inject a little bit of oil outside the eye to ensure proper functioning of the injection mechanism and tight attachment of the blunt cannula to the silicone oil-filled syringe.
- Infuse silicone oil into the vitreous cavity using a large syringe that is attached to the silicone oil pump incorporated within the vitrectomy machine, using the foot pedal for control. Set the vitrectomy machine to viscous fluid injection.
- When silicone oil is first being injected, observe it through the operating microscope and viewing system to ensure correct placement into the vitreous cavity. See Video 18.1.
- While injecting silicone oil through one cannula, use another cannula to vent air from the eye (Fig. 18.1). You can control the venting of air with forceps partially

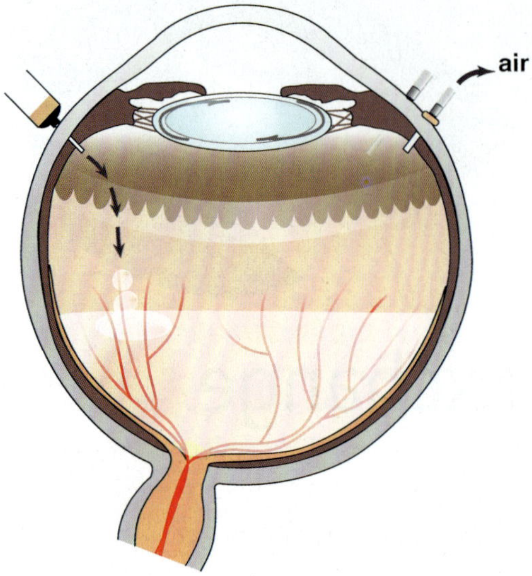

FIGURE 18.1. While injecting silicone oil through one cannula, use another cannula to vent intravitreal air from the eye. A chimney device is inserted into the cannula to vent the air.

placed in the cannula lumen or through the cannula valve. Alternatively, place a chimney device into the cannula to vent the air.

- As silicone oil is injected, lower the air infusion pressure to around 10 mm Hg.
  - Toward the end of the silicone oil infusion, lower the air infusion pressure further and then consider clamping the air line or disconnecting it.
- Maintain a low-normal IOP during silicone oil infusion. If the IOP is too high, silicone oil can be forced into the AC. Through the microscope, watch the silicone oil and stop injecting when the silicone oil begins to enter the infusion line or when it touches the IOL or native lens. Remove any residual air behind the pupillary space to avoid an underfill of silicone oil.
  - Move the eye slightly to the side while slowly adding silicone oil, allowing the air to escape through the vented cannula.
    - Since most cannulas are valved, use a forceps or chimney device to hold the venting cannula open to allow escape of residual air (Fig. 18.2).

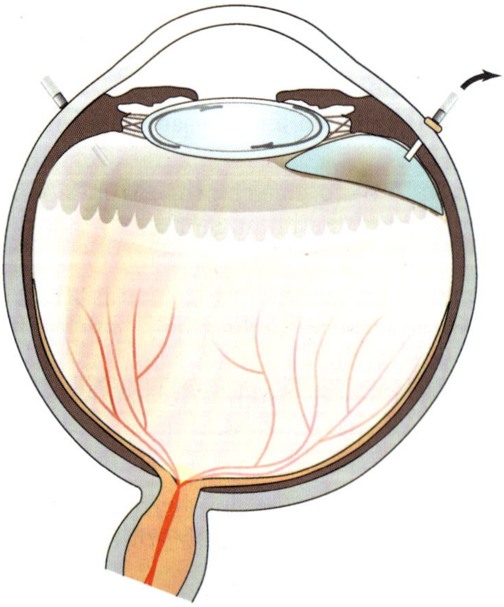

FIGURE 18.2. Use a chimney device to vent the eye through a valved cannula to allow escape of residual air.

- Switching the silicone oil infusion to a different cannula site can also be helpful.
- If a pocket of air remains despite these maneuvers, remove the air with a soft-tip cannula with the silicone soft tip removed, or with the vitrector. Avoid instrument contact with the lens or silicone oil, since the silicone oil may plug the lumen and prevent aspiration of the remaining air.
- If there is concern that air remains, use the light pipe to visualize the small air bubble.

- After the air silicone oil exchange has been completed, palpate the globe gently to check for a "normal" IOP.
- Consider suturing sclerotomies to prevent subconjunctival silicone oil.
- Irrigate the surface of the globe well before closing the conjunctiva.

OIL INJECTION IN AN APHAKIC EYE OR EYE WITH ACIOL

- Inject silicone oil until it reaches the plane of the pupil with the residual air maintained in the AC.
- Make an inferior PI to prevent pupillary block, which could lead to high IOP and misdirect silicone oil into the AC.
- Create the PI using the vitreous cutter when the eye is fluid-filled, before the FAX, so that any bleeding from the iris has time to stop. This will decrease the chance of a postop hyphema and temporary occlusion of the PI.
- Put the PI inferiorly to allow aqueous to pass into the AC during most postop head positions, as the silicone oil remains above the aqueous.

When injecting silicone oil in an aniridic eye, consider placing silicone oil retention sutures using 10-0 Prolene on a 16-mm (STC-6) needle 1 mm posterior to the limbus to provide a barrier to forward migration of silicone oil (Fig. 18.3).

PROBLEMS AND PEARLS

Silicone oil underfill

- Is a risk factor for recurrent RD.
- Aim for a near total silicone oil fill. It is not possible to achieve a 100% silicone oil fill of the vitreous cavity.
- To avoid an underfill, remove the air completely from behind the lens during the air silicone oil exchange, and palpate the globe for a normal IOP at the end of silicone oil infusion.

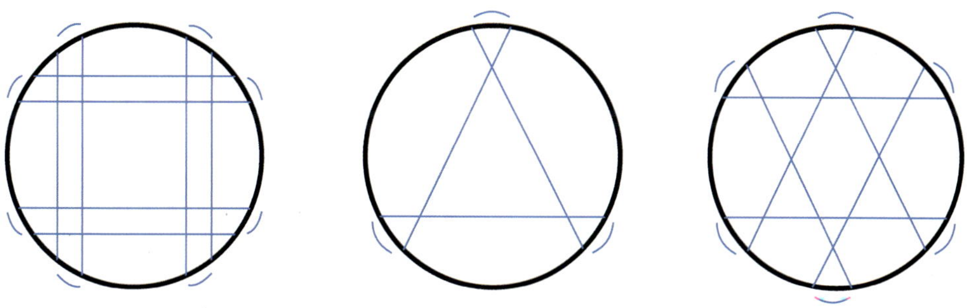

FIGURE 18.3. Various configurations for placing silicone oil retention sutures.

Silicone oil overfill
- Can usually be identified intraop.
- Injecting silicone oil under high pressure can cause silicone oil to move into the AC, even in phakic or pseudophakic eyes.
- Prevent a silicone oil overfill by injecting the silicone oil in a controlled fashion, and monitor the IOP during injection and at the end of the procedure.
- If an oil overfill is determined, oil can be allowed to passively exit through an open cannula.
- If silicone oil enters the AC, efforts should be made to remove it since it can lead to postop complications, such as inflammation, increased IOP, and keratopathy.
  - In a pseudophakic or phakic eye, a limbal incision can be made to allow the exit of an isolated silicone oil bubble from the AC while injecting air slowly from a second limbal site.

Visualization
- If condensation develops on the back of the IOL or the phakic lens feathers, the view will improve dramatically when silicone oil makes contact with the posterior surface of the lens.
- You do not need to observe the retina after the silicone oil infusion starts, but take a peek with the indirect ophthalmoscope when the silicone oil is in. The view may be improved due to the silicone oil-lens optical interface.
- If needed, add additional laser photocoagulation after the silicone oil is in.

CHAPTER 19

Perfluorocarbon Liquid Silicone Oil Exchange

Shelley Day Ghafoori, MD

There are several techniques for instilling silicone oil in the eye. One method is a FAX to remove PFCL followed by an air silicone oil exchange. Another method is a direct PFCL silicone oil exchange in cases at risk of retinal slippage, such as a GRT RD or when there is an extensive retinectomy. Slippage can occur when fluid in the vitreous cavity enters the subretinal space through the GRT during FAX.

STEPS FOR PFCL AIR SILICONE OIL EXCHANGE

- Perform a FAX.
  - As the vitrectomy machine pumps air into the eye through the infusion cannula, aspirate PFCL with a soft-tip cannula. See chapter titled *Vitrectomy Machine Settings*.
  - Keep the tip of the soft-tip cannula within the PFCL bubble until the PFCL is fully removed. Move the tip more posteriorly as the PFCL bubble decreases in size.
- Once the eye is filled with air and all of the PFCL has been removed, inject silicone oil with a viscous fluid injector through a cannula while allowing air to egress passively through an unvalved cannula (or by holding the valved cannula open with a chimney vent or 0.12 forceps). See chapter titled *Air Silicone Oil Exchange*.
- Does not require a chandelier light or lighted infusion.
- Does not require a skilled assistant.

STEPS FOR DIRECT PFCL SILICONE OIL EXCHANGE (VIDEO 19.1)

- Perform a direct PFCL silicone oil exchange with active injection of silicone oil and passive efflux of PFCL with a Charles flute needle (Bausch + Lomb/Synergetics) (Fig. 19.1A) or a backflush cannula (Alcon) (Fig. 19.1B).
  - Instill PFCL to completely fill the vitreous cavity. There should be minimal infusion fluid in the vitreous cavity.

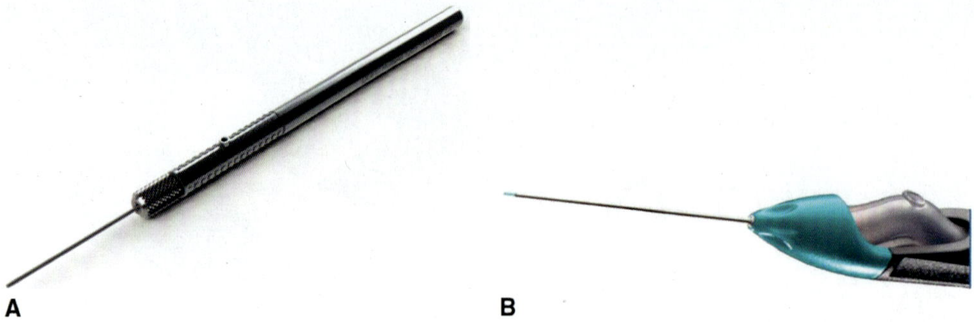

FIGURE 19.1. Direct PFCL silicone oil exchange can be performed with active injection of silicone oil and passive efflux of PFCL using a **A.** Charles flute needle (Bausch + Lomb/Synergetics) or a **B.** backflush cannula (Alcon).

- Remove the infusion line and instill a small amount of silicone oil to make the IOP slightly greater than physiologic.
- Place the light pipe and flute needle or backflush cannula through the ports.
  - Alternatively, you can use chandelier endoillumination or a lighted infusion to free up a port for injection of silicone oil. See chapter titled *Illumination During Vitreous Surgery*.
  - If you use a light pipe, have a skilled assistant hold either the light pipe or silicone oil infusion cannula.
- Place a flute needle or a backflush cannula into the PFCL bubble while injecting silicone oil slowly. As the silicone oil is infused, the IOP increases and the PFCL will be passively aspirated into the flute needle or backflush cannula (Fig. 19.2).
- Since silicone oil is lighter than PFCL, it will remain on top of the PFCL bubble and fill the eye from anterior to posterior as the PFCL bubble decreases in size.
- Keep the tip of the flute needle or backflush cannula within the PFCL bubble as it decreases during direct PFCL silicone oil exchange. If the flute needle enters the silicone oil bubble, it may become clogged resulting in dangerously high IOP with injection of oil.
- Once the PFCL bubble is small, stop injecting silicone oil and allow the PFCL to be passively aspirated. This will prevent the IOP from getting too high, requiring removal of some silicone oil.

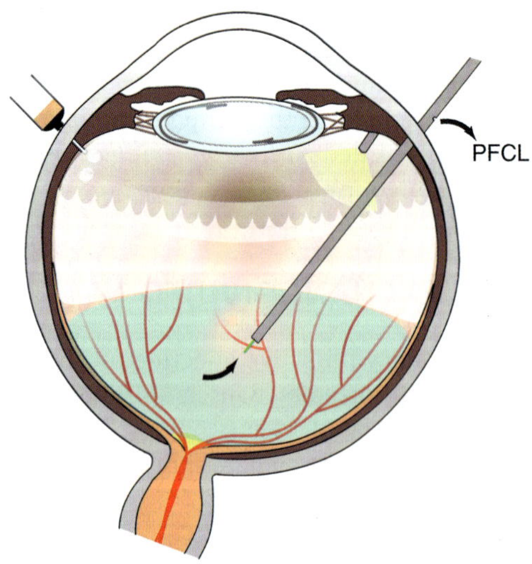

FIGURE 19.2. Place a flute needle or a backflush cannula (pictured here) in the PFCL bubble as silicone oil is slowly injected into the eye through the viscous fluid injector. As the silicone oil is infused, the IOP increases and the PFCL will be passively aspirated into the flute needle or backflush cannula.

- Newer vitrectomy systems may have bimanual modes, which allow simultaneous active infusion of silicone oil and extraction of PFCL. In this situation, active aspiration of PFCL is performed with a soft-tip cannula placed over the optic disc while the silicone oil is actively injected through the infusion cannula.
  - This technique may offer better IOP control since the active aspiration of PFCL is matched with the rate of silicone oil injection.
  - High-pressure tubing is available that allows for injection of silicone oil actively through the infusion line. This frees up a hand allowing you to hold both the light pipe and flute needle or backflush cannula and thus chandelier illumination would not be needed.

Remember to keep checking tactile IOP during a direct PFCL silicone oil exchange. If the flute needle gets clogged with silicone oil, continued silicone oil injection can result in dangerously high IOP.

Remember to place an inferior PI in aphakic eyes or pseudophakic eyes with poor zonular or capsular integrity. If silicone oil ends up in the AC, try injecting viscoelastic or air into the AC to move silicone oil back into the vitreous cavity. If this is unsuccessful, silicone oil can be removed and the eye can be refilled with infusion fluid. The retina can then be reattached with PFCL, and then PFCL silicone oil exchange can be repeated.

Section V

Rhegmatogenous Retinal Detachment

CHAPTER 20

Rhegmatogenous RD vs Exudative RD vs Retinoschisis

Lawrence P. Chong, MD

RD is a separation of the neurosensory retina from the RPE caused by retinal break (*rhegmatogenous*) or secondary to causes other than a break (*exudative*) such as uveitis, uveoscleral outflow obstruction, or hypotony. *Retinoschisis* is a separation within the layers of the neurosensory retina. This separation can be within the inner plexiform layer or the outer plexiform layer.

DIFFERENTIATING FACTORS

- Scotoma
  - Functionally, there is a relative scotoma within the area of RRD or exudative RD, whereas there is an absolute scotoma within the area of retinoschisis.
- IOP
  - The IOP in an eye with RRD is often lower than the fellow eye because of posterior uveal outflow through the open retinal break.
  - IOP is also lower in exudative RD secondary to uveitis or hypotony.
  - Retinoschisis does not affect the IOP.
- Cells
  - Pigmented cells are often visible in the vitreous in the presence of a RRD because the RPE is exposed to the vitreous cavity through the retinal break.
  - Inflammatory cells are seen in exudative RD secondary to uveitis.
  - Pigmented or inflammatory cells are not seen with retinoschisis unless the retinoschisis is also associated with an RRD.
- Retinal surface
  - Undulating and folded or "corrugated" in the setting of a RRD.
  - The surface of retinoschisis or an exudative RD is often smooth and dome shaped.
- Shifting fluid
  - Exudative RD often has "shifting fluid."
    - Test this by moving the patient from an upright to supine position for several minutes or vice versa and reassessing the location of the SRF.

- Demarcation lines
  - Only seen with RRD and never with retinoschisis or exudative RD.
  - RRD with small retinal breaks may similarly present with a smoother, dome-shaped appearance. A demarcation line may be the only differentiating feature.
- PVR
  - Only occurs in the presence of a retinal break.

Indirect ophthalmoscopy or three-mirror contact lens exam may confirm the presence of outer retinal breaks in retinoschisis. This indicates a combined schisis-rhegmatogenous RD.

DIAGNOSTIC IMAGING AND OTHER TECHNIQUES

- Ultrasound
  - May show a thickened sclera in scleritis, thickened choroid in choroiditis, or uveal scleral outflow abnormality in secondary exudative RD.
- FA
  - May identify focal hot spots of leakage in CSR or multifocal spots of leakage in uveitis-related exudative RD.
  - No leakage in RRD.
- OCT
  - RD—separation of the neurosensory retina from the RPE (Fig. 20.1).
  - Retinoschisis—outer layer of the neurosensory retina still attached to the RPE (Fig. 20.2).
  - Direct the OCT toward the suspected retinoschisis or RD to obtain adequate images.
- Laser photocoagulation
  - Retinoschisis—a white laser photocoagulation burn is visualized in the outer retinal adherent to the RPE. No such burn is visualized if it is a RD.

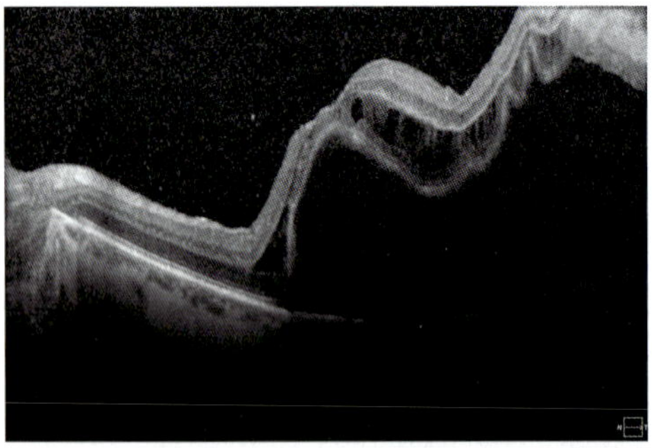

FIGURE 20.1. OCT of RRD. Note that the outer neurosensory retina is not adherent to the RPE.

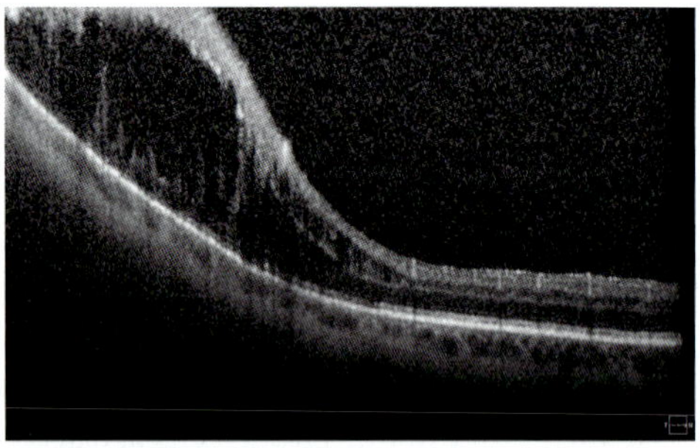

FIGURE 20.2. OCT of retinoschisis. Note the presence of the outer neurosensory retina adherent to the RPE.

CHAPTER 21

Retinal Break Localization

Karen Gehrs, MD

While considerations such as lens status, presence of VH and PVR, the patient's ability to position postop, and air travel requirements influence the approach to RD repair, the size and location of the retinal breaks provide the initial information on which to base a surgical plan.

- **Lincoff's rules for localizing retinal breaks in RRD**
  - Rule 1 (Fig. 21.1A): For superotemporal or superonasal RDs, the primary break lies within 1.5 clock hours of the highest border in 98%.
  - Rule 2 (Fig. 21.1B): For total or superior RDs that cross the 12 o'clock meridian, the primary break is at 12 o'clock or in a triangle, the apex of which is at the ora serrata and the sides of which extend 1.5 clock hours to either side of 12 o'clock, in 93%.
  - Rule 3 (Fig. 21.1C): In inferior RDs, the higher side of the SRF indicates which side of the disc the retinal break lies in 95%.
  - Rule 4 (Fig. 21.1D): Inferior bullous RDs are caused by a superior break.
- **Techniques for localizing retinal breaks**
  - Indirect ophthalmoscopy with scleral depression
    - Equipment
      - 20-, 28-, or 30-D lens
      - Indirect ophthalmoscope
      - Instrument to perform scleral depression (scleral depressor or cotton-tip applicator)
      - Medium for recording findings on paper or electronic record readily available. Prompt recording of findings after the examination maximizes the accuracy of recorded findings.
    - Preparation
      - Patient comfort is essential for the level of cooperation necessary to obtain an adequate fundus exam. Apply topical anesthetic, and use the lowest indirect ophthalmoscope light level that still provides adequate fundus visualization.
      - Lower the room lights to facilitate fundus examination.

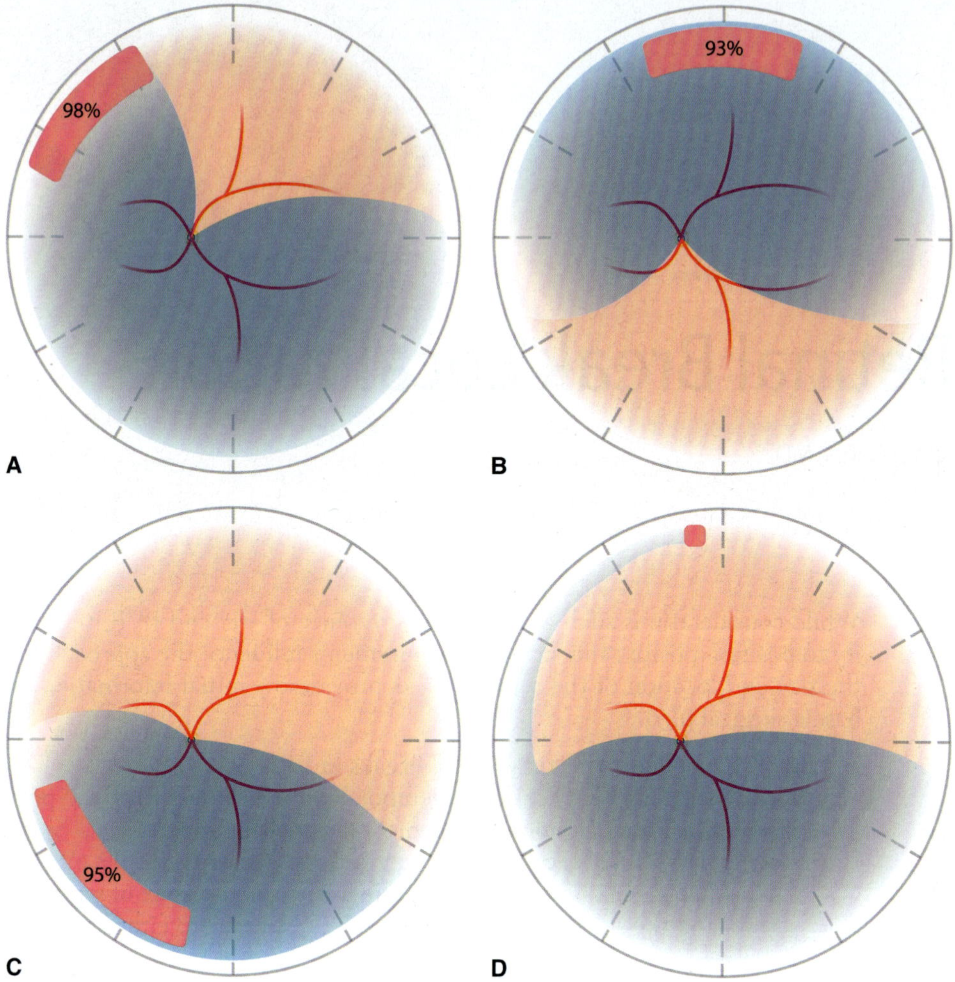

FIGURE 21.1. Lincoff's rules. **A.** For superotemporal or superonasal RDs, the primary break lies within 1.5 clock hours of the highest border in 98%. **B.** For total or superior RDs that cross the 12 o'clock meridian, the primary break is at 12 o'clock or in a triangle, the apex of which is at the ora serrata and the sides of which extend 1.5 clock hours to either side of 12 o'clock, in 93%. **C.** In inferior RDs, the higher side of the SRF indicates on which side of the disc an inferior break lies in 95%. **D.** Inferior bullous RDs are caused by a superior break.

- Method
  - Examine the posterior pole first, then look in each quadrant to get an impression of the extent and location of the RD. In the office setting, ask the patient to gaze in a requested direction. With an anesthetized eye in the OR, rotate the eye into different positions of gaze using a depressor or by applying traction on looped rectus muscles.
  - In the office, place the indenting instrument on the eyelids, although you can place it directly on the sclera as well after administering topical anesthetic eye drops. In the OR with an anesthetized eye (or under general anesthesia), a lid speculum is placed, and scleral depression is performed directly on the sclera.
  - Begin at 12 o'clock and systematically examine each clock hour. Retinal breaks may be present even in areas where the retina is still attached.
  - Place the indenting instrument over the globe and slide in an anterior/posterior direction as far posteriorly as possible (will depend on the level of anesthesia), ensuring visualization of the ora serrata as a landmark (Fig. 21.2). Perform this maneuver for each of 12 clock hours and record abnormal findings.

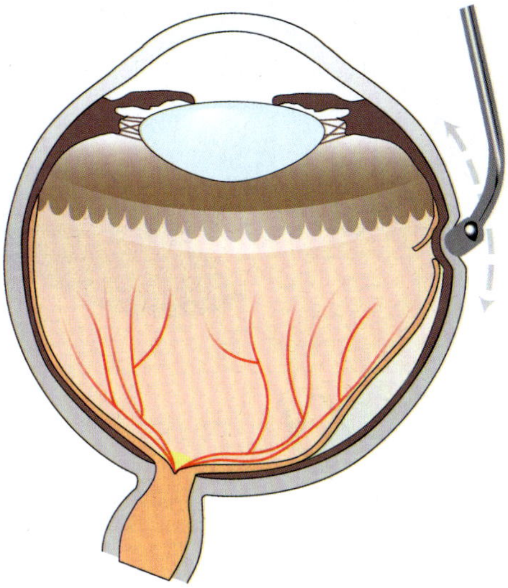

FIGURE 21.2. Place the indenting instrument on the globe and slide in an anterior/posterior direction as far posteriorly as possible (will depend on the level of anesthesia), ensuring visualization of the ora serrata as a landmark in each clock hour.

- Fundus contact lens exam to localize retinal breaks
  - Can provide more magnification to identify small breaks not seen on indirect ophthalmoscopy.
  - Equipment
    - Widefield fundus contact lens or Goldmann three-mirror style fundus contact lens
    - Slit lamp
    - Topical anesthetic eye drops
    - Coupling agent—viscous eye drop to place between the lens surface and eye
  - Method
    - Place the fundus contact lens on the eye and examine the posterior pole—if the macula is detached, evaluate for a FTMH.
    - Systematically examine each clock hour of the mid- and far peripheral retina, and record pathology. In most patients, it will not be possible to see the ora serrata with this technique.

The most common causes of failed RD repair are missed retinal breaks and inadequately supported or treated retinal breaks.

- **Influence of retinal break localization on surgical technique choice and planning for RD repair.**
  - A single break (or multiple breaks within a clock hour) in the superior 8 clock hours qualifies for consideration of a pneumatic retinopexy. See chapter titled *Pneumatic Retinopexy.*
  - Inferior location of retinal breaks, especially multiple inferior retinal breaks with associated lattice degeneration, is a finding that suggests that a SB (with or without a PPV) would be the most appropriate.
  - Posterior location of retinal breaks (at or posterior to the equator, including FTMH) generally requires a PPV with or without a SB for repair.

Even a total RD can be repaired by pneumatic retinopexy alone if the retinal break(s) lies within one of the superior 8 clock hours.

CHAPTER 22

Pneumatic Retinopexy

Michelle Y. Peng, MD • J. Michael Jumper, MD

PREOPERATIVE CONSIDERATIONS

In an eye with a RRD, perform a thorough scleral depressed exam to identify all retinal breaks. See chapter titled *Retinal Break Localization*.

Indications

- Retinal breaks in the superior two-thirds of the retina (8:00-4:00).
- Single or multiple breaks up to 3 clock hours apart (so that all breaks may be tamponaded with the gas bubble in a single position).
- Ability to maintain proper positioning for 1 week postprocedure.

Contraindications

- Breaks located in the lower one-third of the retina (4:00-8:00).
- Presence of significant PVR (grade C or greater).
- Media opacity that prevents adequate identification and treatment of breaks.
- Inability to maintain necessary positioning. See chapter titled *Postop Positioning*.
- Contraindications for the use of intraocular gas (need to travel to high altitude in the postop period). See chapter titled *Gas Tamponade*.

Procedural Planning

- Explain the importance of postprocedure positioning. Manage expectations, and inform patients that new retinal breaks can occur after pneumatic retinopexy.
- Review that the presence of a gas bubble precludes travel to high altitudes.

SURGICAL PROCEDURE

- Perform a thorough retinal exam with scleral depression to identify all retinal breaks.
- Administer anesthetic. The subconjunctival route of administration of 2% lidocaine without epinephrine is often preferred since the patient retains full eye movement to facilitate the treatment of peripheral breaks. Inject the anesthetic where the cryotherapy, gas injection, and AC paracentesis will be performed.

Note that if you opt for a retrobulbar or even a peribulbar anesthetic (see chapter titled *Setting Up for Vitreoretinal Surgery*), there will be minimal resultant eye movement, which may pose difficulty if you need your patient to look superonasally, for example, so you can treat a superonasal break.

- Treat all retinal breaks in the detached retina with cryotherapy. Any breaks or lattice degeneration within attached retina can be treated with laser retinopexy.

For retinal breaks that cannot be treated with cryotherapy because it is within a very bullous RD or located so posteriorly that the cryotherapy probe cannot reach it, consider placing the gas bubble first and treating the retinal break(s) after the retina has reattached, usually with laser retinopexy one to several days later. It is important to carefully photograph or draw the location of the break(s) as it may be more difficult to identify once the retina is reattached and the gas bubble is in place.

- Using a Millipore filter, fill a 1-mL syringe with undiluted perfluoropropane (C_3F_8) or sulfur hexafluoride (SF_6) gas. Place a 27G or 30G needle on the end of the syringe.
- Apply Betadine to the eyelids and lashes. Place an eyelid speculum, and apply topical Betadine to the surface of the eye in a quadrant away from the RD. At this spot, slowly inject 0.3 mL of undiluted C_3F_8 gas or up to 0.6 mL of SF_6 gas into the vitreous cavity through the pars plana, 3.5-4.0 mm from the limbus. See chapter titled *Gas Tamponade.*
- Aim for one large bubble in the vitreous cavity after injection. To achieve this, select a superior location and orient the needle perpendicular to the sclera. Penetrate the needle deep enough to inject into the vitreous cavity but shallow enough that the needle is injecting into the growing bubble. This maneuver will help avoid the creation of multiple small bubbles or "fish eggs" that can possibly find their way through the retinal break and into the subretinal space (Fig. 22.1).

Make sure that the needle is not in the suprachoroidal space prior to injecting the gas into the vitreous cavity (Fig. 22.1).

- Have the patient roll onto their side such that the gas bubble injection site is facing downward. This prevents egress of the gas bubble with removal of the needle. The patient then rolls to a facedown position and then adjusts their head position such that the gas bubble rolls from the macula toward the area of RD. This prevents the gas bubble from pushing SRF into the macula.

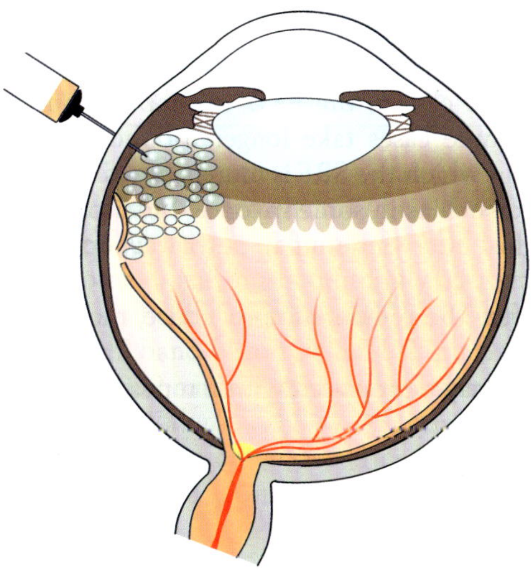

FIGURE 22.1. When injecting intravitreal gas, avoid the creation of multiple small bubbles or "fish eggs" that can possibly find their way through the retinal break and into the subretinal space. Also make sure that the needle is not in the suprachoroidal space.

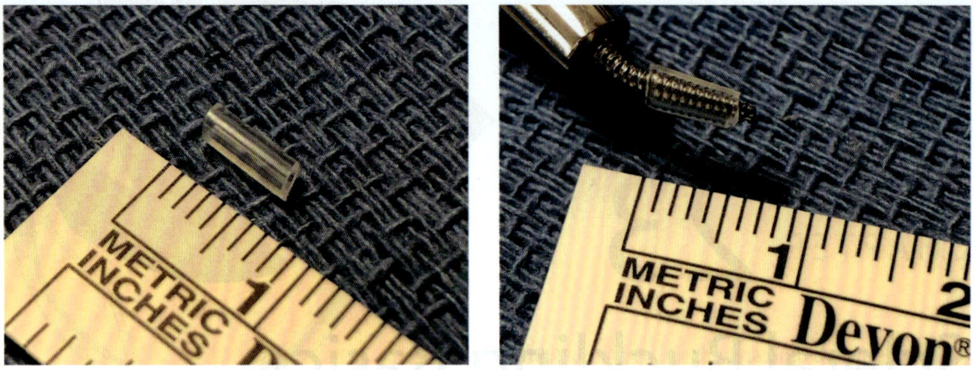

A B

FIGURES 23.1. **A.** The Watzke sleeve is used to secure the encircling band around the eye. **B.** It is placed on the Watzke sleeve spreading forceps.

    - 240 band (2.5 mm wide, 0.6 mm thick)
      - The 40 band and 240 band are narrower and can also be used with tires, grooved strips, and wedges. A variety of tires are available.
        - The 287 wide groove tire can be used with a 41 band in its groove.
  - Use the buckling element to encircle the globe and provide 360 degrees of support to the vitreous base and identified retinal breaks. Secure the encircling element to itself with a Watzke sleeve using the Watzke sleeve spreading forceps (Fig. 23.1A and B).
  - Choose a band to support the vitreous base, any retinal breaks, and also any other vitreoretinal pathology such as lattice degeneration.
  - If needed, place the buckling element in a segmental fashion (discussed below), supporting 1-3 quadrants, or in a radial fashion. See chapter titled *Radial Elements*.
- **Cryo machine setup**
  - Make sure the nitrous oxide exhaust tubing is vented to the outside.
  - Make sure the nitrous oxide cylinders are properly connected and that the foot pedal is properly connected.
  - Connect the cryo probe to the machine. Make sure the cryo probe is locked in place so that it will not disconnect during the procedure (Fig. 23.2).
  - Turn on the compressed gas cylinder. If the pressure does not reach 600 PSI, you will typically want to replace the tank(s).
  - Turn the cryo unit on and adjust the pressure to the desired probe setting (600 PSI).

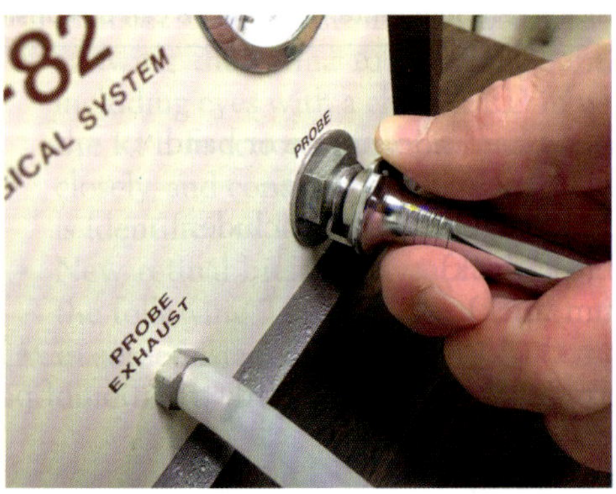

FIGURE 23.2. Make sure the cryo probe is locked in place so that it will not disconnect during the procedure.

- There are a few companies that make cryo units and they all have probes that are specific to that unit.
  - Some of the probes are curved and some are straight.
  - Use a sleeve around the probe to minimize collateral freezing.
- Test it before use.
  - With foot pedal depressed, look for an ice ball to form at the tip of the cryo probe.
  - Typically, the temperature will reach at least −60°C.
  - Once you see ice form on the tip, let up on the foot pedal and you are now ready to use the cryo probe. See chapter titled *Scleral Buckling Steps.*

If you do not see an ice ball forming at the tip, you need to troubleshoot. Usually this is due to the gas in the tank being low or the pressure not turned up high enough, or less commonly, there may be a problem with the probe.

Mistaking indentation from the cryo probe shaft for indentation by the cryo probe tip can result in cryo freezes that are too posterior (Fig. 23.3).

- **Challenging scenarios**
  - Prior strabismus surgery
    - It may not be possible to isolate a recessed rectus muscle. You do not have to isolate all 4 rectus muscles in this situation.
    - If more than one muscle has been recessed, it may be challenging to manipulate the globe to provide exposure for suture placement for the encircling element.
    - It is not necessary to pass the encircling element under a recessed rectus muscle. Instead, that muscle may be skipped and the encircling element is often placed anterior to the new rectus insertion (Fig. 23.4).
    - Learn the details of any prior strabismus surgery to understand where the rectus muscles may be located.
  - Poor view due to opacified peripheral capsule in pseudophakic eye with small rhexis
    - If the RD is low-lying, <3 clock hours, and you cannot visualize a break, consider applying peripheral cryo for the extent of the RD. This will cover the

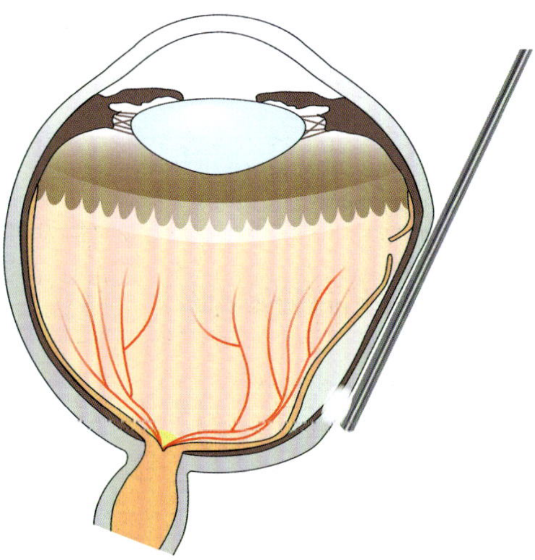

FIGURE 23.3. Mistaking indentation from the cryo probe shaft for indentation by the cryo probe tip can result in cryo freezes that are too posterior.

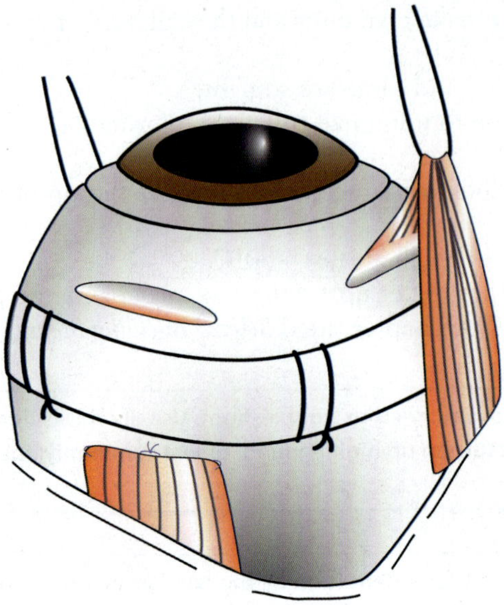

FIGURE 23.4. In an eye with a previously recessed rectus muscle, the encircling element is often placed anterior to the new rectus insertion. That recessed muscle is not isolated with silk suture.

small break in the area of the RD. Giving the patient 125 mg of intravenous methylprednisolone (if the patient is not diabetic and does not have any other contraindications to systemic steroid use) may help decrease the inflammation from the cryo.

- If the RD is not low-lying and/or >3 clock hours, consider adding a PPV. See chapter titled *Scleral Buckle and Vitrectomy for RRD.*

- Presence of a tube shunt
  - Avoid the quadrant where the tube shunt is when performing the conjunctival peritomy.
  - Sometimes, it is not possible to safely isolate the two rectus muscles bordering the quadrant that contains the tube shunt.
  - Placing a segmental scleral buckle in the other 3 quadrants may be an option. If the etiologic retinal break is located in the same quadrant as the tube shunt plate, then SRF drainage in a different quadrant with laser retinopexy to that break may be performed or PPV may be needed.
- Presence of a functioning trabeculectomy
  - Either avoid the quadrant where the trabeculectomy is altogether when performing the conjunctival peritomy or isolate the area of the trabeculectomy and perform a very posterior peritomy in that quadrant with careful closure using running Vicryl suture. Any eye surgery increases the risk of trabeculectomy failure.

Isolating a recently resected rectus muscle may not be advisable since that muscle may be disinserted from the sclera if it has not fully healed following strabismus surgery.

Suturing the encircling element to the tube plate is generally not advisable.

CHAPTER 24

Scleral Buckling Steps

Anne Hanneken, MD

PREOPERATIVE CONSIDERATIONS

- Carefully examine the eye to assess the configuration of the RD and localize the breaks (number, location—anterior, posterior, quadrants). See chapter titled *Retinal Break Localization*.
  - If a break cannot be identified in a RRD, analyze the configuration of the RD to identify the quadrant with the highest probability of harboring a break per Lincoff's Rules.
- Determine if the patient has high myopia, phakia or pseudophakia, visible scleral thinning, diplopia, and refractive error.
- Discuss surgical approaches and expectations. Address the choice of anesthesia (local with sedation or general), visual expectations, refractive error following SB, other surgical risks including diplopia, and redetachment.

SURGICAL PROCEDURE

- Create a conjunctival peritomy for 360 degrees at the limbus using Westcott scissors and 0.12 forceps (Fig. 24.1). Add relaxing radial conjunctival incisions temporally and nasally.
  - Mark the conjunctival surface at the nasal and temporal limbus prior to the peritomy to help reapproximate the conjunctiva at the end of the procedure.
  - Dissect the conjunctiva and underlying Tenon capsule from the scleral surface.

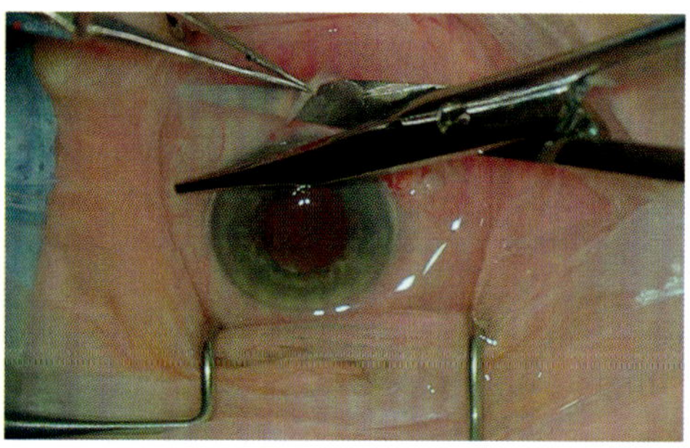

FIGURE 24.1. Perform a 360-degree conjunctival peritomy.

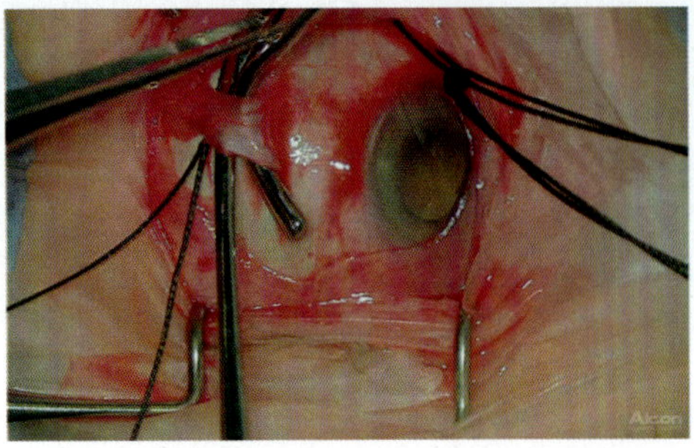

FIGURE 24.2. Pass the muscle hook with 2-0 silk suture under each rectus muscle to isolate the muscle. Attention is paid to engage every muscle fiber.

- Use curved Stevens scissors to clear the Tenon capsule from each quadrant, exposing the bare sclera.
- Isolate each of the rectus muscles by elevating the conjunctiva with 0.3 forceps and pass a muscle hook under each of the rectus muscles. The conjunctiva and Tenon capsule are dissected around each of the four rectus muscle sheaths with a cotton-tip applicator. Thread a 2-0 silk suture into the opening at the tip of another muscle hook, and pass that hook under the rectus muscle to further isolate each rectus muscle and engage every fiber (Fig. 24.2). This reduces postop diplopia. Remove the suture from the muscle hook, so the suture straddles the muscle insertion. Bring the two ends of the suture together to double the suture thickness, and tie the sutures twice, at the end and more proximally near the muscle, to avoid tangling the suture ends while manipulating the four sutures.

Significant bradycardia and even asystole can occur from external traction on the rectus muscles during globe manipulation, known as the oculocardiac reflex. This reflex is reduced with adequate peribulbar or retrobulbar anesthesia. If bradycardia occurs, immediately release traction on the muscle. Ask anesthesia to pharmacologically prevent further bradycardia as you manipulate the muscles.

Approach the superior rectus muscle from the nasal side, anterior to the superior oblique muscle tendon, to avoid trapping the superior oblique as you isolate the superior rectus, and decrease the likelihood of postop diplopia.

- Inspect the sclera in each of the four quadrants to determine whether scleral thinning is present, which appears as a gray-blue area. Avoid areas of scleral thinning when placing scleral sutures. It is not absolutely necessary to pass a scleral suture in each of the four quadrants when placing an encircling element. One and sometimes two quadrants with marked scleral thinning can be skipped.
- *Localization of the breaks.* Examine the peripheral retina with an indirect ophthalmoscope, a 20- or 28-diopter lens, and a scleral depressor to identify the retinal breaks. The assistant orients the globe in the quadrant to be examined using two traction sutures under the rectus muscles opposite the area of the examination. Use the O'Connor depressor to mark the break by placing the marking end over the sclera directly under the position of the break for 5 seconds. Turn on the overhead operating lights or direct the light from the indirect ophthalmoscope to visualize the indentation on the scleral surface, and enhance this mark with a sterile marking pen. If a large horseshoe is present, mark the two anterior horns of the tear, which require strong support.
- Examine the retina for 360 degrees to avoid missing additional breaks.

Tricks for Localizing Breaks

The position of breaks in an RRD can often be predicted by knowing the configuration of the RD and peripheral retinal pathology.

1. **The simple rule is that retinal breaks are often located about one-third of the distance from the most superior aspect of the RD. For example, if the SRF extends from the 1- to 7-o'clock meridian in a clockwise distribution, the break will frequently be localized about one-third from the most superior meridian of the detachment, or about 3 o'clock. See chapter titled *Retinal Break Localization.***
2. **The position of the break in a traumatic RD is often localized to a dialysis in the superotemporal quadrant.**
3. **The position of a break in an eye with lattice is often localized to a patch of lattice.**
4. **The position of a break in an eye with PVR is often localized near the most significant epiretinal traction.**
5. **The position of a break in an eye with old cryotherapy for retinal breaks is often localized near the margin of prior heavy cryotherapy.**

- *Cryotherapy of the breaks.* Treat all of the breaks with cryotherapy using a straight or curved cryoprobe for ~3-4 seconds until whitening is visualized on the edges of the retinal break. Treat the full perimeter of the break, and consider extending treatment one width of the cryoprobe to either side of the break. Breaks in highly bullous RDs may be difficult to reach. In these cases, treat the RPE under the break (if you are able to predict that the retinal break will lay on that exact spot when the retina flattens but this is often not possible), or soften the eye by performing a limbal paracentesis to allow enough indentation with the cryoprobe that the SRF can be pushed away.

Avoid treating the same spot of the retina more than once, the bare RPE within the break, and over-treating as this can increase the risk of PVR.

- Pass the encircling SB under the previously isolated rectus muscles using Nugent or utility forceps. These are designed with a bent angle and a thin profile to grasp the end of the SB and smoothly slide the element under the muscles with minimal difficulty. Grasp the buckling element with the Nugent forceps about 2 mm from the end of the band to allow the band to slide under the rectus muscle while keeping the free end accessible once it emerges from the other side of the muscle. When the free end of the buckling element is visible from the other side of the muscle, use second Nugent forceps to pull the element out from under the muscle (Fig. 24.3). If a tire and its band are placed simultaneously, the band is folded behind the tire to ease the placement of the combined unit under each muscle. The assistant provides essential exposure with the Schepens retractor to facilitate visualization during band placement.

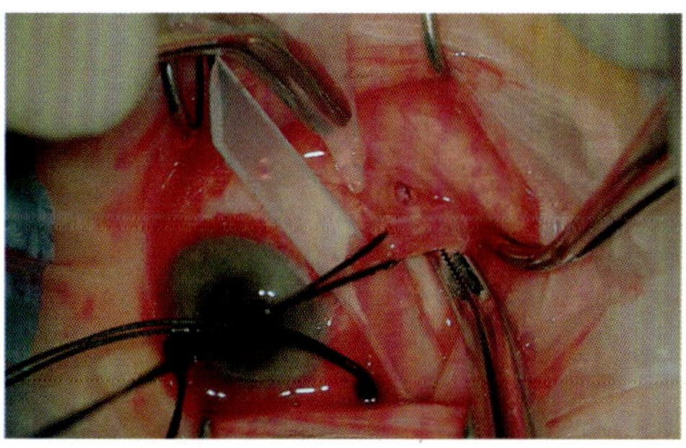

FIGURE 24.3. When the free end of buckling element is visible from the other side of the muscle, use a second Nugent forceps to pull the element from under the muscle.

Make sure there are no twists in the encircling SB.

- *Watzke sleeve.* After an encircling band has been placed under the muscles, secure it in the superonasal quadrant with a Watzke sleeve. The superonasal location hides it under the lids. A Watzke sleeve is a small silicone tube that secures the overlapping segments of an encircling band to maintain the circumference of the band and prevent slippage.
  - The diameter of the Watzke sleeve is selected to accommodate the diameter of the encircling band. A type 71 Watzke sleeve (2.1 mm wide, outer diameter) will accommodate a 240 band or a 41 band. A type 72 Watzke sleeve (2.4 mm wide, outer diameter) will accommodate a 42 band.
  - Cut a 4- to 5-mm segment of the Watzke sleeve, and thread it over the nosepiece of the Watzke sleeve spreading forceps. To secure the band inside the sleeve, hold the spreading forceps with the nosepiece directed away from you. Open the sleeve with the spreading forceps, and thread the proximal end of the band into the sleeve with a Nugent forceps directing the free end of the band toward the distal nosepiece of the forceps (Fig. 24.4). Thread the second end of the band into the sleeve from the opposite direction, placing the second segment over the first segment and toward the base of the spreading forceps. The assistant grabs the top end of the band as it exits the sleeve so the two ends of the band, which are secured in the Watzke sleeve, can be pushed off the spreading forceps by the surgeon using a short Nugent forceps. Tighten the band with a needle holder while straddling the upper segment of the band at the base of the Watzke sleeve with a Nugent forceps. The circumference of the encircling band can be adjusted with this maneuver to create a gentle indentation around the globe, which facilitates positioning of the element. See Video 24.1.

VIDEO

Buckling Element

The location of the retinal breaks and/or the vitreous base is the key factor dictating the position of the buckling element. The success of buckling surgery is dependent on three factors:

1. **The external position of the buckling element**
2. **The placement of the sutures**
3. **The height of the buckling element**

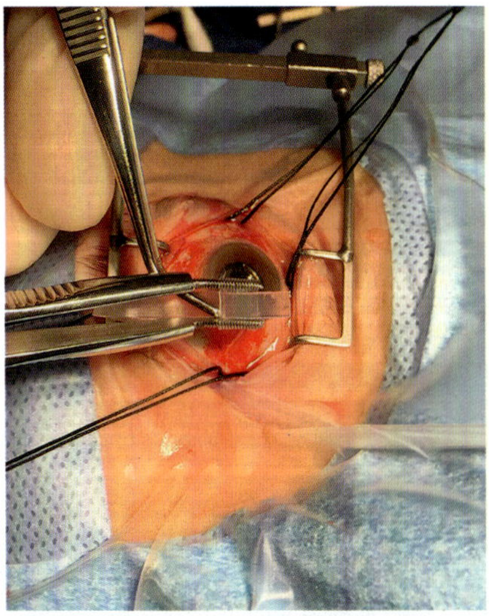

FIGURE 24.4. Open the sleeve with the spreading forceps, and thread the proximal end of the band into the sleeve with a Nugent forceps directing the free end of the band toward the distal nosepiece of the forceps.

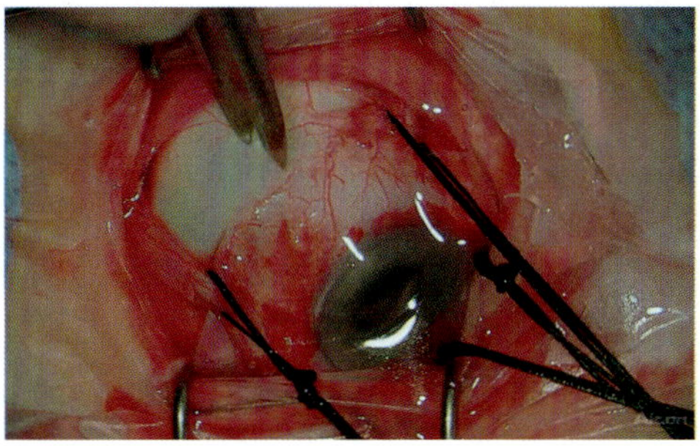

FIGURE 24.5. The encircling element is usually positioned with the anterior edge located about 2-3 mm posterior to the muscle insertions to support vitreous base in a nonmyopic eye.

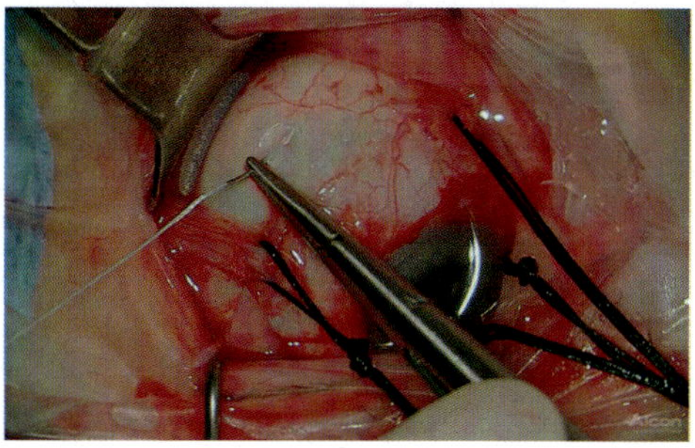

FIGURE 24.6. Place a Dacron or nylon suture parallel to the encircling element about 4 mm in length and about one-half to three-fourths through the depth of the sclera.

- Secure the buckling element to the sclera in the appropriate position to support the retinal breaks and vitreous base. In most RRDs, the retinal breaks are located adjacent to the vitreous base, and placement of the SB supports the breaks and vitreous base simultaneously. As a general rule, an encircling element is positioned with the anterior edge of the band located about 2-3 mm posterior to the insertion of the rectus muscles to support the vitreous base in a nonmyopic eye (Fig. 24.5). In a highly myopic eye, the vitreous base is located more posteriorly, and the anterior edge of the band may need to be positioned 4 mm behind the muscle insertions. In all cases, examine the peripheral retinal to confirm that the SB will support the retinal breaks before the sutures are placed.
- *Sutures.* The buckling element is secured to the sclera using a spatulated needle with 5-0 nonabsorbable polyester (Dacron) or nylon suture placed parallel to the encircling element using a horizontal mattress stitch about 4 mm in length (Fig. 24.6). Place the sutures about one-half to three-fourths through the depth of the sclera while avoiding perforation into the choroid or retina (Fig. 24.7).
  - Consider waiting to permanently tie the sutures to allow revision of anterior or posterior suture placement if the SB needs to be repositioned. Tie sutures with square knots using 3-4 throws (3,1,1,1 for Dacron and 3,1,1 for nylon), and rotate the knots posteriorly (Fig. 24.8).
- *Imbrication.* Use the distance between the placement of the anterior and posterior sutures, one of the two factors, to determine the height of the buckling element. Place sutures in each quadrant 1-2 mm wider than the outer contact diameter of the buckling element. With a larger tire or a radial element, separate the anterior and

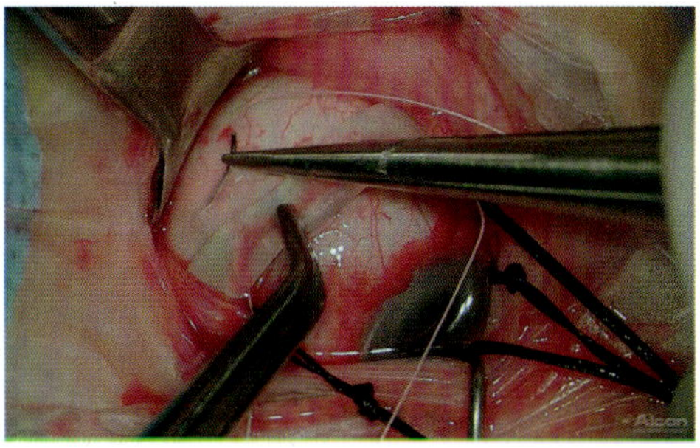

FIGURE 24.7. A second partial-thickness scleral pass as shown forms a horizontal mattress suture. Dacron suture is shown.

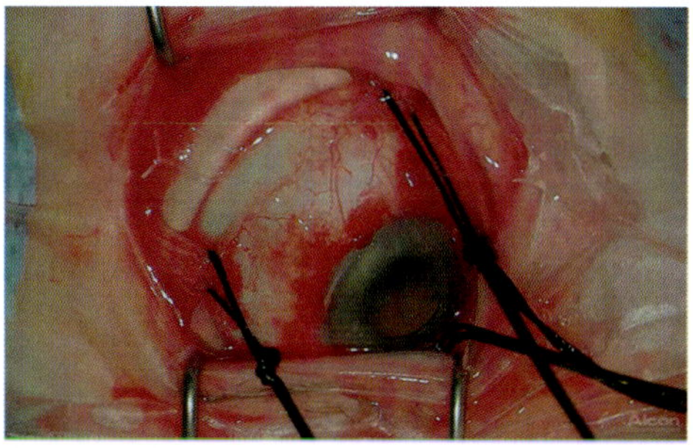

FIGURE 24.8. Tie sutures with square knots (3, 1, 1, 1 for Dacron and 3, 1, 1 for nylon) and rotate the knots posteriorly.

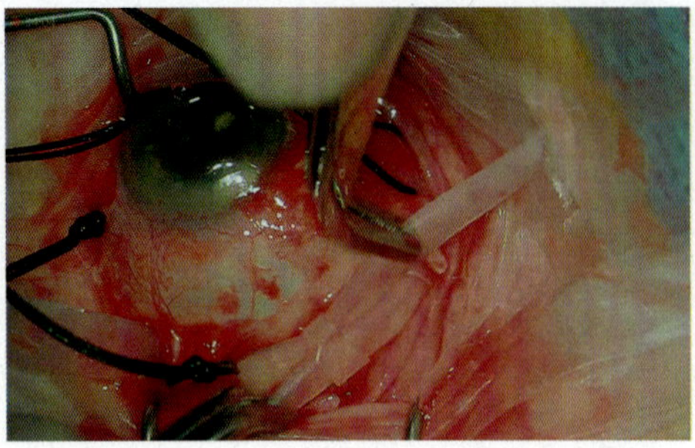

FIGURE 24.9. The band is tightened to contribute to an adequate buckle height.

posterior sutures across the SB at greater widths, up to 3-4 mm wider than the outer contact diameter of the buckling element. With tires, tighten the sutures to imbricate the sclera around the full contact diameter of the buckling element to provide additional height for internal support. Place two sutures in each quadrant around the tires to achieve these goals and create a smooth internal buckle configuration.
  - Only a low-lying scleral indentation is necessary in most cases to support the breaks and vitreous base.
- *Buckle height.* Buckle height is not only a result of mattress suture placement distance in relation to the buckling element but also how tightly the encircling buckle is cinched. Adjust the SB circumference during the placement of the Watzke sleeve to achieve a mild indentation on the scleral surface and avoid excessive laxity while suturing the band to the sclera. Following suture placement, tighten the band ~1 cm with the Nugent forceps to create a mild-moderate internal buckle height and 2 cm to create a moderate-high internal buckle (Fig. 24.9). The same basic rule applies for encircling tires except the circumference of the tire must be cut by 1 cm to oppose both edges of the tire for a mild-moderate buckle height and 2 cm to oppose both edges of the tire for a moderate-high height. Tighten the overlying band to oppose the edges of the tire and prevent slippage. Tires are much less commonly used than bands.
  - Avoid excess height of an encircling element due to risk of anterior segment ischemia, compression on vortex veins, or fishmouthing of large retinal tears.
  - After adjusting the final SB height, cut the excess band length about 0.5 cm from the Watzke sleeve, and thread under the muscle insertion.
- *Tamponade choice.* The simple rule for choosing whether gas tamponade is needed after SB placement depends on whether the break is flat on the SB. See chapter titled *Gas Tamponade.*
  - If the break is flat on the SB, no additional tamponade may be needed.
  - If a break is not flat on the SB, inject a bubble of air or 100% gas through the pars plana to promote break closure during postop positioning. See chapter titled *Postop Positioning.* This provides additional support to breaks that are well positioned on the SB but not completely flat. Use in nondrainage procedures and when fishmouthing of the retinal break occurs in the setting of a large retinal break or high SB.
  - The choice of tamponade includes (1) sterile air, (2) 100% SF_6, or (3) 100% C_3F_8.
    - If the eye is soft after SRF drainage and only a short-term tamponade is needed to flatten the edge of the break(s), air can be injected to support the break and bring the IOP to a normal level.
    - 100% SF_6 will expand to twice its size and 100% C_3F_8 will expand to four times its size. C_3F_8 will be present in the eye for twice as long as SF_6.
    - As a general rule, 0.3 mL of 100% C_3F_8 will expand to a 20% bubble in an emmetropic eye. If the eye is highly myopic and the IOP is quite low, a 0.6-mL volume of gas may be chosen to achieve a similar bubble size. For SF_6, 0.6 mL is often used in an emmetropic eye.

Best Technique

The goal when injecting air or gas is to obtain a single bubble rather than multiple small bubbles, known as "fish eggs," which can migrate under the flap of an open retinal break and prevent reattachment. A single bubble is more likely when the IOP is low and there is less resistance. Grasp the muscle insertion with forceps to stabilize the eye, and inject the intravitreal gas into the most superior pars plana position with a 30G needle on a TB syringe.

  - Assess the IOP after a gas injection, and check for central retinal artery perfusion to reduce the risk of incarceration of the retina after external drainage or central retinal artery occlusion. A limbal paracentesis can be performed using a 30G needle on a TB syringe to decrease the IOP.
- Irrigate the SB with an antibiotic solution often combined with 2-4% lidocaine without epinephrine if desired, remove the silk ligatures from the muscles, close the conjunctival peritomy with absorbable suture, and inject subconjunctival antibiotic and steroid.

CHAPTER 25

Radial Elements

Asad F. Durrani, MD • Thomas R. Friberg, MD, MS

PREOPERATIVE CONSIDERATIONS

Consider a radial element in the following scenarios:

- RRD associated with a single retinal break
- RRD associated with a posterior retinal break and adjacent traction

Advantages of a radial element compared to an encircling SB:

- Faster
- Minimal refractive changes
- Reduces the incidence of postop diplopia
- Avoids fishmouthing of retinal breaks

TYPES OF RADIAL ELEMENTS

Radial elements of different shapes and sizes are available (Fig. 25.1). Selection depends on factors such as size and shape of retinal break, desired buckle effect, and preference.

- Circular silicone sponge
  - Round sponge (5 mm wide/505 styles commonly used)
  - Oval sponge (3 × 5 mm/506 and 5.0 × 7.5 mm/507 styles commonly used)
  - Circular sponge produces higher central buckle height due to its geometry.
- Oblong silicone sponge (508 or 509 styles)
  - Wider buckling effect
- Partial-thickness silicone sponge (510, 511, 515, and 517 styles)
  - Provides similar buckle effect as circular sponges, but reduced sponge thickness decreases the risk of extrusion.
- L-shaped silicone sponge (513 and 514 styles)
  - When fishmouthing occurs, an L-shaped radial element can help augment an encircling buckle to relieve fishmouthing and close the break.
- Piece of hard silicone band (40, 41, 42, 240, 4050 styles)

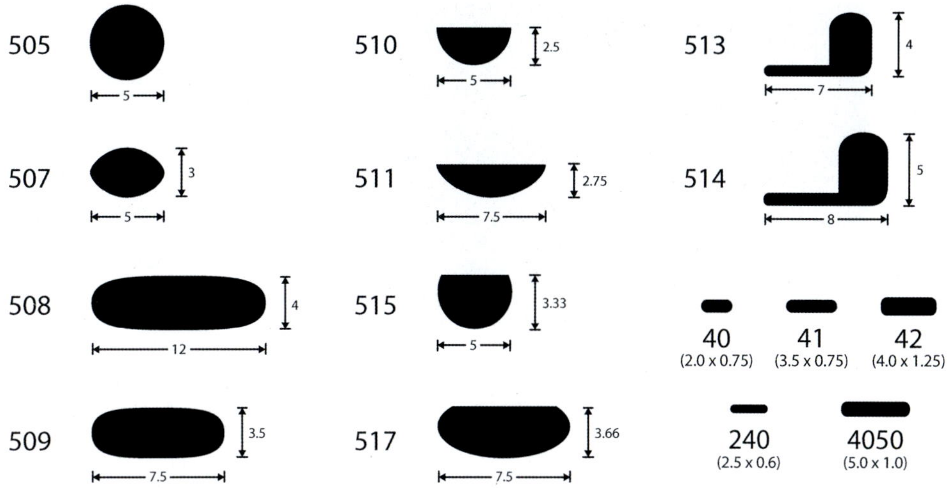

FIGURE 25.1. Radial elements come in different shapes and sizes, including circular silicone sponge, oblong silicone sponge, partial-thickness silicone sponge, L-shaped silicone sponge, and piece of hard silicone band.

SURGICAL TECHNIQUES

- A limited peritomy (often only 180-degree peritomy)
- Visualize, mark, and treat the retinal breaks. See chapter titled *Retinal Break Localization.*
- Select radial element width such that there is 1 mm between the edge of retinal break and edge of radial element.
  - For breaks <4 mm in width, a radial element 5 mm wide can be used (505, 506, or 510 styles).
  - For breaks between 4 and 6 mm, a radial element ≥7 mm in width can be used (8270G, 511G, 509G or 519G styles).
  - If the break is >6 mm, consider placing an encircling SB instead.

Remember buckle height is primarily a function of element width and suture bite distance: greater element width and suture bite distance create a higher buckle effect.

- Place partial-thickness scleral sutures parallel to the long axis of the radial element which should be perpendicular to the limbus (Fig. 25.2).
  - Bite distance a total of 3-4 mm greater than the width of the element creates a higher buckle.
  - Posterior mattress sutures can be challenging; a figure-of-eight suture can be converted to a mattress suture by cutting the suture between the bites.
  - Bites should be taken to create a box configuration of sutures. Avoid sutures that cross each other over the radial element as this decreases buckle height.

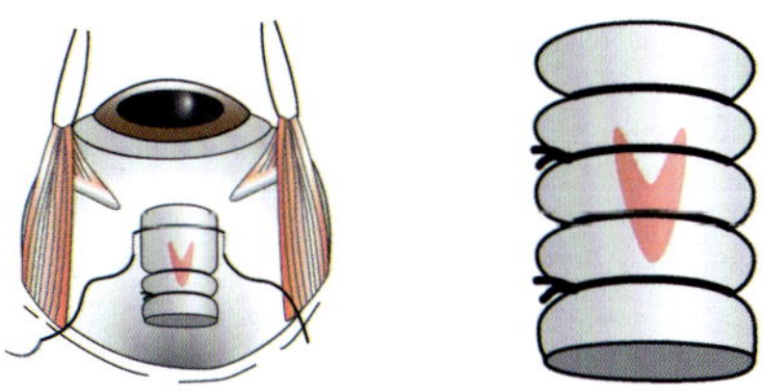

FIGURE 25.2. Place partial-thickness scleral sutures parallel to the long axis of the radial element which should be perpendicular to the limbus. Bite distance a total of 3-4 mm greater than the width of the element creates a higher buckling effect.

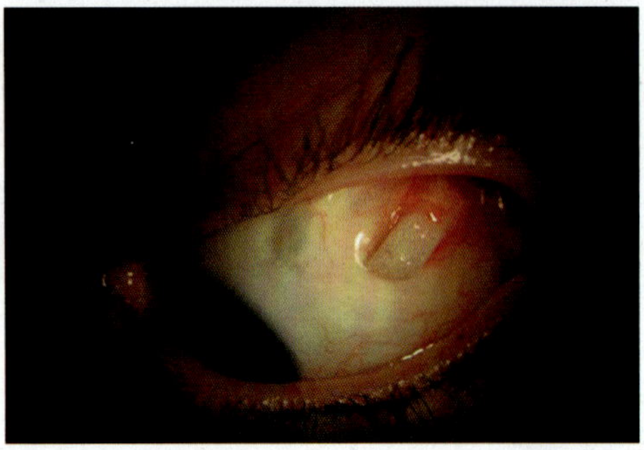

FIGURE 25.3. Element extrusion may occur when silicone sponges are used for RD repair. Minimize the risk by trimming the radial element, rotating knots posteriorly, and closing overlying Tenon capsule prior to conjunctival closure.

The remainder of the surgery is the same as for encircling SB (indirect ophthalmoscopy to confirm adequate buckle height and support of retinal break and perfusion of optic disc, drainage of SRF if planned, normalization of IOP by AC paracentesis if needed, injection of expansile gas if SRF not drained, closure of conjunctival peritomy). See chapter titled *Scleral Buckling Steps.*

POSTOPERATIVE CONSIDERATIONS

- Watch for recurrent RD and/or new retinal breaks.
- Get OCT to look for CME, which can occur 4-6 weeks postop.
- Diplopia and astigmatism may develop. Refractive error is usually unchanged.
- Element extrusion is rare (often associated with infection).
- Element infection often presents with pain, discharge, chemosis, lid edema, and conjunctival hyperemia. Requires radial element removal and culture.
- Rare case reports exist of direct optic nerve injury with radial element use.

CHAPTER 26

External Subretinal Fluid Drainage

Durga S. Borkar, MD

PREOPERATIVE CONSIDERATIONS

- SRF drainage during primary SB surgery for RRD is often considered in these scenarios.
  - Inferior retinal break(s)
  - Chronic RRD, implying more viscous SRF
  - Retinal breaks in ≥3 quadrants
  - Posterior retinal breaks that may not be supported on SB
  - Advanced patient age that may lead to slow SRF reabsorption
  - High myopia with thin sclera
  - Open globe injury that may limit drainage site options
- In a younger patient with an acute RD and anterior-superior retinal break(s) that are supported by a SB, external SRF drainage may not be necessary. Without intravitreal gas, the young patient can lay supine so the vitreous can tamponade the break(s) as the SRF reabsorbs postop. Or, gas tamponade can be used. See chapter titled *Gas Tamponade*.

SURGICAL PROCEDURE

- Intraop timing of SRF drainage
  - Treat all retinal breaks with cryo and place the SB element.
  - Place suture in all quadrants. In the drainage quadrant, pass the suture in this quadrant before SRF drainage since the eye typically becomes hypotonous afterward. It is more difficult to pass scleral sutures in a hypotonous eye and carries an increased risk of scleral perforation during suture pass. Place the suture so that it will not interfere with the drainage site.
  - Tighten the SB if encircling. Instead, you could preplace a 2-0 silk traction suture on the SB 180 degrees away from the planned drainage site. Having a tightened SB or traction suture on the SB during drainage increases the IOP and helps decrease the risk of intraop SRH.

- Location of drainage site
  - Perform drainage in the bed of the SB so that the drainage site will ultimately be well supported on the SB.
  - Choose a site where significant SRF exists but away from known retinal breaks. Avoid the vortex veins.
    - Drainage near a vortex vein may increase the risk of SRH.
    - Drainage near a retinal break may increase the risk of:
      - The drainage needle entering the vitreous cavity and draining liquefied vitreous, leading to more marked hypotony
      - Vitreous incarceration in the drainage site
      - Retinal incarceration in the drainage site
- SRF drainage

  There are two main ways to drain SRF.
  - External needle SRF drainage
    - Obtain a 25G, 26G, or 30G ½ inch needle.
    - Put a piece of no. 270 silicone tubing over the needle to create a guard (Fig. 26.1).
    - Connect the needle to a 3-mL syringe with the plunger removed.
    - Position the needle at the planned drainage site at a 45-degree angle with the bevel facing away from the sclera.
    - Under visualization with the indirect or with a widefield viewing system and chandelier illumination, the needle is advanced into the subretinal space (Fig. 26.2). See chapter titled *The Chandelier Buckle.*
    - With traction on the SB or pressure on the eye, SRF is passively drained.
      - Do not actively aspirate fluid from the drainage site since this will increase the risk of retinal or vitreous incarceration.
    - Slowly retract the needle from the eye as SRF drains into it, to avoid contact between the needle and retina, until the needle is completely removed from subretinal space.
    - Gently massage the drainage site with a cotton tip to prevent further egress of SRF and decrease the risk of retinal or vitreous incarceration.
  - Cut-down SRF drainage
    - Create a linear scleral incision in the bed of the SB, radial to the limbus, using a no. 57 blade, and cauterize the edges with external cautery.
    - Apply gentle diathermy to the choroid.
    - Insert a 30G ½ inch needle or a tapered needle (removed from an 8-0 Vicryl suture and loaded backhand on a locking needle driver) through the scleral incision and diathermized choroid to enter the subretinal space, and then remove the needle. The 30G needle may be more appropriate for a chronic RD with viscous SRF than the tapered needle.
    - Gently massage the adjacent sclera to facilitate the drainage of SRF.

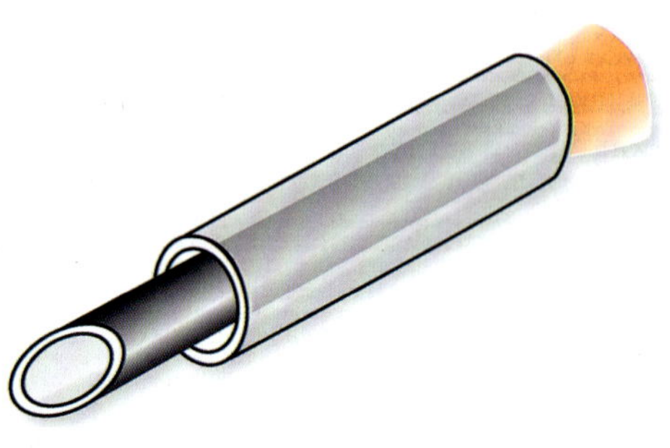

FIGURE 26.1. A piece of no. 270 silicone tubing may be placed over the needle to create a guard.

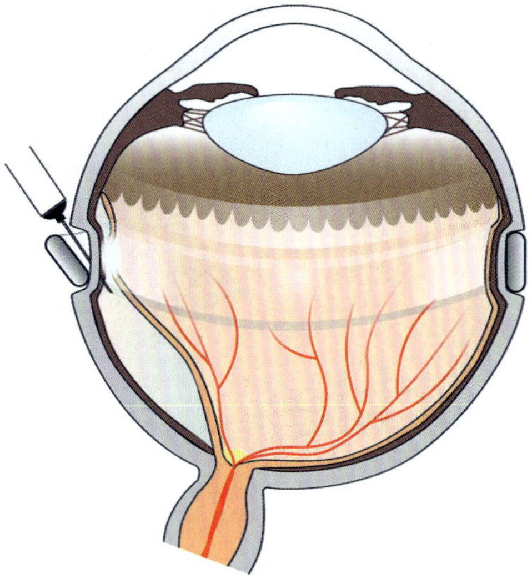

FIGURE 26.2. Under visualization with the indirect or with a widefield viewing system under chandelier illumination, the needle is advanced into the subretinal space.

  - Once SRF stops passively draining out or pigment clumps are noted in the egressed SRF, the drain is likely adequate.
  - Confirm adequate drainage and lack of SRH with indirect ophthalmoscopy.
  - Suture the scleral drainage incision with absorbable suture if preferred.
- Inject an intravitreal expansile gas bubble in the usual fashion through the pars plana if planned. See chapter titled *Gas Tamponade*.
  - If gas injection is not planned but the eye is hypotonus, inject filtered air instead into the vitreous cavity to pump up the eye.
- Suture down the SB in the quadrant of the drainage site.

POSTOPERATIVE CONSIDERATIONS

- You may note SRH at the drainage site or, less commonly, retinal or even vitreous incarceration after external SRF drainage is performed. Usually, the SRH is localized and extrafoveal and can be observed. In some cases, retinal or vitreous incarceration may require PPV. See chapter titled *Retinal Detachment in Open Globe Injury*.
- Avoid these postop challenges by draining SRF slowly and gently and not repeatedly entering the drainage site during SRF drainage.

CHAPTER 27

The Chandelier Buckle

Eric W. Schneider, MD

Chandelier-assisted SB utilizes contemporary direct widefield viewing systems with chandelier illumination to replace binocular indirect ophthalmoscopy in primary SB surgery.

PREOPERATIVE CONSIDERATIONS

Traditional SB surgery requires the intraop examination and treatment of retinal breaks utilizing indirect ophthalmoscopy, which provides limited magnification and inverted images of the retina.

Indications

- Traditional indications for primary SB surgery include RRD with attached hyaloid, young phakic myopes, and retinal dialysis.
- Chandelier-assisted SB may be especially beneficial in the following circumstances:
  - Small pupil
  - Residual dense peripheral capsular opacity
  - Operating with trainees
  - Presbyopic surgeons since it allows completion of the entire SB procedure under the surgical microscope

Advantages

- More magnified view of retinal pathology
- Direct image of the retina
- Familiarity of viewing system for vitrectomy-trained surgeons
- Improved surgeon posture and ergonomics

Disadvantages

- Introduction of transscleral incision
  - Endophthalmitis risk
  - Risk of vitreous prolapse during scleral depression and band tightening if chandelier is removed and sclerotomy not closed and plugged
  - Vitreous incarceration in chandelier sclerotomy

- Limited illumination immediately below the chandelier position
- Suboptimal view if the eye is rotated away from transaxial orientation of the pupil and widefield lens

SURGICAL PROCEDURE: CHANDELIER-ASSISTED SCLERAL BUCKLE (VIDEO 27.1)

- Review detailed preop exam findings.
- Create a 360-degree conjunctival peritomy. See chapter titled *Scleral Buckling Basics.*
- Dissect the Tenon tissue in oblique quadrants with curved Stevens scissors.
- Isolate all four rectus muscles on a 2-0 silk ligature. See chapter titled *Scleral Buckling Steps.*
- Place 23G or 25G transscleral cannula for seating of a cannula-based chandelier.
  - In pseudophakic eyes, place the cannula ~180 degrees away from pathology.
  - In phakic eyes, place the cannula ~90 degrees away from pathology to avoid chandelier fiber-lens touch.
- Use standard contact or noncontact widefield viewing with chandelier endoillumination to examine retinal periphery and treat breaks with external cryotherapy (Fig. 27.1). See chapter titled *Lenses and Viewing Systems.*
- Mark breaks externally using viewing system as above. See chapter titled *Retinal Break Localization.*
- Remove chandelier. Place 7-0 Vicryl suture in sclerotomy if needed.

Use a valved cannula or nonvalved cannula with associated plug to house the chandelier. Selectively remove the chandelier for portions of procedure when endoillumination is not required (eg, SB placement/tightening), and place a plug to prevent vitreous prolapse through a nonvalved cannula or bare sclerotomy. If these options are not available, the cannula can be removed and the sclerotomy temporarily sutured when the chandelier is not in place.

- Place selected SB element(s) to support causative breaks, and secure buckle with mattress sutures and Watzke sleeve. See chapter titled *Scleral Buckling Steps.*
- Tighten the buckle to obtain appropriate buckle height.

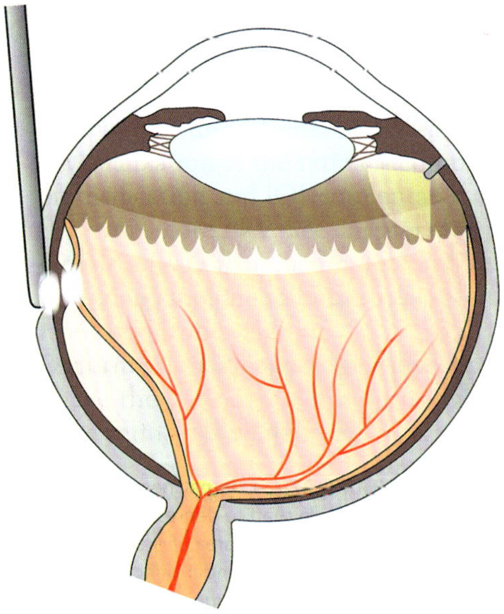

FIGURE 27.1. Use standard contact or noncontact widefield viewing with chandelier endoillumination to examine the retinal periphery and treat retinal breaks with external cryotherapy.

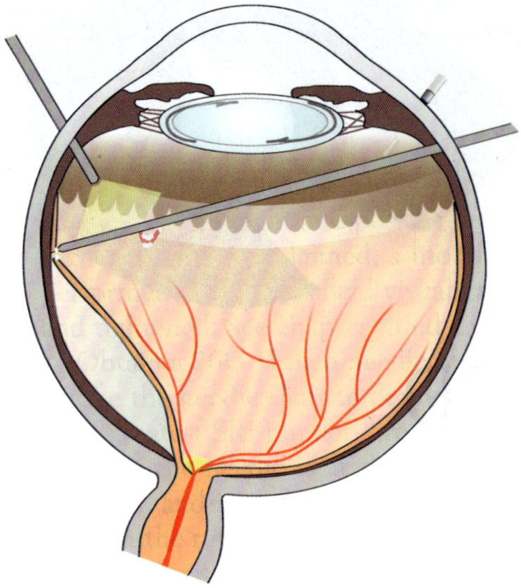

FIGURE 28.1. Mark all retinal breaks with endodiathermy.

- Mark all retinal breaks with endodiathermy (Fig. 28.1).
- To reattach the retina, drain SRF internally with or without the use of PFCL. See chapter titled *Posterior SRF During Vitrectomy for RRD.*
  - SRF drainage without PFCL (Video 28.2)
    - Create a drainage retinotomy using endodiathermy nasal to the optic disc if the RRD involves the nasal retina. Touch the tip of the endodiathermy instrument to the detached retina at the selected retinotomy site. The retina will whiten. Repeat endodiathermy at that same site to create a retinal hole at that site, which will allow egress of SRF into the vitreous cavity (Fig. 28.2). The soft-tip cannula can also be used to engage the diathermized retina in order to create a retinal hole at that site and drain SRF.
    - During the FAX, drain the remaining SRF using a soft-tip cannula through the drainage retinotomy. Use low magnification to improve visualization.
      - Perform a direct fluid-fluid exchange before the FAX using the soft-tip cannula or vitreous cutter on aspiration to drain SRF through the drainage retinotomy or an existing retinal break.
  - SRF drainage with PFCL
    - Use a dual bore cannula (MedOne Surgical, Inc.) to inject PFCL slowly over the optic disc to allow the retinal break(s) to lie flat on the eye wall. See chapter titled *Perfluorocarbon Liquid.*

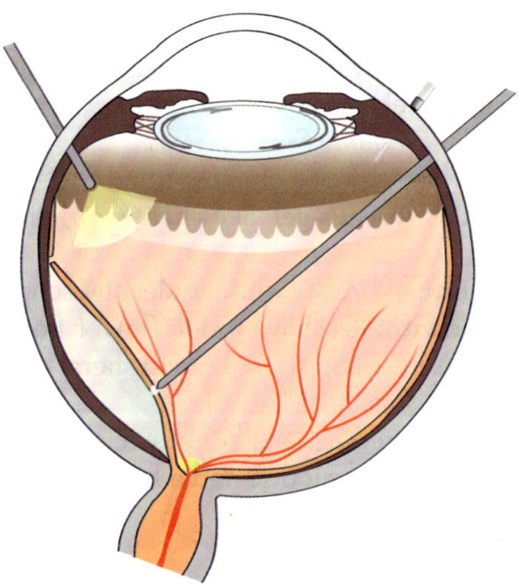

FIGURE 28.2. Touch the tip of the endodiathermy instrument to the detached retina at the selected retinotomy site preferably nasal to the disc. The retina will whiten. Repeat endodiathermy at that same site until a retinal hole develops, which will allow egress of SRF into the vitreous cavity.

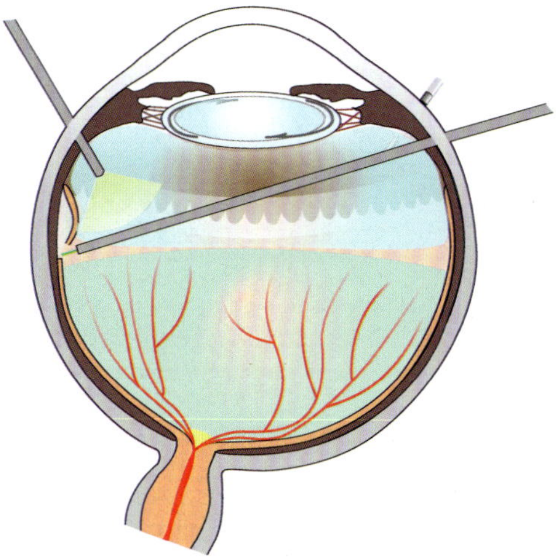

FIGURE 28.3. The Sandwich Technique. PFCL reattaches the posterior retina as air reattaches the anterior retina while you aspirate SRF through the retinal break using a soft-tip cannula.

- Keep the cannula tip within the PFCL bubble to prevent the formation of small "fish egg" PFCL bubbles. Any small bubbles may inadvertently enter the retinal break(s) and subretinal space. See chapter titled *Subretinal Perfluorocarbon Liquid*.
- Continue to inject PFCL and fill the vitreous cavity to the level of the posterior edge of the most anterior retinal break. The PFCL can cover the retinal break if the break lies flat on the eye wall. This will allow endolaser retinopexy to the retinal break(s) in a fluid-filled eye.
- If the retinal break(s) do not lie flat on the eye wall during PFCL placement, make sure all vitreous and membranous traction on the break has been removed. Then, perform a FAX while draining SRF through the retinal break with a soft-tip cannula. This is referred to as The Sandwich Technique, where the PFCL reattaches the retina posterior to the retinal break as air reattaches the retina anterior to the retinal break while SRF is aspirated (Fig. 28.3).

All traction on retinal break(s) must be relieved (Fig. 28.4) before PFCL placement; otherwise, the PFCL may enter the retinal break(s) and the subretinal space.

A dual-bore cannula allows injection of PFCL through its tip while also allowing egress of infusion fluid from one or more separate openings on the shaft. This prevents overpressurization of the eye during PFCL injection when using valved cannulas for PPV.

- Laser retinopexy can be placed under PFCL and infusion fluid or after the sandwich technique described above.
- Once the retinal breaks are flat on the eye wall, apply endolaser to surround all retinal breaks. You can apply 360 degrees of laser retinopexy to the retinal periphery at the vitreous base to cover any occult peripheral breaks if needed.

If performing 360 degrees of peripheral laser retinopexy, consider treating lightly or avoiding the 3:00 and 9:00 periphery altogether to spare the long ciliary nerves.

- After applying endolaser retinopexy, use the soft-tip cannula to remove any fluid or PFCL in the vitreous cavity and any residual SRF.
  - Remove any infusion fluid over the PFCL during FAX and drain through a retinal break, trying not to touch the edges of the break or the bare RPE in the bed of the break, to remove any residual SRF.
  - Remove the PFCL. See chapters titled *Fluid Air Exchange* and *Air Silicone Oil Exchange and Perfluorocarbon Liquid Silicone Oil Exchange*.

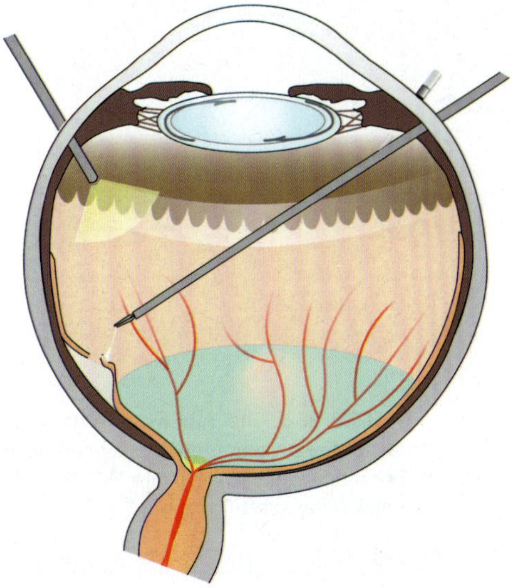

FIGURE 28.4. Relieve all traction on retinal breaks before instilling PFCL; otherwise, the PFCL may enter the subretinal space through the retinal break. See chapter titled *Subretinal Perfluorocarbon Liquid.*

- A tamponade of choice is prepared and placed in the vitreous cavity.
  - If gas is used, make sure the gas is diluted to the appropriate nonexpansile concentration (20% SF_{6s} and 14% C_3F_8). See chapter titled *Gas Tamponade*.
    - Clamp the infusion line.
    - Attach the syringe containing the prepared diluted gas to the infusion line.
    - Place a chimney vent in another cannula or use a 0.12 forcep to keep the valve in the venting cannula open to allow gas flushed into the eye to escape.
    - 25 mL of gas diluted in a 30-mL syringe is cycled through the eye, which will result in the desired nonexpansile concentration to fill the vitreous cavity.
    - 25G or 27G sclerotomies generally do not need to be sutured. 23G sclerotomies may need to be sutured.

Completely filling the vitreous cavity with undiluted, expansile gas can cause permanent visual loss due to marked elevation of IOP in the postop period.

  - If silicone oil is used as the tamponade, do not overfill the eye with silicone oil. See chapters titled *Air Silicone Oil Exchange* and *Perfluorocarbon Liquid Silicone Oil Exchange*.
    - A silicone oil overfill can lead to IOP elevation that would require another surgery to extract excess oil.
    - For aphakic eyes or eyes with ACIOL, make an inferior PI to avoid pupillary block glaucoma in the postop period. See chapter titled *Silicone Oil Tamponade*.
    - Suturing sclerotomies when silicone oil is used is suggested.

POSTOPERATIVE CONSIDERATIONS

- Educate your patient about proper positioning to maximize the tamponade and improve surgical success and decrease tamponade-related complications. See chapter titled *Postop Positioning*.
  - Allow the gas bubble to tamponade the retinal break(s).
  - Avoid supine positioning until tamponade is gone.
  - Avoid changes in altitude, including airplane travel, while the gas bubble is in the eye. Plane flight is permissible in silicone oil-filled eyes.
  - Minimize eye rubbing, particularly in aphakic eyes with silicone oil.

CHAPTER 29

Posterior SRF During Vitrectomy for RRD

Christopher L. Haupert, MD

There are three general approaches to dealing with posterior SRF during PPV for RRD (Video 29.1).

LEAVE THE SRF IN PLACE AND POSITION THE PATIENT FACEDOWN

See chapter titled *Postop Positioning*.

- Advantages
    - Shortens and simplifies the operation by avoiding extra steps such as a drainage retinotomy or use of PFCL.
- Disadvantages
    - Risk of inadvertent macular translocation and/or macular fold with poorer visual outcomes. See chapter titled *Postop Retinal Fold*.
- Technique pearls
    - The patient must be compliant; the importance of strict facedown positioning must be strongly emphasized, citing inadvertent macular translocation with possible macular fold, significant distortion, and loss of visual acuity as possible permanent consequences.

CREATE A POSTERIOR DRAINAGE RETINOTOMY

- Advantages
    - Reduces likelihood of inadvertent macular translocation and/or macular fold
    - More cost-effective
- Disadvantages
    - Can predispose to ERM formation and/or PVR
    - Can cause bleeding that could migrate beneath the macula
    - If the operative view worsens late in the case, the retinotomy can be difficult to visualize for laser treatment.
    - Rarely can cause a scotoma
    - Rarely can cause CNV

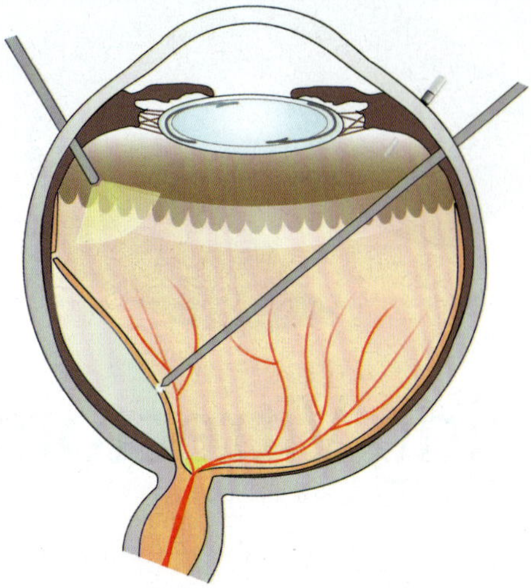

FIGURE 29.1. Mark the site of the retinotomy using endodiathermy, usually outside the vascular arcades but relatively posterior and often nasal to the disc.

- Technique pearls
  - Mark the site of the retinotomy using endodiathermy (Fig. 29.1).
    - This reduces bleeding and allows visualization of the retinotomy subsequently under air to facilitate laser treatment.
  - Create the retinotomy outside the vascular arcades but relatively posterior, often nasal to the disc and ideally in the same clock hour as the causative retinal break.
    - Superonasal (approximately 3 DD superonasal to the disc, well clear of retinal vessels) is the ideal location to maximize distance from the macula and facilitate coverage by the gas tamponade with minimal positioning.
  - Minimize laser treatment around the retinotomy. One row of confluent treatment is sufficient.
    - Excessive laser treatment of a drainage retinotomy can predispose to the sequelae mentioned previously.

USE PFCL

- Advantages
  - Avoids possible complications related to drainage retinotomy as described above
- Disadvantages
  - Expensive
  - Can be difficult to remove completely. Retained PFCL in the subretinal space or vitreous cavity may cause inflammation, migration to the AC, a central scotoma if subfoveal, and/or "bubbles" as floaters visible to the patient.
  - Fast injection through a small-bore cannula could cause a retinal break or FTMH and even subretinal PFCL.
- Technique Pearls
  - Inject PFCL through a soft-tip cannula or dual-bore cannula (MedOne Surgical Inc.) (Fig. 29.2).
  - Consider placing a chandelier to allow for bimanual handling of the PFCL syringe, which maximizes control during injection. See chapter titled *The Chandelier Buckle*. Alternately, a skilled assistant can manipulate the syringe.
  - If a dual-bore cannula is not available, consider reducing the infusion pressure and inserting a short needle into one of the cannulas to vent the eye and allow for easier PFCL injection with less resistance. Inserting such a needle could cause IOP fluctuation during injection with sudden bursts of infusion fluid causing PFCL bubbles or "fish eggs."

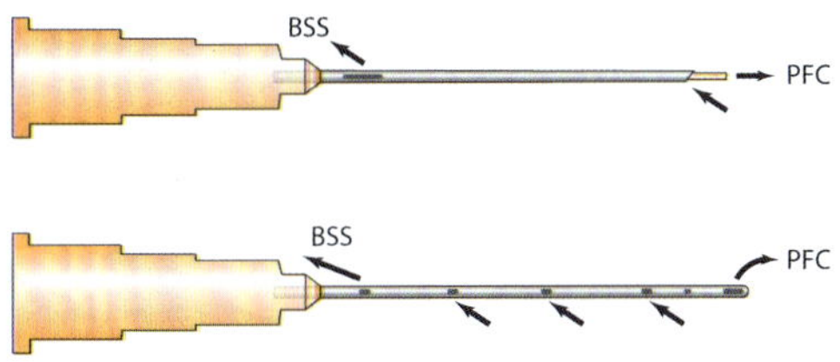

FIGURE 29.2. A soft-tip cannula demonstrated on top and dual-bore cannula shown on the bottom. Both may be used for injecting PFCL. The dual-bore cannula allows for more IOP control by allowing infusion fluid to egress while PFCL is injected.

- Inject PFCL slowly and keep the cannula tip immersed in the PFCL to minimize small bubble formation, which can increase the risk of subretinal PFCL. Keep the stream of PFCL directed toward the optic nerve to avoid inadvertent FTMH formation and subretinal PFCL.
- Position the tip of the cannula opposite the location of a peripheral break where you plan to drain SRF so that the SRF will be displaced toward that break.
- Fill the vitreous cavity with PFCL up to the posterior margin of the most anterior break, through which SRF will be drained.
- Perform a FAX, placing the tip of the soft-tip cannula connected to extrusion tubing over the peripheral break where you plan to drain SRF. This is called The Sandwich Technique (Fig. 29.3).
- Drain SRF through the peripheral break as infused air displaces anterior SRF posteriorly.
- Drain SRF well through the peripheral break, as any residual SRF will migrate posteriorly.
  - Once you have drained all SRF anterior to the break, remove some PFCL, and then go back to the peripheral break and drain through the soft-tip cannula again. Repeating this maneuver 2-3 times helps to ensure thorough SRF drainage and helps to avoid posterior migration of any residual fluid.
- Once you have aspirated nearly all of the PFCL, carefully aspirate over the disc to ensure complete removal.
  - To prevent PFCL from refluxing back out of the soft-tip handpiece when PFCL aspiration is complete, continue aspirating until after you have removed the soft-tip instrument from the eye.
  - While under air, inject a few drops of infusion fluid over the macula and optic disc at this step, and then aspirate the residual infusion fluid with the soft-tip cannula over the disc. This thereby ensures all PFCL has been removed along with the infusion fluid. Caution must be utilized during this latter maneuver to avoid getting any infusion fluid near the retinal break(s).

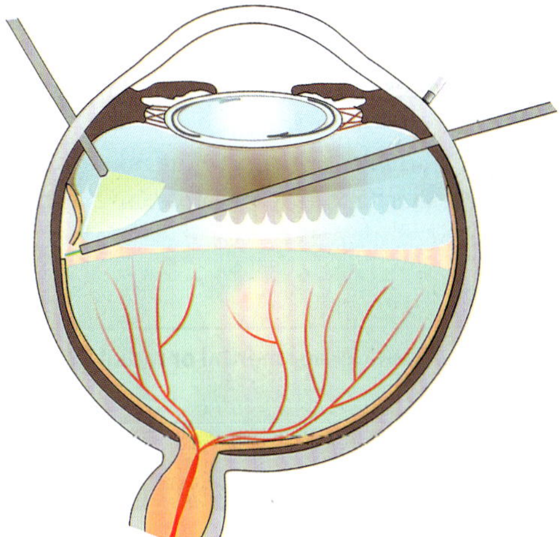

FIGURE 29.3. The Sandwich Technique. Perform a FAX, placing the tip of the soft-tip cannula connected to extrusion tubing over the peripheral retinal break where you choose to drain SRF. In this figure, air is superior in the vitreous cavity, fluid is subretinal and PFCL is inferior and filling the vitreous cavity to the posterior edge of the retinal break.

Section VI

Macular Surgery

CHAPTER 32

Epiretinal Membrane

Pouya N. Dayani, MD

PREOPERATIVE CONSIDERATIONS

- A PVD is present in up to 90% of eyes with idiopathic ERMs.
- Trauma, ocular inflammation, retinal vascular disease, a retinal break, retinopexy, and prior ocular surgery are risk factors for ERM formation.
- PPV with ERM removal is the treatment of choice for visually symptomatic membranes.
- The optimal time for surgical intervention has not been standardized, and the decision for surgery is primarily based on the extent of visual symptoms and loss of VA.
  - The majority of ERMs remain stable after several months without further progression or improvement.
- Preop prognostic factors that have been reported to affect visual outcome following ERM surgery include integrity of the inner segment/outer segment junction of the photoreceptors, VA, duration of symptoms, severity of metamorphopsia, integrity of cone outer segment tips, central foveal thickness, and extent of RPE changes on fundus autofluorescence.
- Concurrent ILM peeling may reduce the rate of ERM recurrence (11% without ILM peeling vs 2% with ILM peeling).
  - Postop VA and central macular foveal thickness do not appear to be consistently improved with ILM peeling.
- Potential surgical complications include cataract formation, retinal break or RD, FTMH, endophthalmitis, retinal phototoxicity, and direct toxicity from ICG. See chapter titled *Intraoperative Visualization Agents*.

SURGICAL PROCEDURE (VIDEO 32.1)

- Perform a PPV with the creation of a PVD if needed. See chapter titled *PVD Induction*.
- Triamcinolone diluted with normal saline solution (often in a 1:4 ratio) can help highlight the vitreous, hyaloid, and ERM. See chapter titled *Intraoperative Visualization Agents*.
  - This can be particularly helpful in cases of vitreoschisis or anomalous vitreous separation.

  - Settled triamcinolone crystals can also help delineate peeled from unpeeled areas of ERM with the crystals highlighting ERM tissue.
- ICG (or brilliant blue G) may be utilized to facilitate ILM peeling.
- To prepare the lyophilized ICG (25 mg/vial) for use, reconstitute it with 20 mL of preservative-free D5W to get a 1.25 mg/mL solution. Withdraw 2 mL from the ICG vial in a 3-mL syringe. Attach two green 0.22-µm filters to the 3-mL syringe. Attach a 22G needle to the filters. Inject 1 mL through both filters into TB syringe for the final product. Use promptly.
  - Mixing ICG with D5W makes the ICG "heavy."
  - ICG can alternately be mixed with BSS but will need to be injected, usually under air after FAX, closer to the macula to allow for contact and staining.
- Inject the ICG-D5W mixture with a soft-tip cannula (or 25G needle) over the desired area under fluid.
- With valved cannulas, the ICG will settle posteriorly, and sufficient ILM staining can be attained without significant delay prior to removal.
  - ICG staining is better in areas without ERM (Fig. 32.1).
- Use a pinch-and-grab technique to create an ILM edge. Intraop OCT may be helpful.
  - Often there is a 'break' in the ILM adjacent to a retinal vessel.
- In certain cases, such as in eyes with significant media opacities or myopic degeneration, a Tano Diamond Dusted Membrane Scraper (Synergetics), a barbed MVR blade or needle, or the Finesse Flex Loop (Alcon) may facilitate creation of an ILM flap instead of using a pinch-and-grab technique.
  - The Tano scraper is a silicone-tipped device coated with diamond particles that can engage the ERM.
    - Insertion of a Tano can be challenging when using valved cannulas. Retractable scrapers may facilitate insertion.
    - To minimize iatrogenic retinal trauma when using a Tano, it is essential to orient it so that the ERM is engaged with the natural bent edge of the instrument, bevel down (Fig. 32.2).
  - The Finesse Flex Loop can similarly be used to create an ILM edge.
    - The thin loop allows for optimal visibility of the contacted area.
    - The tines are designed to penetrate no deeper than 85% of the ILM, thereby minimizing unintended trauma to the retina.
    - Adjust the retractable tip to control the length of the loop and, thereby, its stiffness.

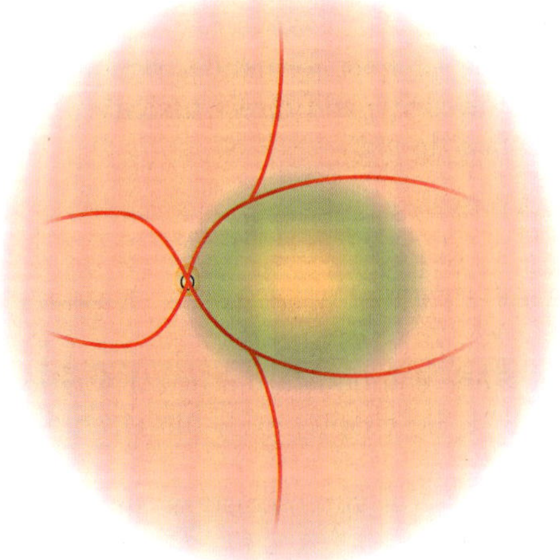

FIGURE 32.1. ICG staining is better in areas without an ERM.

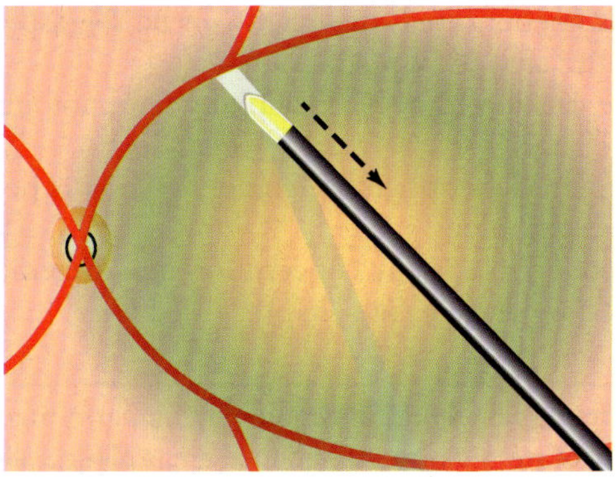

FIGURE 32.2. To minimize iatrogenic retinal trauma when using a Tano Diamond Dusted Membrane Scraper (Synergetics), it is essential to orient it so that the ERM is engaged with the natural bent edge of the instrument, bevel down.

  - Alternatively, use a barbed MVR blade to engage the edge of the membrane and elevate an edge from the macular surface.
- Engage the ILM away from the macular center (1-2 DD from fovea) in an area without significant ERM.
  - This will ensure complete removal of the central ERM along with ILM.
  - It will also reduce the possibility of inadvertently peeling the hyaloid (that can stain with ICG in cases of anomalous PVD) instead of the ILM, thus ensuring adequate ERM removal.
- Once an adequate flap in the ILM has been created, use forceps or a Tano to extend the peel circumferentially around the macula.
  - Use tangential motion during peeling instead of anterior pulling, which may lead to foveal traction or loss of the ILM flap (requiring repeated peeling attempts).
  - Both the ERM and ILM can be simultaneously peeled together.
  - When using a Tano to extend the peel (prior to using forceps), place it over the folded flap created earlier to create an additional barrier against retinal trauma.
- ILM forceps are ideal for membrane peeling.
- When peeling (particularly temporally), ensure forceps remain in view to avoid iatrogenic trauma to the retina. Slightly lift forceps away from the macula to create distance from the retinal surface as the eye wall curves.
- Avoid tearing the ERM (or losing the flap created), thereby minimizing repeated attempts at regrasping.
- The area of the peel should involve at least 1 DD beyond the fovea, preferably extended to the arcade.
- In cases of a thick, mature ERM, peel it first prior to staining and peeling the ILM.
  - Otherwise, staining from the ICG will be limited and lead to unnecessary repeated use of ICG.
  - Combined peeling of both the ILM and ERM can also be challenging with a mature ERM, requiring repeated regrasping.
- If the macula has significant distortion and folds, even following adequate ERM removal, retinal striae may create the false impression of persistent ERM. Remain aware of areas where ERM peeling has been performed.
  - If there is a question, consider repeat staining with ICG or diluted triamcinolone.
  - Significant traction can also lead to fluffy, white-appearing inner retina (or cotton wool spots) that may be mistaken for ERM. Avoid initiating membrane peeling in such areas.

Bleeding from iatrogenic trauma or firm adhesions to retinal vessels is typically self-limited and does not require prolonged elevation of IOP or diathermy.

- If an area of unusual adherence is encountered, the ERM can be regrasped in another location and peeled toward the area of firm adhesion.
- When peeling over the fovea, take caution to peel tangentially (and not anteriorly) to avoid creation of an iatrogenic FTMH.
- Once ERM peeling has been completed, peripheral scleral depression is performed to ensure absence of any peripheral pathology.
- Air or short-acting gas may be used if there is any concern for an iatrogenic FTMH or in cases of VMT with ERM or lamellar hole. See chapter titled *Gas Tamponade*.

If there is associated CME, a subtenon or intravitreal steroid injection may be performed at the conclusion of the case in eyes without a history of steroid response or open angle glaucoma.

POSTOPERATIVE CONSIDERATIONS

- Visual recovery is dependent on a number of factors, most importantly, baseline VA and duration of symptoms.
- Most of the visual recovery will occur in the first 3 months, but gradual improvement can be seen for 6-12 months postop.
- Patients can typically expect to regain roughly ½ of the visual loss due to the ERM.
  - Eighty to 90% of eyes with idiopathic ERM will experience 2 or more lines of visual gain.
- Noncystic macular thickening will improve gradually over time, sometimes up to 12 months typically without additional therapy.
  - This will take longer in cases of increasing preop traction and CME.
- Inner nuclear cystic changes seen on the postop OCT do not appear to affect visual recovery and may not need to be treated.

CHAPTER 33

Macular Hole

Charles Wilson, MD

PREOPERATIVE CONSIDERATIONS

- Evaluate the FTMH on OCT.
  - Determine the maximum diameter of the FTMH, the maximum thickness of the retina adjacent to the FTMH, the status of the vitreous (attached, unattached), and the presence or absence of an ERM.
  - Favorable characteristics include:
    - Absence of other macular pathology
    - A small FTMH (<400 μm)
    - Edge retinal thickness equaling or exceeding the diameter of the FTMH
    - These eyes are most likely to experience anatomical hole closure with improvement in VA.
  - Unfavorable characteristics include:
    - RPE pigmentary changes suggesting chronicity
    - Flat open configuration
    - Large FTMH size (>400 μm)
    - FTMHs with less favorable characteristics are not necessarily excluded from surgical consideration, but they close less often with less VA improvement.
- Evaluate media opacities
  - FTMH surgery can often wait until a problematic cataract is removed. Some prefer to combine both surgeries. A YAG or surgical capsulotomy may be needed in pseudophakic eyes.
- Evaluate the vitreous
  - If the vitreous is attached, there is no ERM, and the FTMH is small, the eye is potentially a candidate for enzymatic vitreolysis with ocriplasmin (Jetrea, Thrombogenics) or pneumatic vitreolysis. The most common and usually transient side effects of ocriplasmin use include floaters in 17%, decreased VA in 17%, and photopsias in 17%. Ocriplasmin can only be used once.
- Other
  - Is the patient willing and able to maintain facedown positioning? See chapter titled *Postop Positioning*.
  - What is the status of the fellow eye?
  - Does the patient's livelihood depend on good binocular vision?

- Are there other macular comorbidities such as AMD?
- For how long has the patient been symptomatic?
  - Presence of symptoms for <6-12 months portends a more favorable prognosis.

SURGICAL PROCEDURE

- Set up for a standard, 3-port PPV. See chapter titled *Vitrectomy Surgery Steps*.
- Detach and remove the posterior hyaloid, if attached. See chapter titled *PVD Induction*.
  - Use triamcinolone, 40 mg/mL (TRIESENCE, Alcon), to visualize the vitreous during its removal.
- Remove any ERM that may be present.
  - Remove ERM before or after staining ILM. See chapter titled *Epiretinal Membrane*.
- Stain the ILM with one of the staining agents. See chapter titled *Intraoperative Visualization Agents*.
  - Trypan blue 0.06% (VisionBlue, DORC).
    - First, perform FAX and then place 0.5 mL of the dye on the posterior pole. Staining is only fair.
  - Brilliant blue G 0.125 mg/0.5 mL (ILM-Blue, DORC).
    - Produces more intense ILM staining
    - Can be used in BSS-filled eyes and will sink to the macula
  - ICG (25 mg reconstituted with 20 mL of preservative-free D5W for a final concentration of 1.25 mg/mL. Withdraw 2 mL from the ICG vial in a 3-mL syringe. Attach two green 0.22-μm filters to the 3-mL syringe. Attach a 22G needle to the filters. Inject 1 mL through both filters into TB syringe for the final product. Use promptly.).
    - Provides intense staining of the ILM and will sink to the macula in BSS infusion fluid
  - Triamcinolone in small amounts can indirectly identify the ILM during peeling. Peeling without staining may produce less consistent results. Dyes are removed after 30 seconds or so of sitting on the macula. Timing the dye exposure is recommended.
- Next, the ILM is peeled.
  - General considerations
    - Most prefer to peel the ILM around the FTMH, knowing that the chances of anatomic closure are better with than without it. Small FTMH may not require ILM peeling.
    - ILM removal may injure the inner retina. Despite concerns about this and the potential toxicity of dyes used to highlight ILM (particularly ICG), ILM peeling remains a widely accepted practice.
    - There is no consensus on how wide to extend the peel, but it is felt that larger FTMHs require wider peeling.
    - ILM peeling is usually done with the use of a macular contact lens which offers the greatest magnification without loss of depth perception. The field of view and depth of field, however, are limited with such a contact lens, and thus, your instruments may only come into view when they are very close to the retinal surface.
      - Given the limited field of view and depth of field, instruments can unknowingly contact and damage the retina.
      - When you first start using a macular lens, first increase the magnification and focus on the retina.
      - Next, remove all magnification and bring your instruments into view in the mid-vitreous cavity.
      - Next, increase zoom and slowly advance your instruments until they are in focus close to the retinal surface.

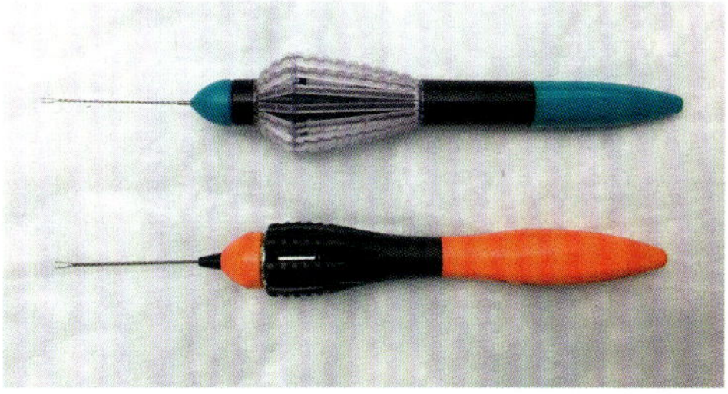

FIGURE 33.1. ILM forceps. These represent the first generation of ILM peeling instrumentation. It requires the greatest degree of dexterity and is felt to have the greatest potential of trauma, especially if multiple regrasps are needed. Some restrict use of ILM forceps to elevated flaps of ILM.

- Peeling procedure. Video 33.1
  - There is no consensus as to the best way to initiate peeling.
  - Some prefer a direct pinch-and-peel approach with ILM forceps.
    - Using ILM forceps (Fig. 33.1), create a fracture in the ILM by pinching the ILM. Next, release the pinched area of ILM to ensure that only ILM was grasped by the forceps. Next, use the edge of fractured ILM to initiate your ILM peel.

ILM peeling tip 1. Generally, ILM is most susceptible to fracture near a major retinal vessel or near the edge of the optic disc. These are good places to start to fracture the ILM and form the initial flap.

  - You can raise a small flap of ILM first.
    - Use either a bent needle or bent MVR blade, Finesse Flex Loop (Alcon, Fig. 33.2), or Tano Diamond Dusted Membrane Scraper (Bausch and Lomb/Synergetics, Fig. 33.3, Video 33.2).
    - Once the ILM has been fractured and a flap has been created, use ILM forceps to peel the ILM in a circular motion around the FTMH, regrasping as needed to direct the peel (as is done in capsulorrhexis during cataract surgery).
  - Restaining the ILM and starting a second flap are methods to deal with flaps that tear away incompletely.
  - When an ERM is also present, it can often be removed along with the ILM, by starting the ILM peeling in an area peripheral to the ERM. The ERM will be represented by negative staining when using ICG and positive 'staining' when using triamcinolone. Intraop OCT may be helpful.

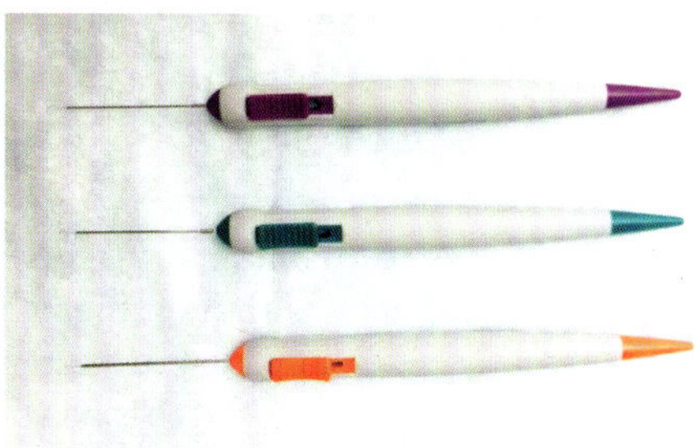

FIGURE 33.2. Finesse Flex Loop. This is a third generation tool for peeling membrane, specifically the ILM. The loop is extensible, so the ratio of pressure exerted by the surgeon to force on the retina can be changed—full extension of the loop provides the "lightest touch." The loop is roughly shaped to resemble the form of a snowshoe. "Walk" the snowshoe on the ILM by planting it, then drawing along the retina surface. Do not push it toward the tip. The wider contact with the retina allows a more generous fracture of the ILM with little trauma. In complex cases of FTMH, when the ILM is checkered with overlying ERM, and particularly when ILM is peeling in small fragments, this tool can be used to roll the ILM over unpeeled retina successfully, similar to rolling up a carpet.

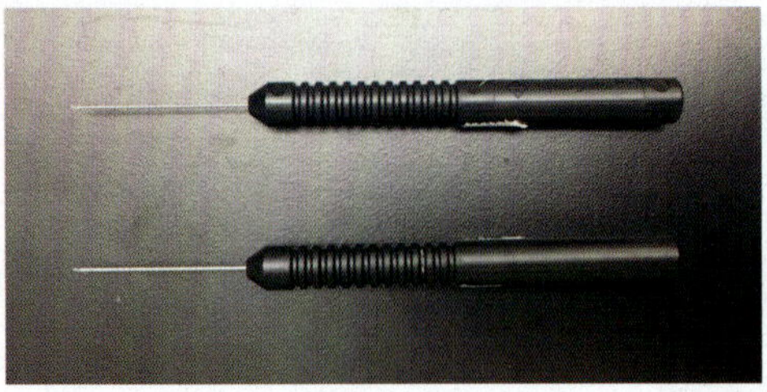

FIGURE 33.3. Tano Diamond Dusted Membrane Scraper. This is a second generation tool for peeling the ILM. It is useful in fracturing the ILM and engaging organized ERM. It is two-sided. The curved side is more flexible and is often the side of choice for ILM peeling. As far as technique, the Tano is used very much like the Flex Loop.

ILM peeling tip 2. Do not expect the ILM to peel the same way in any two cases. Sometimes, it will come off in small pieces. At other times, it will peel as a more integral sheet.

ILM peeling tip 3. If an ERM has formed around the FTMH, there will often be cellular continuity between the ERM and neural retina. You will see this material everting from the FTMH and will note that manipulation of it will cause the FTMH to deform. There is no way to know where the ERM ends and neural tissue begins. Occasionally, this material has lutein pigment and is more clearly a part of the FTMH that should remain. Consider minimally debulking redundant tissue with the high-speed cutter or leaving some or most if it behind, letting it position itself under the gas bubble.

- Complete a peripheral retinal exam and peripheral vitreous shaving.
- Perform a complete FAX. See chapter titled *Fluid Air Exchange*.
- Infuse gas tamponade using gas of choice. See chapter titled *Gas Tamponade.*
  - Silicone oil tamponade may be considered in patients who need to get on a flight or those who are unable to position facedown postop.

Special Considerations

- Recurrent/failed FTMH: Repeat surgery can often be successful. Recommendations include peeling the ILM, if that was not done initially. A wider excision of the ILM and longer facedown positioning (up to 2 weeks) might be helpful. Other techniques have been reported which are discussed in other chapters in this book. See chapters titled *Autologous Retinal Transplant*. A long-acting gas mixture may also be considered (eg, 14% C_3F_8) if a shorter acting one was used the first time (20% SF_6).
- Lamellar holes: Most lamellar holes are associated with good VA and tend to retain it. The few exceptions with decreasing VA may be treated as a FTMH. Although it is not technically necessary to perform a FAX and use gas tamponade in these cases, some may prefer it in the hopes of accelerating the transition to a more normal foveal contour.

POSTOPERATIVE CONSIDERATIONS

Most surgeons ask their patients to maintain a facedown position for 45 minutes out of every hour while away for 5-7 days, although many ask for longer and some ask for shorter. Patients can sleep on the side opposite the operative eye during this time and not on their back until the tamponade is gone. Success has been reported with no facedown positioning and avoidance of faceup, which might be helpful for patients who cannot maintain a facedown position due to other medical issues such as severe arthritis.

CHAPTER 34

Advanced Vitrectomy Techniques for Macular Holes

Cindy X. Cai, MD • Cynthia A. Toth, MD

See chapter titled *Macular Hole.*

PREOPERATIVE CONSIDERATIONS

Successful anatomic closure of FTMH with a single surgery is around 90% with conventional PPV, ILM peeling, gas, and postop positioning. However, some FTMH require more advanced techniques for successful closure. These challenging cases include larger FTMH (although traditionally defined by the International Vitreomacular Traction Study Group as FTMH >400 µm in diameter, the Manchester Large Macular Hole Study suggests that the cutoff should be 650 µm with modern techniques), chronic FTMH >6 months, myopic FTMH, and recurrent FTMH after prior surgical repair. In these more challenging cases, successful closure of the FTMH might be facilitated by the use of more advanced techniques.

INVERTED ILM FLAP (VIDEO 34.1)

- Perform a core PPV and stain the ILM. See chapter titled *Intraoperative Visualization Agents.*
- Peel ERM if present. See chapter titled *Epiretinal Membrane.*
- Peel ILM in a circular fashion for ~2DD around the FTMH but leave it attached to the FTMH.
- Trim the ILM so that only a small central portion remains attached to the FTMH (Fig. 34.1).
- Massage the flap of ILM 360 degrees over the FTMH such that it is now "upside down" or inverted—the side of the ILM that previously faced the vitreous now faces the RPE.
- Perform a FAX. See chapter titled *Fluid Air Exchange.*
- Perform an air gas exchange. See chapter titled *Air Gas Exchange.*
- Keep the patient in the prone position. See chapter titled *Postop Positioning.*

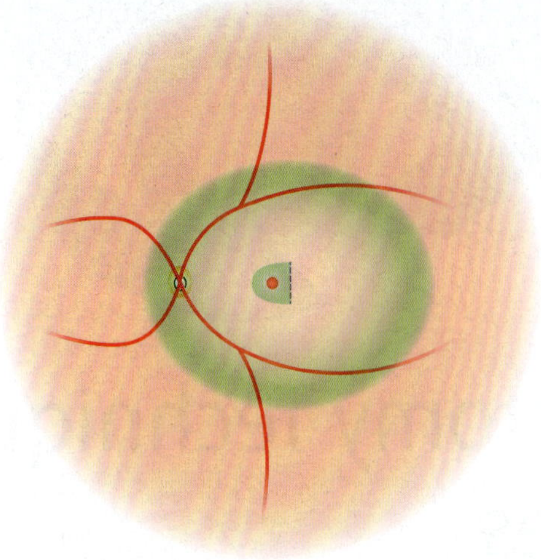

FIGURE 34.1. Inverted ILM flap. Trim the ILM so that only a small central portion remains attached to the FTMH.

- **Inverted ILM flap may detach spontaneously during the FAX. Use the soft-tip cannula to gently massage it back into place.**
- **When drying the macula, aspirate over the area where the ILM has been peeled to prevent inadvertent aspiration of the ILM flap.**

Modifications

- Temporal inverted ILM flap technique: Create an asymmetric ILM flap where the temporal aspect of the flap is wider than the width of the FTMH, and only use the temporal aspect of the flap to fold over the FTMH.
- A temporally hinged flap may be helpful as drying nasally over the nerve is less likely to cause inadvertent flap aspiration and the fluidics may help maintain flap inversion over the FTMH.

INTERNAL LIMITING MEMBRANE RETRACTING DOOR

- Perform a PPV and stain the ILM.
- Create a large flap of ILM starting nasal to the FTMH (a Finesse Flex Loop may be useful to initiate the large flap).
- Carry this flap temporally over the fovea and area of FTMH.
- Leave the flap attached temporally and drape it back over the area of the FTMH (Fig. 34.2).
- Perform a FAX, followed by air gas exchange, and keep the patient in the prone position.
- This is a good technique for myopic macular holes where the presence of a posterior staphyloma and very fragile ILM might make the inverted ILM flap technique more difficult to perform.

- **This technique is less prone to ILM flap displacement during FAX since there is only one large flap.**

RELAXING RETINOTOMIES

- Perform core vitrectomy, stain ILM, and peel ILM.
- Create superior and inferior 120-degree relaxing retinotomies just outside of the superotemporal and inferotemporal vascular arcades under PFCL.

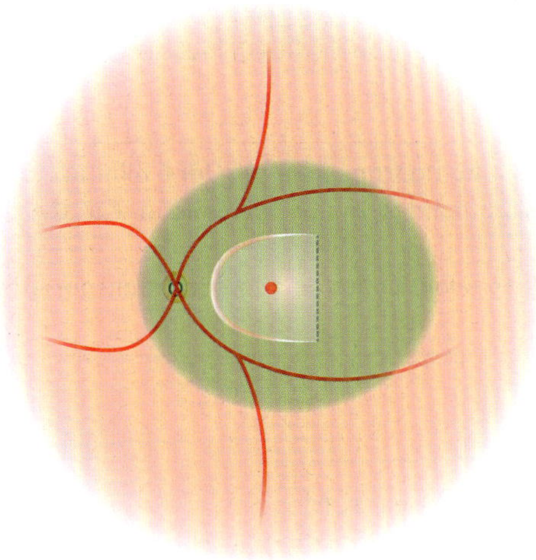

FIGURE 34.2. ILM retracting door. Leave the flap attached temporally and drape it back over the area of the FTMH.

- Control bleeding with diathermy.
- Massage the retina around the FTMH under PFCL until the FTMH closes.
- Perform a FAX, followed by air gas exchange, and postop positioning.
- This is a good technique when the rigidity of the retina, (for instance due to FVP) surrounding the FTMH prevents hole closure, even after ILM peeling.

PLATELET-RICH PLASMA

- Prepare the platelet-rich plasma.
  - Before surgery, place a second IV to facilitate peripheral blood draw.
  - As soon as the decision is made to proceed with platelet-rich plasma, obtain autologous whole blood from the patient under sterile conditions by venipuncture via the second IV.
  - Transfer 10 mL of the autologous whole blood into the double syringe of the Arthrex Autologous Conditioned Plasma (ACP) Double Syringe System (Naples, FL). Anticoagulant citrate dextrose (ACD) is not needed as an anticoagulant if the sample will be used within 20 minutes.
  - Using the Arthrex Rotofix 32A machine and the single centrifugation technique, centrifuge the whole blood to separate the plasma from the cellular components at 1500 rpm for 5 minutes.
  - This will separate the whole blood into red blood cells and white blood cells at the bottom and a supernatant containing platelets in the bottom one-third and platelet poor plasma in the top two-thirds. See Figure 67.2 in the chapter titled *Optic Pit Maculopathy*.
  - Push down on the outer syringe to extract the plasma layer into the inner syringe, taking care not to disrupt the red blood cell layer. Now the inner syringe containing about 1-2 mL of plasma can be removed and used.
  - On the sterile field, 1 mL of the plasma is drawn into a TB syringe attached to extension tubing and a soft-tip cannula and is now ready for use. If ACD is not added, you have 20 minutes to use the plasma.
- Perform core vitrectomy, stain ILM, and peel ILM.
- Perform a FAX and meticulously yet carefully dry the FTMH using a 33G or 34G extrusion cannula.
- Using the soft-tip cannula, instill several drops of the platelet-rich plasma over the FTMH, and let it stand for 5-10 minutes.

- Remove the excess fluid but let a thin residual layer cover the macula.
- Add an internal tamponade and have the patient position facedown for 2 weeks. See chapter titled *Gas Tamponade.*

> - **Various centrifuge settings may be effective, ranging from 4000 rpm for 5 minutes to 3000 rpm for 10 minutes. Use whatever setting is recommended by the manufacturer of the centrifuge machine and your facility's laboratory.**
> - **Prepare the platelet-rich plasma in the OR to avoid contamination and transportation of the platelet-rich plasma.**

INDUCING MACULAR DETACHMENT

- Perform a core vitrectomy, stain ILM, and peel ILM.
- Create a puncture retinotomy in each quadrant of the macula using a 41G rigid subretinal cannula.
- Infuse infusion fluid into the subretinal space through the retinotomies to create a subretinal bleb until it connects with the FTMH, at which time it will stop enlarging, to achieve total macular detachment.
- Perform a FAX but leave the SRF in place—do not drain it.
- Add an internal tamponade and have the patient position facedown.
- This is a good technique in cases of recurrent FTMH where intrinsic rigidity of the retina prevents it from mobilizing.

> - **Infuse the infusion fluid into the subretinal space either manually with a syringe and cannula connected by extension tubing or via the viscous fluid injection function on your vitrectomy machine at a setting of ~18-20 mm Hg. Would recommend testing the infusion set-up prior to entry into the eye.**
> - **The extent of total macular detachment can be variable in size but roughly aim for detachment up to the temporal vascular arcades.**

Modifications

- Additional massage of the macular retina can be done with a Tano Diamond Dusted Membrane Scraper (Synergetics) to further mobilize the retina.

CHAPTER 35

Autologous Retinal Transplant

Tamer H. Mahmoud, MD, PhD

PREOPERATIVE CONSIDERATIONS

Possible Indications

- Primary FTMH: high myope, Alport syndrome, large >400 µm, or chronic
- Persistent or recurrent FTMH, irrespective of etiology
- Myopic FTMH RD
- FTMH associated with RD and PVR
- FTMH associated with GA or disciform scar

SURGICAL PROCEDURE (VIDEO 35.1)

- Use Finesse Flex Loop (Alcon) to get an idea of the size of the FTMH.
- Identify a donor location in superior retina (which allows for easier tamponade) to harvest the autologous retinal tissue. Locate an area that allows easy access to cut the graft.
- Put four dots of diathermy at thin blood vessel crossings (avoid large vessels) to delineate graft size (Fig. 35.1).
- Fill the eye with PFCL just beyond donor site. This stabilizes the retina where you will be working, avoids bimanual techniques, and reduces bleeding while cutting the graft.
- Use pneumatic vertical scissors to cut the graft. The graft should be at least 25% larger than the size of FTMH (Fig. 35.2).
- Perform endolaser around the donor site, but do not place the laser spots on the graft edges. See chapter titled *Endolaser Types and Settings.*
- Use MaxGrip forceps (Alcon), Finesse Flex Loop, or similar instrument to move the autologous graft to cover the FTMH.
- In highly myopic eyes, use longer myopic forceps, and gently drag the autologous transplant tissue over the edge of the staphyloma so that it stays flat against the retina.
- Slightly stretch the transplant over the FTMH without pushing down.

In highly myopic eyes, avoid pulling the transplanted tissue straight toward the FTMH as this may cause the autologous graft to wrap around the forceps. If this happens, return the transplant to the donor area, open the forceps to unwrap the transplant in place under PFCL, and try again to relocate the tissue.

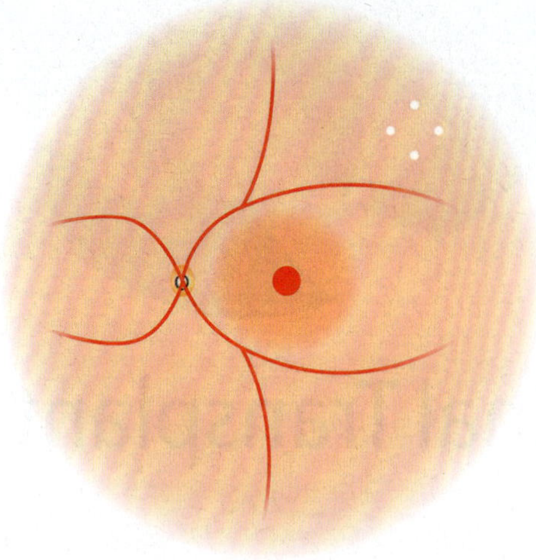

FIGURE 35.1. Identify a donor area in superior retina (which allows for easier tamponade) to harvest the autologous retinal tissue. Locate an area that allows easy access to cut the graft. Put four dots of diathermy at thin blood vessel crossings (avoid large vessels) to delineate graft size.

- Make sure all edges of the FTMH are covered including any eccentric holes. Covering all FTMH edges is crucial in Alport syndrome where the graft may need to be 50% larger than the FTMH size to avoid progression to a larger FTMH.
- Fill the eye with PFCL, which will remain in the eye at the end of the case.
- Before suturing sclerotomies, infuse air so that air and not fluid will overlie the PFCL. This decreases the amount of PFCL that may egress during closure of the sclerotomies.
- Advise patients to assume any position except facedown.
- Use topical prednisolone and follow closely for inflammation or rise in IOP.
- Remove the PFCL in about 1-2 weeks and ideally closer to 2 weeks if no PFCL-related complications are detected.

Special Scenarios

For cases of myopic MH RD

- Follow steps above under PFCL. Drain any SRF pushed to peripheral retina through the superior donor site after removing some PFCL or using The Sandwich Technique with air infused over the PFCL. See chapter titled *Fluid Air Exchange.*
- After the SRF has been removed, fill the eye with PFCL and follow the steps above.

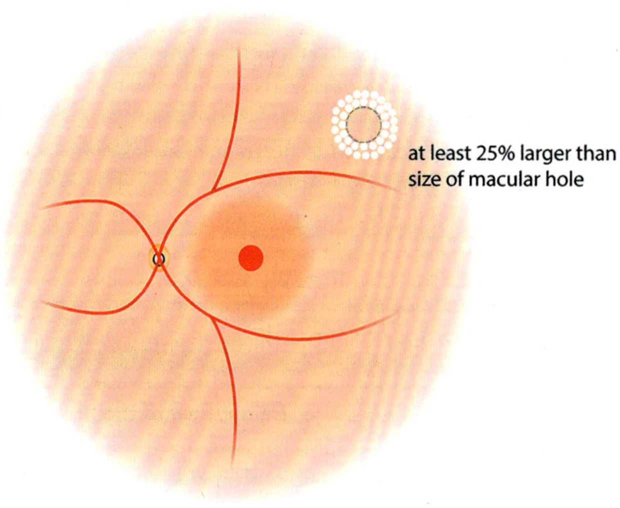

FIGURE 35.2. The autologous graft should be at least 25% larger than the size of MH.

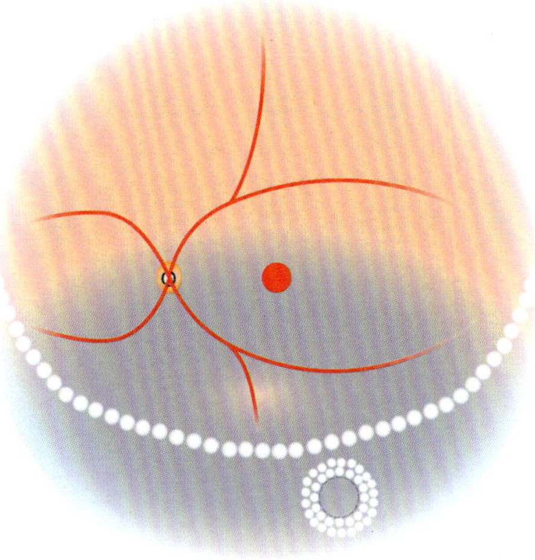

FIGURE 35.3. If a large retinotomy and retinectomy are required, delineate with diathermy a retinal graft of appropriate size peripheral to the retinotomy.

For MH associated with RD and PVR

- Peel all PVR membranes first, then instill PFCL, and follow steps as for the myopic MH RD. See chapter titled *Proliferative Vitreoretinopathy Surgery.*
- If a large retinotomy and retinectomy are required, delineate with diathermy a retinal graft of appropriate size peripheral to the retinotomy (Fig. 35.3).
- Using bimanual techniques (chandelier needed for those cases; see chapter titled *The Chandelier Buckle*), move the autologous graft either preretinal or subretinal and adjust in or under the FTMH, inject PFCL to flatten the retina, endolaser, and then follow steps as above.
- At 2 weeks, exchange PFCL with silicone oil in PVR cases for longer tamponade. See chapter titled *Perfluorocarbon Liquid Silicone Oil Exchange*.

For MH associated with GA of disciform scar

- Autologous retinal transplant is combined with RPE and choroidal transplant.
- Follow same steps as above but with a deeper cut involving RPE and choroid at donor site. For cases associated with disciform scarring, the scar can be peeled and removed under high infusion pressure, to prevent intraop bleeding, prior to transplantation.

Section VII

Lensectomy and Secondary IOL Placement

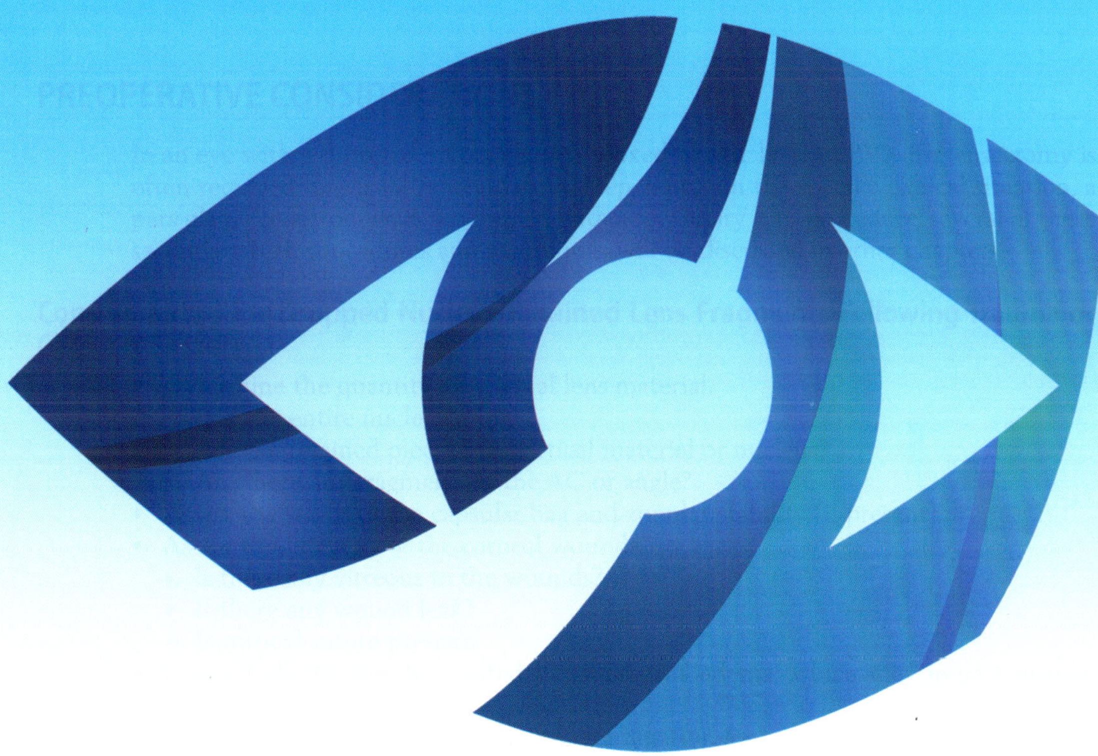

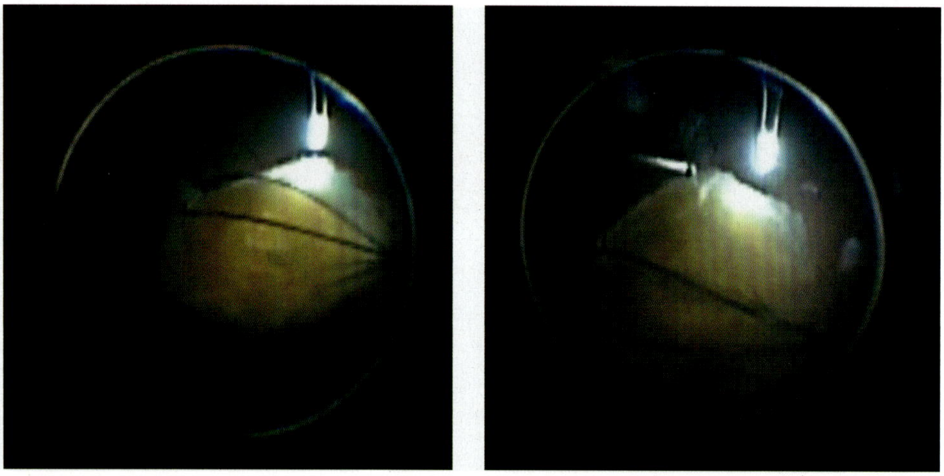

FIGURE 36.2. The Frag Bag is a 1-cm basket in the 1.5-French NCircle Nitinol Tipless Stone Extractor (Cook Medical) that can stabilize the entire dislocated nucleus in the mid-vitreous cavity to facilitate removal.

- Disassemble the nucleus into small pieces so that they can be more easily aspirated using the fragmatome. The light pipe can be used to both steady the nucleus and break the nucleus into smaller fragments.

You may elect to use a Frag Bag (1.5-French NCircle Nitinol Tipless Stone Extractor [Cook Medical]) that fits through a 23G cannula to secure the entire nucleus in the mid-vitreous cavity to allow it to be fragged within the 1-cm nitinol basket (Fig. 36.2).

- In addition to not touching the fragmatome to the metal such as the metal cannula, also be careful not to allow the light pipe to come into contact with the metal tip of the fragmatome when it is active as this metal-to-metal contact can cause the release of small metal shavings into the vitreous cavity.
- Be careful to monitor the sclerotomy site where the fragmatome is in contact with the sclera. Scleral burns have been known to occur in cases where the shaft of the fragmatome heats the sclerotomy. Irrigating the shaft with topical BSS and occasionally pausing to allow the instrument to cool can avoid this.
- Once all retained lens fragments have been removed, carefully inspect the peripheral retinal for any breaks.
- Close the enlarged sclerotomy using 7-0 Vicryl and the overlying conjunctiva with 6-0 plain or suture of choice.

SURGICAL PROCEDURE NO. 2: PARS PLANA LENSECTOMY FOR SUBLUXED CATARACT

- The initial steps to approach a subluxed cataract can be done in a similar fashion to a dropped cataract as described above. Again, surgical steps may be adjusted depending on whether concurrent secondary IOL placement is planned.
- Depending on the degree of subluxation and density of the lens, disassemble the subluxed cataract using either the vitrector or fragmatome while it is still in an anterior position.
- Penetrate the equator of the lens nucleus using a sharp blade such as an MVR, butterfly needle, or the trocar itself to allow access to the cataract.

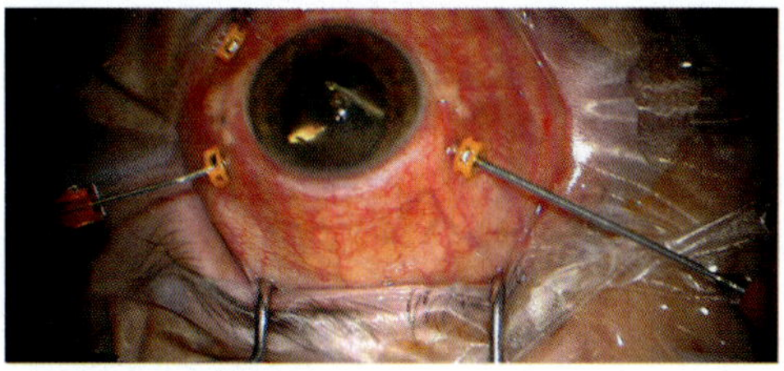

FIGURE 36.3. A second instrument such as a butterfly needle inserted through the cannula can be used to stabilize the lens during removal.

- A second instrument such as a light pipe or even a butterfly needle inserted through the cannula can be used to stabilize the lens during removal (Fig. 36.3).
- If the lens material is too dense, use the fragmatome to remove the lens once the sclerotomy is enlarged (as described above).
- Perform a complete vitrectomy prior to using the fragmatome. Remove all anterior vitreous to avoid traction on the retina. See chapter titled *Vitrectomy Surgery Steps.*
- Alternatively, the subluxed lens can be intentionally dislocated to allow for disassembly and removal in the vitreous cavity. Use the vitrector to cleave the zonular attachments to the capsular bag and allow the lens to drop posteriorly. Removal can then be conducted as described above for a dropped nucleus.

CHAPTER 37

Dislocated IOL

R. Keith Shuler Jr, MD

PREOPERATIVE CONSIDERATIONS

- Perform a complete ophthalmic exam, and rule out concurrent VR pathology, including pseudoexfoliation, Marfan syndrome, Ehlers-Danlos syndrome, or homocystinuria.
- If visualization of the peripheral retina is limited, perform a B-scan.
- Obtain medical records to determine the specifications of the IOL. This facilitates the determination of secondary IOL power needed and determination of optic size and length of the corneoscleral incision for removal.
- Manage postop expectations, including refractive changes as well as sequelae of some secondary IOLs such as chronic ocular inflammation, UGH syndrome, CME, or glaucoma. See chapter titled *The Preoperative Discussion*.

VIDEO SURGICAL PROCEDURE (VIDEO 37.1)

- Position the wrist rest lower than the usual position to allow maneuvers in the AC and anterior vitreous cavity. See chapter titled *Setting Up for Vitreoretinal Surgery*.
- Locate the previous corneal incision associated with prior cataract surgery.
- Create a limited peritomy in the area of the planned corneoscleral incision.
    - Create the corneoscleral incision temporally or superotemporally or possibly superiorly.
    - Avoid areas of extensive corneal scarring or thinning as well as recent corneal incisions.
- Achieve hemostasis with wet-field cautery.
- Use the curved corneal blade to create the corneoscleral incision ~1.5 mm posterior to the limbus. Stay anterior in the corneal tissue so as not to enter the AC prematurely. This is one of the maneuvers that requires the lower wrist rest position. The AC is not entered at this time.
- Insert the cannulas 3.5 mm posterior to the limbus in the inferotemporal, superotemporal, and superonasal quadrants as usual. Placement of the cannulas may need to be adjusted depending on the corneoscleral incision location. See chapter titled *Gauge Selection and Cannula Placement*.

- Perform a complete PPV. See chapter titled *Vitrectomy Surgery Steps*.
  - Shave the vitreous base to prevent an IOL haptic from pulling on peripheral vitreous, creating iatrogenic retinal breaks.
  - Induce a PVD if not present; however, in certain cases of extraordinary VR adherence, the hyaloid may be left attached in order to avoid iatrogenic injury. See chapter titled *PVD Induction*.
  - Use intravitreal triamcinolone to highlight the vitreous to improve its visualization and facilitate PVD induction and thorough vitreous removal. See chapter titled *Intraoperative Visualization Agents*. During vitrectomy, care should be taken to prevent retinal injury due to trauma associated with excessive IOL movement.
  - Only increase the infusion pressure during PPV if absolutely needed to prevent excessive movements of the IOL and possible retinal injury.
- Once the vitrectomy is complete, the noncontact widefield viewing system is kept in place. See chapter titled *Lenses and Viewing Systems*.
- Engage the dislocated IOL.
  - Use forceps
    - Insert the light pipe through the temporal cannula.
    - Place MaxGrip forceps (Alcon) through the nasal cannula, regardless of which eye is the operative eye, and grasp one of the IOL haptics.
    - Choose an accessible haptic that is not near the fovea or optic nerve. Aim for the haptic, even when the IOL is still within its capsule.
    - Avoid grasping the Soemmering ring (lens capsule) alone since your control of the IOL will be limited.
    - Rarely use PFCL to facilitate atraumatic lifting of the IOL from the retinal surface or to protect the macula during PPV. Lift the IOL into the mid-vitreous cavity.
  - Use the soft-tip cannula.
    - Position the soft-tip cannula over the center of the IOL optic.
    - Start extrusion and use the suction to lift the IOL into the mid-vitreous cavity.
    - Remove the light pipe and widefield viewing system. Use the operating microscope alone to view the anterior segment. While still engaging the IOL with the cannula, grasp the IOL with the MaxGrip forceps.
- Fill the AC with viscoelastic and enter the AC through the previously created shelved corneoscleral incision.
  - Alternatively, create a paracentesis and insert a Sinskey hook and forceps to grab the IOL and prolapse it into the AC. Inject Miochol-E (Bausch + Lomb) into the AC to constrict the pupil. Leave the IOL resting on the iris while the corneoscleral incision is enlarged. Cut the IOL in the AC using special IOL cutting scissors, if needed.
- Make the corneal incision long enough to accommodate removal of the IOL.
  - If the IOL is being removed in toto, make the interior opening of the corneal entry wound wider than its external aspect to facilitate removal of the IOL.
  - If the IOL is going to be cut in half, a shorter corneal wound may suffice.
  - The approach is dependent on what secondary IOL may be placed. See subsequent chapters.
    - If a foldable IOL is being placed, a small corneoscleral wound is preferable with cutting of the dislocated IOL.
    - If a rigid IOL is being placed (ACIOL), use a large corneoscleral wound to remove the dislocated IOL as a single piece.
- Alternatively, the corneoscleral incision can be enlarged prior to elevating the IOL into the mid-vitreous cavity.
  - Gaping of the corneoscleral incision and deformation of the AC and cornea may significantly limit visualization. If this occurs, place one or two temporary 10-0 nylon sutures in the corneoscleral wound.

SURGICAL PROCEDURE: ACIOL

- Make a conjunctival periotomy from 10 to 2 o'clock.
- Diathermize the episclera and sclera to achieve hemostasis.
- Make a scleral incision 1-2 mm posterior to the limbus and 6 mm wide with a bent crescent blade.
- Use a Super Sharp blade and make a side port at the limbus.
- Tunnel the scleral incision toward the cornea with a crescent blade until about 1-2 mm into clear cornea (without entering the eye).
- Extend lateral edges of incision into clear cornea with the crescent blade for ease of ACIOL insertion (Fig. 38.1).
- Inject Miostat or Miochol through the side port to constrict the pupil, and then fill the AC with viscoelastic to protect the corneal endothelium.
- Enter the AC through corneal wound using a keratome for the full length of the wound.
- Refill the AC with viscoelastic as needed.
- Position the sheets glide over the iris and across the pupil until it reaches the inferior angle (Fig. 38.2). Make sure that the inferior iris is not bunched up under the sheets glide but instead that the sheets glide sits on top of the iris.
- Insert the first haptic of the ACIOL into the AC over the sheets glide using an angled McPherson forceps. Remove the sheets glide and then insert the second haptic under the lip of the scleral wound.

Insert the ACIOL into the AC in a specific orientation. Confirm that the proximal haptics and optic do not form an "S" shape. "S is for stop" (Fig. 38.2).

- Locate the distal elbow of the IOL in the angle using a Sinskey hook or Kuglen push/pull instrument, and rotate so the ACIOL is free of iris capture.
- Make a PI using the vitreous cutter or forceps and small Vannas scissors. If planning to use silicone oil, then the PI must be inferior.
- Remove viscoelastic with the vitreous cutter.
- Suture the wound with 10-0 nylon and make sure that it is watertight.
- Suture the conjunctiva with 7-0 Vicryl.

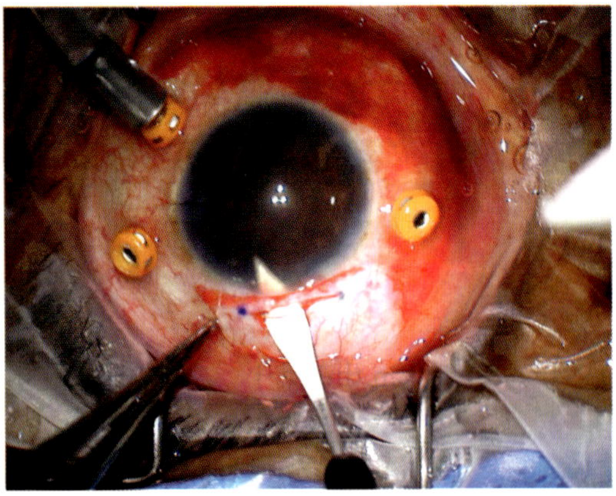

FIGURE 38.1. Extend lateral edges of incision into the clear cornea with crescent blade for ease of ACIOL insertion. The wound will likely need to be bigger than shown herein.

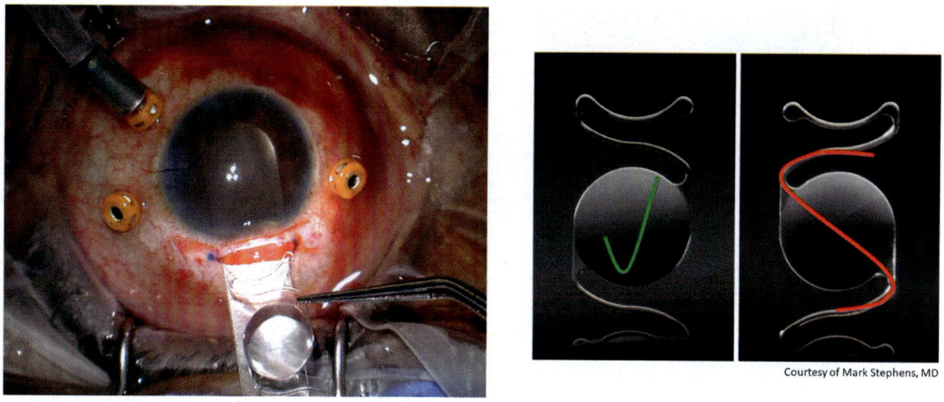

Courtesy of Mark Stephens, MD

FIGURE 38.2. Insert ACIOL into the AC in a specific orientation. Confirm that the proximal haptics and optic do not form an "S" shape. "S is for stop." (Courtesy of Mark Stephens MD.)

SURGICAL PROCEDURE: IRIS-FIXATED IOL

- Perform PPV to remove the vitreous and free the dislocated or subluxed IOL so that it rests on the retinal surface. See chapter titled *Dislocated IOL*.
- Grab a haptic in order to retrieve the IOL from the vitreous cavity using an end gripping or other forceps and place the optic in the AC. Use Miostat or Miochol to induce miosis and a nondispersive viscoelastic to protect the corneal endothelium.

Lift the dislocated IOL off the retinal surface using a soft-tip cannula with active extrusion. If using a chandelier light, lift the IOL into the anterior vitreous cavity using the soft-tip cannula through the nasal cannula and a forceps in the temporal cannula (allowing for greater AP rotation) to push and capture the IOL into the AC (Fig. 38.3).

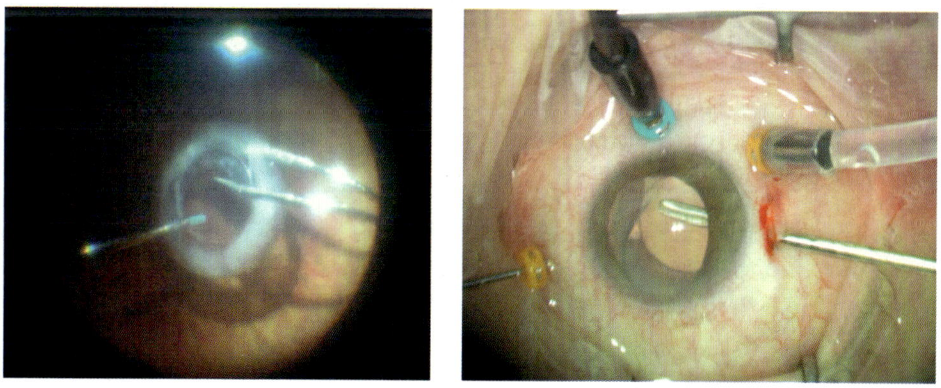

FIGURE 38.3. If using a chandelier light, lift the IOL into the anterior vitreous cavity using the soft-tip cannula through the nasal cannula and a forceps in the temporal cannula (allowing for greater AP rotation) to push and capture the IOL into the AC.

- Use a modified Siepser slip knot or McCannel suture to secure both haptics to the posterior iris (Fig. 38.4).
    - Modified Siepser (Video 38.1)
    - Use the Super Sharp blade to make an AC paracentesis.
    - Place the CIF-4 (10-0 Prolene) needle through the paracentesis→ then through the proximal iris→posterior to haptic→ through the distal iris→ out through the distal clear cornea.

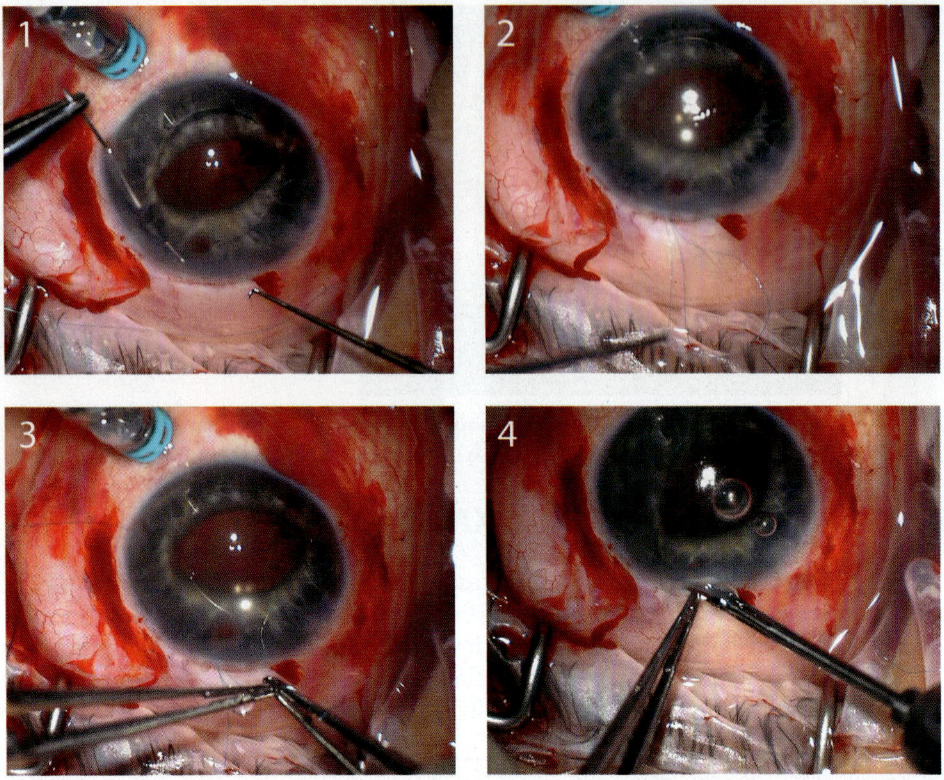

FIGURE 38.4. Modified Siepser slip knot or McCannel suture to secure both haptics to posterior iris. 1. Place the CIF-4 (10-0 Prolene) needle through the paracentesis→ then through the proximal iris→posterior to haptic→ through the distal iris→ out through the distal clear cornea. 2. Pull and externalize the distal end of suture through the paracentesis using a Kuglen hook to form an external loop of suture. 3 and 4. Slip knot: Tie the free end of the suture OVER the side of external loop coming from the IRIS twice and pull on both ends.

- Pull and externalize the distal end of suture through the paracentesis using a Kuglen hook to form an external loop of suture.
- Slip knot: Tie the free end of the suture *OVER* the side of external loop coming from the IRIS twice and pull on both ends.
- Retrieve the distal end of suture and externalize loop through AC paracentesis again.
- Locking knot: Tie the free end *UNDER* the side of the loop that extends to the iris and back under free end, and secure knot by pulling on both ends again.
- Repeat to secure other haptics.
- Push the optic into posterior chamber using Sinskey hook.

CHAPTER 39

Sutured Scleral Fixated IOL

Frank Brodie, MD, MBA • Durga S. Borkar, MD • Dilraj S. Grewal, MD

PREOPERATIVE CONSIDERATIONS

A report by the American Academy of Ophthalmology reviewing a range of secondary lens choices and implantation techniques in the absence of capsular support did not find any one lens or technique universally superior. Rather, they suggest customizing the approach to the patient. In selecting a secondary IOL and implantation technique, there are several factors to consider.

- Patient suitability: Does the patient have visual potential to merit a secondary lens? Are there any contraindications to the lens, technique, or location for placement such as a history of corneal pathology, uveitis, or glaucoma that would preclude an ACIOL, or a history of multiple glaucoma procedures that may make conjunctival manipulation challenging.
- This chapter discusses two secondary IOL techniques.
    - VIDEO Scleral Sutured: Akreos AO60 (Bausch and Lomb) (Video 39.1)
        - Pros: 4-point fixation allowing for good centration, larger sutures that are easy to manipulate making it technically easy, small corneal incision.
        - Cons: Hydrophilic lens with reports of opacification with tamponade following air gas exchange as well as with anterior chamber gas in endothelial transplants. Optic may warp with over-tightening or sutures inducing irregular astigmatism. Requires a conjunctival peritomy.
    - VIDEO Scleral Sutured: MX60 Envista lens (Bausch & Lomb) (Video 39.2)

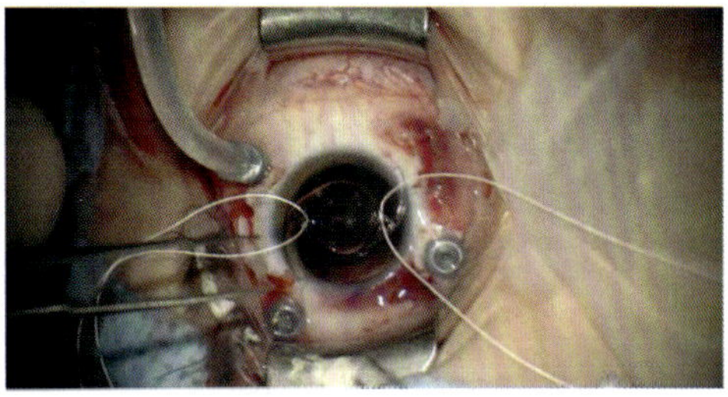

    - Pros: No risk of opacification under gas as it is a hydrophobic, aspheric, acrylic lens. Does not warp under tension from sutures.
    - Cons: Requires a peritomy.
- Lens calculation
  - With placement 3 mm posterior the limbus, "in the bag" calculations can be used.
  - If unavailable through optical biometer, Barret 2 Universal lens calculator can be found at http://calc.apacrs.org/barrett_universal2105/

SURGICAL PROCEDURE

- General information
  - Akreos AO60 lens
    - Fits through 3-4 mm incision without injector
    - Available in +0 to +30 diopters
    - A-constant 118.5
    - Acrylic hydrophilic lens
  - MX60 Envista lens
    - Fits through 3-4 mm incision without injector
    - Available in +0 to +34 diopters
    - A-constant 119.1
    - Acrylic hydrophobic lens
- Incision placement.
  - Using a toric marker, place 2 marks 180 degrees away at the limbus.
    - Consider superonasal and inferotemporal placement for ease of access.
  - Make a local peritomy in both locations to reveal sclera at least 3 mm posterior to the limbus.
  - Mark 3 mm posterior to the limbus and 2 mm on either side of this posterior mark—these are the insertion sites.
  - Cauterize any vessels in the area with bipolar wet-field cautery.
  - If performing concurrent vitrectomy, place either 25G or 27G cannulas in the superior insertion site on either side and make the sclerotomy at the inferior insertion sites with the trocar alone or 25G needle.
- Make clear corneal incision of 3-4 mm superiorly or in the axis of steep corneal astigmatism.
- Preloading the lens
  - The Akreos has two islets on either side. Envista has one.
  - Remove the needles and pass the suture from posterior to anterior then anterior to posterior on each side (Figs. 39.1A and B).

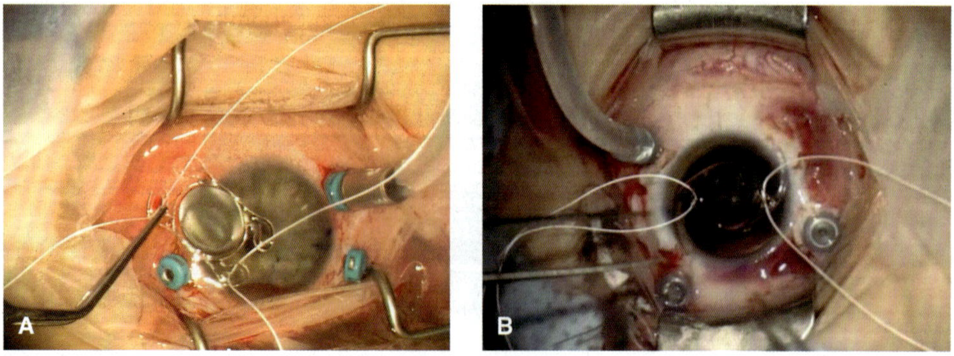

FIGURE 39.1. A. Intraop photograph showing the Gore-Tex suture passed through the four islets of the Akreos AO60 IOL prior to insertion in the eye. **B.** Intraop photograph of the MX60 Envista IOL prepared for suture fixation with Gore-Tex sutures passed through the two islets outside the eye prior to insertion through the corneal incision.

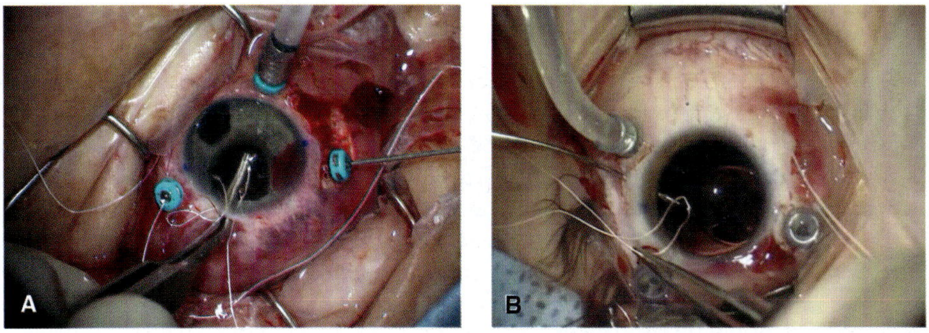

FIGURE 39.2. A. Intraop photograph of the Akreos AO60 IOL with the trailing Gore-Tex suture being passed through the sclerotomy using the handshake technique. **B.** Intraop photograph of the MX60 Envista IOL showing the Gore-Tex suture being removed from the scleretomy using end-grasping forceps.

    - This minimizes the risk of iris chafing as the suture force is directed posteriorly.
    - For the Envista lens, make sure the suture travels over, not under, the-haptics.
  - Choice of suture
    - 9-0 Prolene suture
      - Approved for intraocular use and has a long track record of stability and safety. Reports of breakage over time.
    - Gore-Tex CV-8 suture
      - Gore-Tex suture (W.L. Gore & Associates, Newark, DE) is a nonabsorbable polytetrafluoroethylene (PTFE) monofilament suture used in cardiac valve repair surgery for over 25 years.
      - Greater tensile strength than Prolene and easier to manipulate.
      - Not approved by the FDA for use in the eye.
- Securing the IOL before insertion
  - Keeping the IOL oriented outside of the eye, the suture is passed through clear corneal wound using MST forceps.
  - Using a handshake technique, grasp the suture with retinal forceps inserted through the respective sclerotomy (Fig. 39.2).
  - Repeat for all four sclerotomies and take care to ensure correct orientation and placement.
  - Secure the nasal and temporal sutures with a triple throw without any additional ties to allow for adjusting tension as needed.
- Insertion of the IOL
  - Fold the IOL using IOL forceps and insert through the clear corneal wound taking care to ensure correct orientation.
- Securing and centering the IOL
  - Cannulas are removed as needed.
  - Tighten sutures to ensure centration under equal tension.
  - Complete the locking throws (3,1,1).
  - Trim the excess suture and rotate the knot internally through the sclerotomy.
  - Close the peritomies.
    - To minimize risk of conjunctival erosion, Tenon should be closed separately and then conjunctiva.

Opacification and the Akreos IOL

The Akreos IOL offers many advantages for secondary IOL placement including 4-point fixation and ability to secure sutures prior to IOL insertion; however, there have been reports of IOL opacification with exposure to intraocular air, gas, or silicone oil, with both AC (in corneal transplants) or posterior chamber air or gas and has also been reported with routine in-the-bag placement of the IOL. The mechanism of opacification is unknown, but biochemical analysis shows calcium and phosphate deposition. Although the rate of opacification is likely low, consider not using an Akreos IOL in an eye that might undergo concurrent or subsequent retinal or corneal surgery requiring tamponade.

A Transconjunctival Approach

An alternate transconjunctival approach without peritomy can be performed with additional cannulas. 25G cannulas are placed at all four insertion sites and an infusion cannula is placed inferiorly. The suture is attached to the IOL and sutures are externalized in a similar fashion. Cannulas are removed and retinal forceps is inserted between the conjunctiva and sclera to grasp the suture tip at the fellow sclerotomy site, so both ends of suture are exiting the conjunctiva at the same site. The suture is then tightened, tied down, trimmed, and rotated (As described by Drs. Mitchell Fineman and Chris Aderman, Wills Eye Hospital).

CHAPTER 40

Sutureless Scleral Fixation Techniques

Nicholas Saba, BS • Scott D. Walter, MD, MSc

If no capsular support, consider scleral fixation of a secondary IOL implant, particularly when an ACIOL is contraindicated due to glaucoma and/or corneal decompensation risk (eg, pseudoexfoliation or decreased endothelial cell counts). Sutureless scleral fixation techniques may have benefits compared to sutured IOLs due to their relative technical ease and procedural simplicity.

- Potential advantages
  - Minimally invasive wound construction
  - Decreased suture-induced astigmatism
- Potential disadvantage
  - Uncertainty regarding the long-term stability

PEARLS

- Remove all vitreous from the AC before beginning.
- Concurrent PPV may be performed (eg, retained lens material or posteriorly dislocated IOL).
- Use a viscoelastic to protect the corneal endothelium while performing AC maneuvers.
- All techniques can be performed with a foldable three-piece IOL. The Prolene haptics of these IOLs are prone to bending and/or breakage.

The haptics of the Zeiss (CT Lucia 602) three-piece IOL may be sturdier than those of the Alcon (AcrySof MA60AC) three-piece IOL.

If attempting to rescue a dislocated three-piece IOL and fixate it, be sure to have a backup IOL available in case the haptics break or kink during surgical maneuvers.

- The total diameter of a three-piece IOL from haptic to haptic is 13.0 mm and the lens optic vaults 10 degrees forward. Stretching the haptics beyond 13.0 mm will reduce the lens vault and the effective dioptric power of the lens.
- Consider performing a vitrector-assisted PI at the time of surgery to minimize the risk of lens-induced pupillary block.

Many prefer to secure the haptics near the 3 and 9 o'clock position due to favorable exposure in the horizontal meridian. However, in patients with horizontal corneal diameters >12.5 mm, the haptics should be fixated at the 6 and 12 o'clock position, because the vertical diameter of the cornea is less.

SURGICAL PROCEDURE NO. 1: THE "GLUED IOL TECHNIQUE"

- Use a toric marker to mark the corneoscleral limbus at two points, 180 degrees apart.
- Create a conjunctival peritomy and apply wet-field cautery to the episcleral vessels immediately posterior to the corneal marks.
- Place the infusion (either an AC maintainer or a pars plana infusion cannula).
- Using a scleral crescent blade, create two partial-thickness scleral flaps (~2.5 × 2.5 mm). The flaps are limbal-based (Fig. 40.1A) and centered exactly 180 degrees apart.
- Using a 26G needle, create an intrascleral tunnel beginning within the flap and extending ~3.0 mm into full-thickness sclera (Fig. 40.1B). The tunnels should be antiparallel to accommodate the orientation of the IOL haptics.
  - Dab the needle with a sterile violet marking pen to help visualize the tunnels during the case.
- Using a 22G needle, create a nonbeveled, full-thickness sclerotomy 1.0 mm posterior to the hinge of each flap.
- Using a 2.8-mm keratome blade, create a clear corneal incision.
- Using a B cartridge and a foldable three-piece IOL, introduce the IOL with the leading haptic in the sulcus and trailing haptic in the AC.
- Pass a 23G or 25G intraocular forceps (such as the Grieshaber MaxGrip [Alcon]) through the sclerotomy. Inside the eye, grasp the tip of the leading haptic with your forceps and externalize the haptic through the sclerotomy.
- Have an assistant gently hold the tip of the leading haptic to prevent slippage back inside the eye.
  - A small vascular clamp may be used in lieu of an assistant to stabilize the externalized haptic.
- Dunk the trailing haptic into the sulcus with a Sinskey or Kuglen hook. Grasp the tip of the haptic with forceps and externalize it through the other sclerotomy site.
  - Alternatively, use another intraocular forceps to transfer the haptic from one hand to the other using the "handshake technique."
- Tuck the externalized tip of each haptic inside the scleral tunnel (Fig. 40.1C).
- Using a cellulose sponge, check each sclerotomy site for vitreous incarceration. Carefully remove any vitreous from the sclerotomy site with Westcott microscissors or vitreous cutter.
- Remove the infusion.
- Inject sterile air to fill the AC.
- Dry and seal the scleral flaps and conjunctiva by applying fibrin glue tissue adhesive (Fig. 40.1D).

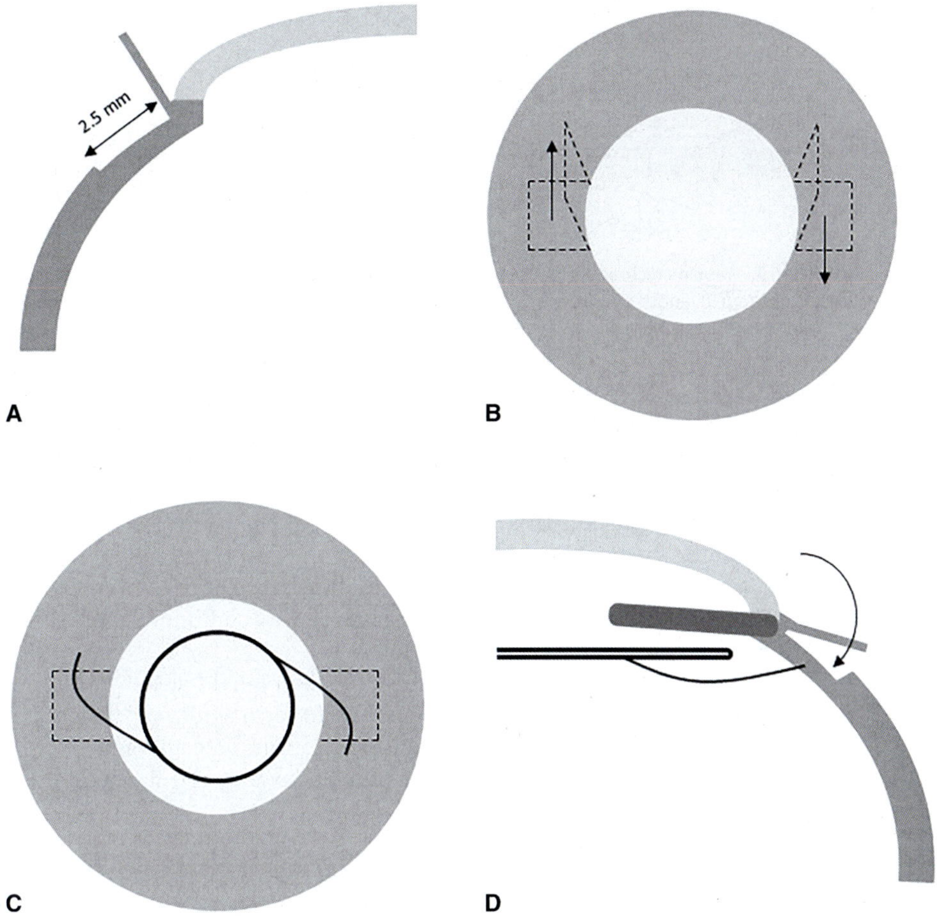

FIGURE 40.1. Glued IOL technique. **A.** Create a partial-thickness scleral flap measuring 2.5 × 2.5 mm. **B.** Create intrascleral tunnels beginning at the edge of the scleral bed with a 26G needle. **C.** Tuck the externalized haptics into the scleral tunnels. **D.** Seal the scleral flap with a fibrin glue.

SURGICAL PROCEDURE NO. 2: THE "YAMANE TECHNIQUE," IOL FIXATION WITH FLANGED HAPTICS (VIDEO 40.1)

- Use a toric marker to mark the corneoscleral limbus at 3 and 9 o'clock.
- Place the infusion (either an AC maintainer or a pars plana infusion cannula).
- Using a 2.8-mm keratome blade, create a clear corneal incision.
- Create a AC paracentesis on each side of the main clear corneal incision.
- Using a B cartridge and a foldable three-piece IOL, introduce the IOL with the leading haptic in the sulcus and the trailing haptic outside the eye.
- Using a 30G TSK ultra–thin-walled needle made in Japan, create an angled sclerotomy through the conjunctiva and sclera (Fig. 40.2A).
  - Begin 2.0 mm posterior to the limbus and 2.0 mm superior to the 3:00 mark, tunneling parallel to the limbus at a 30-degree angle.
  - Once you reach the mark, adjust the angle of the needle to 90 degrees to enter the posterior segment.
- Using 25G MST Snyder Grasper or 23G MST Ahmed Micro-Tying forceps, thread the leading haptic into the lumen of the needle.

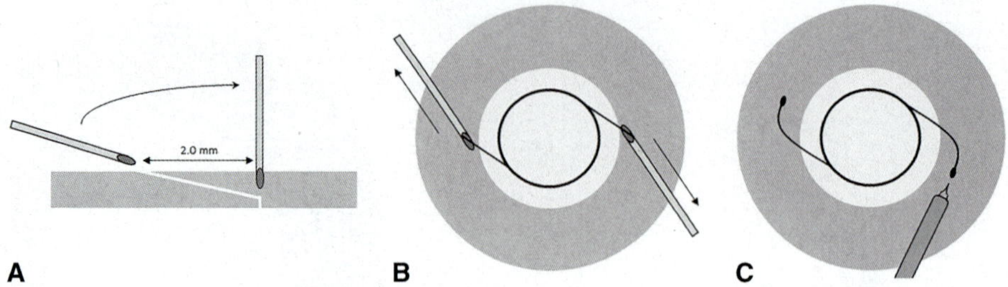

FIGURE 40.2. "Yamane technique." **A.** Use the ultra–thin-walled 30G TSK needle to create an angled scleral tunnel measuring 2 mm in length prior to entry into the eye. **B.** After docking both haptics into the needles, externalize both haptics simultaneously. **C.** Use low-temperature cautery to flange the externalized haptics.

- Using another 30G TSK ultra–thin-walled needle, create an angled sclerotomy through the conjunctiva and sclera, antiparallel to the first needle track.
  - Begin 2.0 mm posterior to the limbus and 2.0 mm inferior to the 9:00 mark, tunneling parallel to the limbus at a 30-degree angle.
  - Once you reach the mark, adjust the angle of the needle to 90 degrees to enter the posterior segment.
- Using the same MST forceps, thread the trailing haptic into the lumen of the needle.
- Externalize both haptics onto the surface of the conjunctiva by simultaneously withdrawing both needles (Fig. 40.2B).
- Using a handheld low-temperature fine-tip cautery, held about 1.0 mm away from the haptic, lightly melt the tips of each haptic to form a bulb or "flange" (Fig. 40.2C).
  - Do not shorten the haptics by more than 1.5 mm on each end.
- Push the haptics back into the scleral tunnels, so that the flange is flush with the sclera.

SURGICAL PROCEDURE NO. 3: THE "BEAUMONT TECHNIQUE," 27G TRANSCANNULAR SUTURELESS INTRASCLERAL FIXATION

- Use a toric marker to mark the limbus exactly 180 degrees apart in the inferotemporal and superonasal quadrants.
- Using valved 27G vitrectomy cannulas, create inferotemporal and superonasal sclerotomies (Fig. 40.3A).
  - The sclerotomies are created exactly 2.0 mm posterior to the limbus and exactly 180 degrees apart. Both intrascleral tunnels should be constructed with a counterclockwise orientation.
  - A 30- to 45-degree beveled entry into the sclera is preferred.
    - These cannulas are to be used for externalization of the IOL haptics. Minimize manipulation of these sclerotomies in order to maintain wound architecture.
- Place an infusion line in the inferotemporal cannula.
- Create a third sclerotomy in the superotemporal quadrant, 3.0-4.0 mm posterior to the limbus.
  - This sclerotomy is not used for haptic externalization and should be used as the dominant working sclerotomy for vitrectomy, lensectomy, etc. as dictated by the needs of the case. Once the vitrectomy is complete, relocate the infusion from the inferotemporal cannula to the superotemporal cannula.
- Using a 2.8-mm keratome blade, make a clear corneal incision at the superior limbus.
- Using a B cartridge and a foldable three-piece IOL, inject the IOL so that the leading haptic is oriented clockwise in the sulcus. Temporarily suspend the trailing haptic anterior to the iris to prevent the IOL from falling into the vitreous cavity.

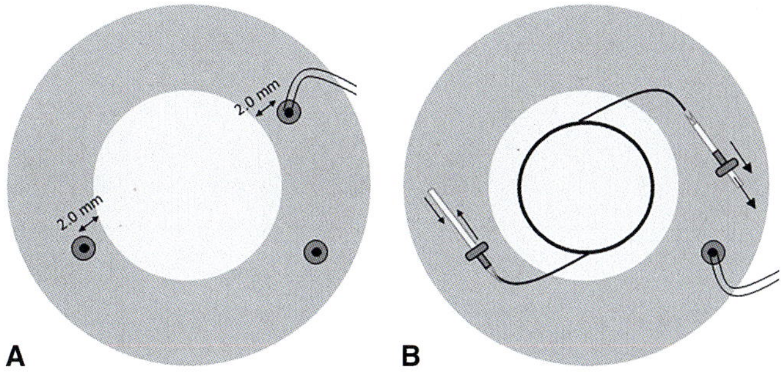

FIGURE 40.3. "Beaumont technique." **A.** Location of 27G cannula insertion in a right eye. **B.** Move the infusion to the superotemporal cannula and externalize the haptics with end-grasping forceps.

- Place a 27G end-grasping forceps through the inferotemporal cannula. Grasp the very tip of the leading haptic with the forceps. With the haptic engaged, carefully withdraw the closed forceps into the cannula.
  - The jaws of the forceps can break if too much force is applied.
- Nugent forceps are used to retract the cannula over the shaft of the MaxGrip forceps, with the haptic still engaged. Gently externalize the haptic through the sclerotomy before releasing with the forceps (Fig. 40.3B).
- Repeat the same technique with the trailing haptic 180 degrees away.
  - Temporarily suspending the trailing haptic on the iris allows you to use only one pair of forceps.
- Adjust each haptic to center the IOL optic.
- Using nontoothed forceps, gently lift the conjunctiva to reposition the haptics under the conjunctiva.
  - The flanged haptic technique (using low-temperature cautery to melt the haptic tips as described in detail above) can also be applied before securing the haptics in the scleral tunnel.

COMPLICATIONS

Reported surgical complications of sutureless scleral fixated IOLs include hypotony, IOL dislocation, intraocular hemorrhage, RD, endophthalmitis, and secondary glaucoma. Patients should be counseled about potential refractive issues including lenticular astigmatism, glare, and other higher-order aberrations. Patients may also be at risk for complications, including iris optic capture, secondary pigment dispersion, and UGH syndrome. Perform a PI intraop with the vitrector to reduce the risk of developing pupillary block. The risk of developing postop CME is likely greater than with intracapsular IOL fixation.

Section VIII

Diabetic Vitrectomy

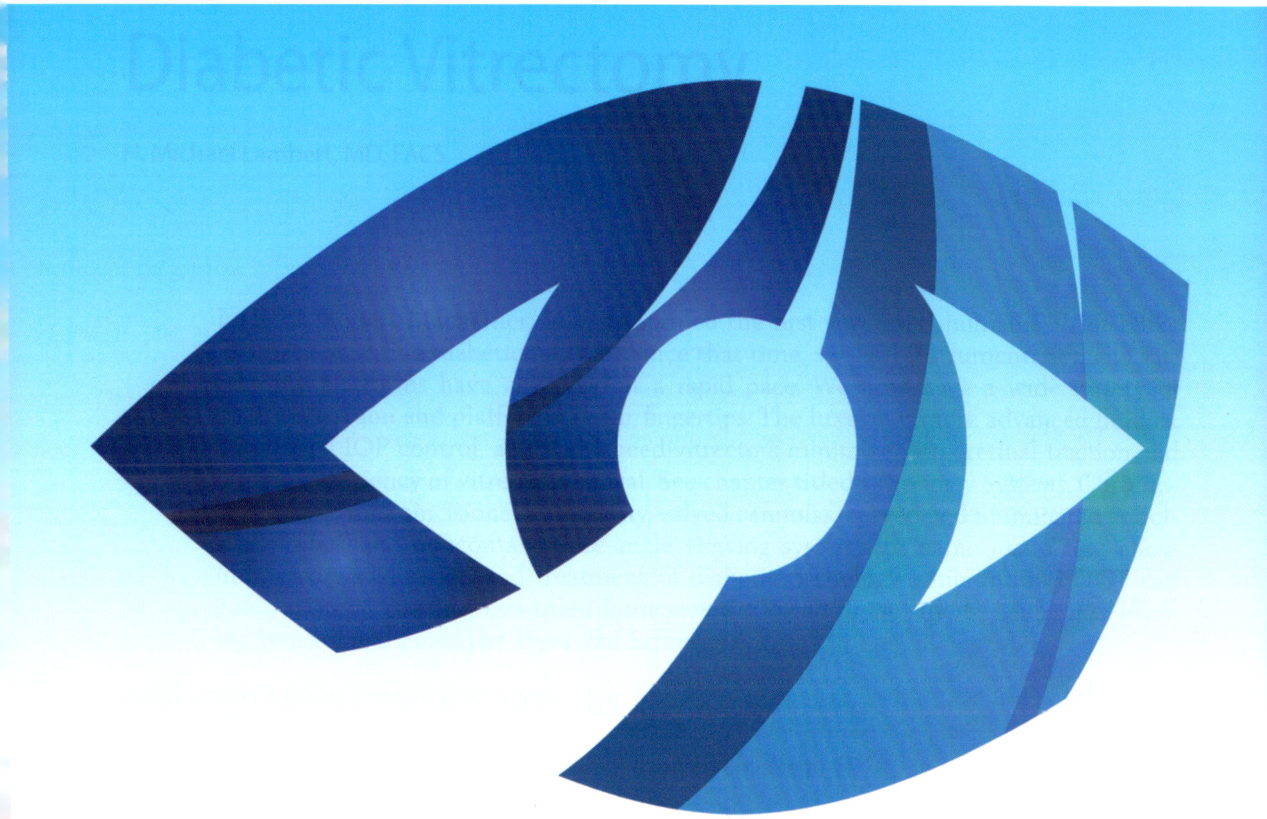

- RD
  - TRD threatening or involving the fovea
  - TRD/RRD
- Postvitrectomy
  - Ghost cell glaucoma
  - Recurrent NCVH that does not clear with anti-VEGF
  - Reproliferation
  - RD

- Patient discussion. See chapter titled *The Preoperative Discussion*.
  - Explain both ocular and systemic risks of VR surgery and guarded visual prognosis given retinal ischemia in PDR.
  - Emphasize collaboration by internist colleagues (eg, medical clearance, anticoagulation, glucose management if steroids used, HTN management, dialysis schedule).
  - Explain gas and silicone oil tamponade and possible need for facedown positioning. See chapter titled *Postoperative Positioning*.
  - Consider having a third person in the room during the discussion and document such.
- Systemic optimization to minimize anesthetic risk since PDR is a marker for systemic vascular disease.
- Evaluation by internal medicine physician and anesthesiologist.
  - Medical clearance for planned anesthetic
    - Optimize BP, glucose, lipids, and renal status.
  - Antiplatelet/anticoagulant requirement
  - Periop hospitalization
  - Dialysis schedule
  - Postop care
- Ophthalmic evaluation and optimization
- Document preop VA, APD status, retinal perfusion on FA or OCT angiography, and B-scan.
- Consider preop fundus photography.
- Glaucoma consultation
- Cataract consultation
- Media opacity and surgical view
  - Obtain B-scan
  - Consider anti-VEGF 1-3 days preop.

INTRAOPERATIVE CONSIDERATIONS

- Think about your surgical approach and plan before you start.
  - Presence of a preop PVD
  - Vitreoschisis
  - Sclerotomy placement
  - Delamination vs segmentation vs *en bloc* dissection
  - Chromo-assisted PPV
  - Plan for lens opacity
  - Incising posterior hyaloid
  - Clearing subhyaloid blood
  - TRD? Combined TRD/RRD? (See chapter titled *Diabetic TRD*.)
  - Iatrogenic break with adjacent residual traction
  - Hemostasis
  - Tamponade choice

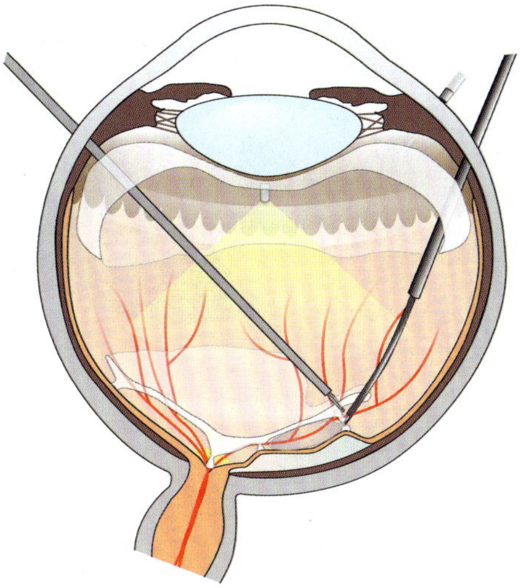

FIGURE 41.1. Viscodissection. Viscoelastic is injected under the fibrovascular proliferation plaques to create space for further dissection.

- Surgical instrumentation
  - Vitrectomy platform
  - Gauge selection
  - Lenses and viewing system
  - Buckling elements
    - Encircling vs radial
  - Iris hooks
  - Fragmatome
  - Phaco machine
  - Visualization agents
  - Intraop OCT
  - Vertical scissors (20G or 23G pneumatic or 23G or 25G manual)
  - Horizontal scissors
  - Viscodissector and viscoelastic (Fig. 41.1)
  - Lighted pick
  - Special forceps
  - PFCL
  - Diathermy
  - Endolaser probes
  - Humidified air
  - Anti-VEGF agent
  - Gas
  - Silicone oil

POSTOPERATIVE CONSIDERATIONS

- Manage expectations regarding outcome
- Positioning instructions
- Gas precautions
- IOP management
- NVG
- DME
- Eye drop instructions
- Collaborate with internist
- Follow up appointment schedule
- Emergency contact number
- Plan for the fellow eye

CHAPTER 42

Nonclearing Vitreous Hemorrhage

Wenlan Zhang, MD

PREOPERATIVE CONSIDERATIONS

Consider the etiology of VH: vascular (DM, CRVO, PCV, RAM), tractional, trauma, etc. Keep in mind the age of patient (eg, nonaccidental trauma in a baby with hemorrhage in the fellow eye, adult with NCVH from PDR, etc.). If there is any view at all, an ultra-widefield FA may highlight pathology in this or the fellow eye, which can help narrow the diagnosis to a potential vascular etiology.

Perform B-scan ultrasonography to evaluate for possible etiologies that would change management (eg, retinal break, RD, mass, open globe injury, IOFB).

B-SCAN PEARLS

- Perform transverse B-scans and radial/longitudinal scans at all clock hours to assess for retinal breaks and possible areas of vitreoretinal traction.
- Keep in mind that heme on posterior hyaloid can be highly echogenic, which can make it difficult to differentiate it from a RD, even when using concurrent A-scan. Perform a dynamic B-scan and use motility of that interface to help decide if it is retina or heme on the hyaloid.
- Look for findings of SRH, which appears hyperechoic (if present, consider wet AMD, PCV, RAM, trauma), as this will affect patient counseling.
- Assess PVD status.

MANAGEMENT OPTIONS

- Consider discontinuing antiplatelet or anticoagulant agents in consultation with an internist.
- Discourage Valsalva and eye rubbing.
- Elevate HOB to help VH settle.
- If no retinal break, RD, IOFB, anterior segment NV without prior PRP laser, or globe trauma, consider monitoring to see if VH will clear on its own.
- If there is a mass, consider the differential of peripheral exudative hemorrhagic chorioretinopathy, vasoproliferative tumor, choroidal granuloma, choroidal melanoma,

choroidal mass, etc., and discuss with an ocular oncology specialist regarding the next steps.

- If the eye has known PDR without evidence of prior or current extensive NV or traction on ultrasound, cautiously consider anti-VEGF. In some eyes with PDR, use of intravitreal anti-VEGF can contribute to TRD formation.

SURGICAL PLANNING

- Manage patient expectations about VA recovery and residual VH that will still take time to resolve, even after PPV.
- Let the OR team know if you need set-up and instrumentation for the following:
  - RRD repair
  - TRD repair. See chapter titled *Instruments and Considerations During Diabetic Vitrectomy*.
  - Open globe and IOFB. See chapter titled *Intraocular Foreign Body*.
  - Cryotherapy unit. See chapter titled *Scleral Buckling Basics*.
  - Subretinal tPA. See chapter titled *Submacular Hemorrhage*.
- Keep in mind the lens (phakic/pseudophakic/aphakic) status.
- If there is a retinal vascular etiology of VH, consider anti-VEGF injection or PRP (sectoral or 360 degrees depending on etiology and presence of NV) at the end of the case.

SURGICAL PROCEDURE (VIDEO 42.1)

- Consider repeating B-scan ultrasonography in the OR if there has been a time lapse since prior ultrasound.
- Carefully cut the vitreous just inside the cannula opening to decrease vitreous traction with instrument insertion and removal (Fig. 42.1).
- Slower instrument movement is essential in eyes with very dense VH to prevent vitreoretinal traction that may result in retinal breaks.
- If unable to see cutter tip in a phakic eye, point instruments toward optic nerve, and cut within the cannula and just as you enter the vitreous cavity until visualization improves enough to slowly insert instruments further toward the mid-vitreous.
- Start the PPV centrally and move more peripherally slowly. See chapter titled *Vitrectomy Surgery Steps*.
- If there is no PVD, consider inducing a PVD or relieving AP traction by incising the vitreous for 360 degrees. In diabetic VH, you may find some vitreous separation in the midperiphery.

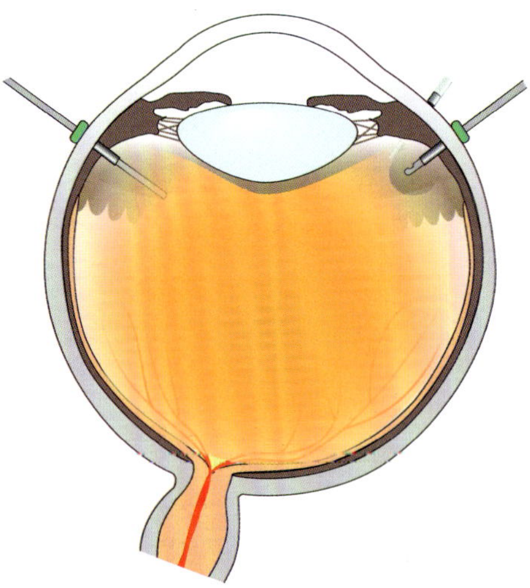

FIGURE 42.1. Cut the vitreous just inside the cannula opening to decrease vitreous traction with instrument insertion and removal.

- For clot on the retinal surface, use a combination of gentle aspiration followed by cut mode.
- Use reflux on the vitrector to move or disrupt layered hemorrhage; when refluxing, point the cutter port down toward layered blood.
  - Can also use soft-tip cannula or backflush cannula to reflux or to gently aspirate.
- Look for the source of VH including vitreous attachments, NVE, sclerotic vessels, and retinal breaks, and address any areas of identified traction.
- Perform careful scleral depression.
- Avoid aggressive maneuvers aimed at hemorrhage on the posterior capsule in phakic eyes.
- Consider FAX.
- Consider anti-VEGF or PRP at the end of the case if the VH is due to a VEGF-mediated process and NV is present.

POSTOPERATIVE CONSIDERATIONS

Remind the patient that there will always be residual VH at the end of surgery and that it will take time to clear.

PERFORMING FAX FOR NCVH IN THE VITRECTOMIZED EYE IN CLINIC

- Administer subtenon, peribulbar, or retrobulbar anesthetic.
- Position patient supine and turn head sideways with operative eye in the dependent position.
- Place chuck or towel strategically to catch any fluid.
- Insert one 25G needle and syringe with filtered air (10-mL syringe) through the nasal pars plana (Fig. 42.2).
- Insert a second 25G needle through the temporal pars plana. No syringe is attached.
- Inject filtered air slowly nasally while intraocular fluid from the vitrectomized vitreous cavity passively drains out through the temporal needle.

Instead of a revision PPV or FAX in clinic, consider intravitreal anti-VEGF to promote clearing of a persistent or recurrent VH.

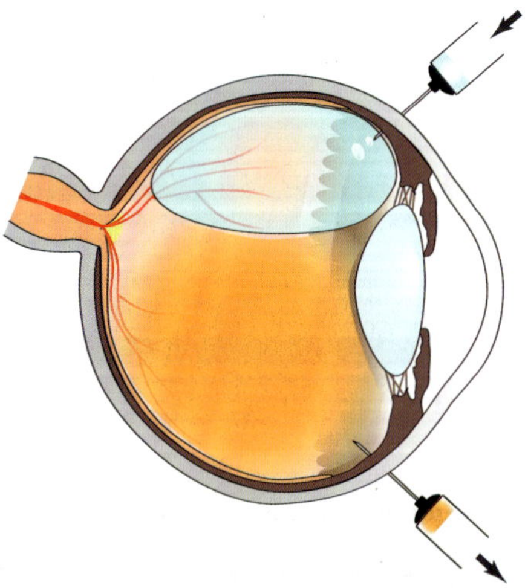

FIGURE 42.2. FAX in the clinic setting in a vitrectomized eye with a NCVH.

CHAPTER 43

Diabetic TRD

Akosua Nti, MD • Adrienne Scott, MD

DIFFERENTIATING A TRD FROM A COMBINED TRD/RRD

- FVP, traction, and contraction may lead to a TRD or combined TRD/RRD with stretch holes located posteriorly, paravascularly, or immediately adjacent to vitreoretinal traction and areas of retinal elevation.
- A convex appearance to the retina is often seen in a combined TRD/RRD, with SRF often extending to the ora vs a concave appearance in a TRD without a rhegmatogenous component.

PREOPERATIVE CONSIDERATIONS

- Obtain medical clearance and optimize the patient medically for surgery as diabetic patients may have significant cardiovascular and renal disease concurrent with retinopathy.
- Consider preop use of an anti-VEGF agent.
  - May decrease intraop bleeding, surgery time, iatrogenic retinal breaks, silicone oil use, and need for a relaxing retinotomy.
  - Consider injecting 1-5 days before surgery, which may contribute to better postop outcomes at 6 months such as improved VA and fewer persistent/recurrent VH.
- Consider preop PRP laser.
  - Reduces the risk of further NV or FVP.
  - Provides counter traction at time of intraop membrane peeling.
  - Consider earlier PPV in eyes with PDR and NCVH that have not had prior PRP laser, even in the absence of a TRD.

SURGICAL PROCEDURE

- Consider adding 3 mL of dextrose 50% to infusion fluid to prevent intraop and postop crystalline lens opacification in phakic diabetic eyes. See chapter titled *Vitrectomy Machine Settings*.

- Clear media. See chapter titled *Getting and Maintaining Your View.*
  - Remove any visually significant lens opacities that impede your intraop view; however, sparing of the crystalline lens is preferred when possible. Note that risk of NVI, NVA, and NVG is greater in aphakic and pseudophakic eyes.
    - Progression of cataract is common following PPV, particularly with use of gas or silicone oil tamponade. Cataract surgery can often be deferred until the retina is stable following TRD/RRD repair.
  - Phacoemulsification may be combined with PPV. However, corneal edema from ultrasound energy can make visualization during complex retinal surgery suboptimal.
  - Pars plana lensectomy decreases the occurrence of corneal edema associated with phaco energy. However, a secondary surgery for IOL implantation may be needed. See chapter titled *Pars Plana Lensectomy.*
- Remove any vitreous hemorrhage with the vitreous cutter.
  - Clear all vitreous near the ports to avoid vitreous incarceration.
  - Proceed with core vitrectomy just posterior to lens, while maintaining a safe distance from detached retina and posterior lens capsule. See chapter titled *Vitrectomy Surgery Steps.*
- Relieve AP traction.
  - Eliminate scaffold for retinal NV and vitreoretinal adhesions by completely separating the hyaloid from the retina. See chapter titled *Physiology of Vitreous Surgery.*
  - Incise the posterior hyaloid if elevated in the midperiphery, and extend this posterior hyaloid opening for 360 degrees peripherally before turning attention to preretinal posterior and macular membrane dissection.
  - Eyes with the TRD component from PDR will have a taut posterior hyaloid with multiple focal or broad areas of hyaloid/fibrovascular tissue tightly adherent to the retina resulting in retinal traction.

Rapid stripping of posterior hyaloid (as often performed with nondiabetic vitrectomy, eg, VMT or FTMH cases) is discouraged, as iatrogenic breaks may occur.

  - Careful segmentation of the posterior hyaloid with instruments such as curved horizontal scissors, small-gauge vitrector, or vertical scissors may be necessary. See chapter titled *Considerations and Instruments During Diabetic Vitrectomy.* Triamcinolone is helpful to visualize the vitreous to ensure complete removal. See chapter titled *Intraoperative Visualization Agents.*
- Dissect FVP causing tangential traction (segmentation and delamination) to relieve traction on retina.

Segmentation refers to isolating islands of FVP so that they are not causing any residual tangential traction, whereas delamination refers to gross removal of FVP.

  - Instrumentation: small-gauge cutter, membrane peeler cutter (MPC) scissors (20, 23 gauges), ILM or MaxGrip (Alcon) forceps, lighted pick, blunt spatula, vertical scissors, horizontal scissors, curved scissors. See chapter titled *Considerations and Instruments During Diabetic Vitrectomy.*
  - Identify surgical planes using flat contact lens (disposable or reusable quartz) or noncontact high-magnification viewing system. Consider intraop OCT. See chapter titled *Lenses and Viewing Systems.*

- Start membrane dissection at the nerve and work your way peripherally (inside-out approach). You are less likely to create iatrogenic breaks, and planes are more often easily discernible posteriorly.
- Segmentation can be achieved with the vitreous cutter or scissors.
  - For unimanual dissection, use a small-gauge vitreous cutter (or vertical scissors) and light pipe.
    - Use high cut speeds (up to 10 000 cpm), smaller 25G/27G instruments. Closer proximity of port opening to tip allow for precise segmentation and delamination without the need of a second instrument. This technique can be difficult if very adherent plaques are present.
  - Widen the space between the FVP and retina with slow blunt dissection with the vitreous cutter, spatula, or viscodissection.
    - To perform viscodissection, gently inject viscoelastic into the potential space between FVP and retina to gently separate the tissue planes.

For viscodissection, use a 27G cannula with a bent tip attached to a syringe of viscoelastic. A more viscous viscoelastic may be preferred. Other instruments for viscodissection include the Hubbard Visco Dissector (Synergetics) or the BD Visitec Vitreoretinal Viscodissector 90 (Beaver-Visitec International). Remove any residual viscoelastic from the eye when finished.

  - Feed the FVP into the cutter with the vitrector oriented 90 degrees from the underlying retina.
  - Be careful as you approach the more anterior edge of the FVP as the retina is often drawn up along this edge and you may inadvertently create an iatrogenic break.
- Delamination
  - Once islands of FVP have been segmented, you may choose to delaminate the FVP. Sometimes, the entire FVP may be so tightly adherent that delamination may be required from the outset.
  - To delaminate tissue, reflect the edges of FVP and sever the fibrovascular pegs and points of vitreoretinal adhesion with the cutter or scissors.
  - Alternatively, place the vitrector directly over the FVP with the cutter port up or slightly rotated towards the FVP. Allow the suction from the cutter to draw the FVP into the cutter (fold-back delamination). This technique minimizes the risk of creating iatrogenic breaks.
  - Not all FVP needs to be delaminated if the island of FVP has been completely isolated so as to release all tangential traction. The exception to this rule is if there is an adjacent break, in which case the nearby FVP should be delaminated.
- VIDEO Bimanual dissection (Video 43.1)
  - For tightly adherent plaques that require significant manipulation to relieve retinal traction
  - Use chandelier endoillumination and/or lighted pick as lighting source. See chapter titled *The Chandelier Buckle.*
  - Elevate tissue planes during membrane dissection to minimize iatrogenic retinal breaks. Use forceps or lighted pick to reflect FVP away from the retina to create space for vitrector or scissors to sever fibrovascular pegs or vitreoretinal adhesions (Fig. 43.1).
- Consider peeling ICG-stained ILM to relieve tangential traction in select cases and to ensure complete removal of posterior hyaloid. See chapter titled *Intraoperative Visualization Agents.*

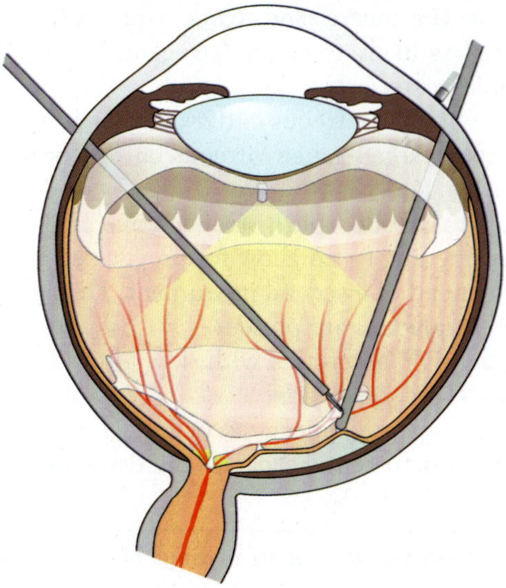

FIGURE 43.1. Delamination. Use forceps or lighted pick to reflect FVP away from the retina to create space for vitrector or vertical scissors to sever fibrovascular pegs or vitreoretinal adhesions.

- Role of retinotomy/retinectomy or SB.
  - Consider in re-ops or eyes with significant anterior hyaloidal FVP where membrane dissection cannot successfully relieve retinal traction, or when the retina is thin and prone to iatrogenic breaks during membrane dissection.
  - Diathermize retinal blood vessels to ensure hemostasis prior to retinectomy/retinotomy. In retinectomy, remove anterior retina to prevent fibrosis and traction of remaining retina or detachment of ciliary body, which may result in hypotony. Residual anterior retina is source for VEGF, so if it cannot be removed, ablate it with laser. See chapter titled *Proliferative Vitreoretinopathy Surgery.*
  - In phakic eyes with remaining peripheral AP traction, consider SB to support vitreous base, which may obviate the need for a retinectomy.
- Endolaser. See chapter titled *Endolaser Types and Settings.*
  - Apply full PRP with scleral depression to encourage regression of NV and to create adhesions around retinal breaks, retinotomies, and retinectomies.
  - Consider a curved laser in phakic eyes to decrease chance of lens trauma, and straight laser in pseudophakic or aphakic eyes.
- Tamponade agents. See chapters titled *Gas Tamponade* and *Silicone Oil Tamponade.*
  - If no breaks are noted, a tamponade agent may not be necessary.
  - You may choose to use gas tamponade despite the absence of visible breaks because sometimes thin ischemic retina can act like a sieve allowing accumulation of SRF, in the absence of tamponade.
- Role of intraop antiVEGF
  - Use in cases of persistent active NV as adjuvant to reduce postop VH or in cases with comorbid DME.

SPECIAL CONSIDERATIONS FOR COMBINED TRD/RRD

- In cases of combined TRD/RRD, start membrane dissection away from detached retina for better countertraction.
- PFCL can stabilize detached retina to allow for countertraction during membrane dissection, but there may be an increased risk of subretinal PFCL with posterior retinal breaks if traction remains when the PFCL is injected.
- Remove all vitreous and FVP around retinal breaks.

- In cases of peripheral retinal breaks with associated dense membranes, peripheral membrane dissection may not be possible, especially in phakic eyes. In such cases, consider a retinectomy or SB.
- Use bimanual tissue dissection to separate FVP overlying detached retina.
- A rhegmatogenous component necessitates a tamponade agent (SF_6, C_3F_8, silicone oil). See chapters titled *Gas Tamponade* and *Silicone Oil Tamponade.*
  - Consider silicone oil if repeat surgery, retinectomy, or poor vision in fellow eye.

POSTOPERATIVE CONSIDERATIONS

- Postop positioning is important to achieve tamponade of retinal breaks.
- Recurrent VH may make postop monitoring difficult, necessitating serial B-scans or reoperation. Reoperation rates after TRD range from 24% to 47%. Intravitreal anti-VEGF may be useful in clearing postop VH following PPV and obviate the need for a reoperation.
- Consider removing silicone oil at 6 weeks to 3 months depending on the case. See chapter titled *Silicone Oil Tamponade.*

Section IX

Pediatric Vitreoretinal Surgery

CHAPTER 44

Indications and Unique Surgical Considerations for Pediatric Vitreoretinal Surgery

Karl Olsen, MD • Antonio Capone Jr, MD, FACS

- Examining a child's retina is often challenging.
  - An EUA will allow you to completely examine an uncooperative patient.
  - It is an essential part of the pediatric retinal examination.
  - EUA is often performed with laryngeal mask anesthesia and conversion to endotracheal anesthesia with or without paralysis if surgery is required.

> **Eye protection with polycarbonate safety glasses is recommended for all children with any retinal condition.**

PREOPERATIVE CONSIDERATIONS

- **Sclerotomy Placement**
  - The pediatric eye is not fully grown until 3 years of age.
    - Modify sclerotomy placement anteriorly in the child's eye.
    - In neonates, enter 1-1.5 mm posterior to the limbus for lens-sparing vitrectomy. See chapter titled *Pediatric RRD*.
    - Transilluminate the globe to outline the ciliary body and confirm the anatomy (Fig. 44.1).
  - Avoid creating iatrogenic retinal breaks when putting in the sclerotomies, especially in eyes with elevated retina.
    - In eyes with anterior segment dysgenesis, use intraop OCT to help clarify where the ciliary body is located, allowing safer entry.
    - In eyes where a lens-sparing vitrectomy is not possible (ie, retina adherent to lens with cataract formation), try a translimbal approach with lensectomy.

Section X

Vitreoretinal Surgery for Tumors and Uveitis

CHAPTER 47

Diagnostic Vitrectomy

Sruthi Arepalli, MD • Phoebe Lin, MD, PhD

PREOPERATIVE CONSIDERATIONS

- Consider a diagnostic PPV in an eye with vitreous inflammation without clear etiology, especially if concerned about an infectious, malignant, or atypical uveitic presentation, and in eyes with primary vitreoretinal lymphoma, vitreoretinal metastasis, and presumed infectious endophthalmitis.
- A diagnostic PPV may rarely help debride the vitreous load or accelerate clearance of inflammatory markers or cells. There may be an adjunctive role to chemotherapy in cases of intraocular lymphoma.
- If an indolent fungal, viral, or mycobacterial infection is suspected, a vitreous needle biopsy may be sufficient. If there is concurrent concern for lymphoma or vitreoretinal metastatic disease, perform a diagnostic vitrectomy instead.
- Instead of a clinic-based needle vitreous biopsy, consider diagnostic PPV in pediatric patients or those unable to follow instructions.
- PPV in an inflamed eye may lead to increased risk of hypotony, uncontrolled postop inflammation, or PVR from disturbing the blood-ocular barrier.
- If lymphoma is suspected, promptly obtain a brain MRI and consider a lumbar puncture to rule out intracranial involvement.
- Relative contraindications include hemorrhagic choroidals, retinoblastoma, uveal melanoma, or severe systemic illness.

SURGICAL PLANNING

- If media opacities prohibit preop visualization of the retina, perform a B-scan ultrasound to rule out RD or choroidals and assess for posterior masses and pathology.
- If the patient is on oral steroids but lymphoma is suspected, consider stopping steroids (both topical and/or oral) at least 2-3 weeks before the diagnostic PPV to avoid lysis of lymphoma cells and increase yield.
- Alert the lab and pathologist of the possibility of intraocular lymphoma so that the sample can be processed immediately and appropriately. Communicate with the flow cytometry lab, cytology lab, and molecular diagnostic lab if PCR or cytokine analysis is planned.

SURGICAL PROCEDURE: DIAGNOSTIC VITRECTOMY (VIDEO 47.1)

- Set up a three-port PPV with 23G, 25G, or 27G valved cannulas. Valved cannulas reduce reflux of undiluted vitreous.
- Place 3 cannulas in the standard pars plana sclerotomy locations, unless alternative placement of ports is needed. See chapter titled *Gauge Selection and Cannula Placement.*
- Either draw air into the vitrectomy handpiece line or do not prime the vitrector handpiece by using the "skip prime" function on the vitrectomy machine. See chapter titled *Vitrectomy Machine Settings.*
- Place the infusion line, verify placement, but do NOT turn on infusion. See chapter titled *Endophthalmitis.*
- Connect a 10-mL Luer-Lok syringe to the vacuum/aspiration tubing attached to the vitrectomy handpiece (Fig. 47.1) and manually aspirate (with aid of an assistant) during foot-pedal–controlled vitrectomy to collect the undiluted sample, usually 2 mL or until the eye softens (Video 47.1).
  - Aliquot the collected sample to different capped syringes.
  - If primary vitreoretinal lymphoma is suspected, send one aliquot for flow cytometry in Roswell Park Memorial Institute 1640 medium (RPMI, Gibco, Life Technologies) and transport to the lab within 20 minutes.
  - If either primary lymphoma or metastasis is suspected, fresh vitreous should be sent to cytopathology if they are able to process the sample immediately or sent in liquid cytology fixative (CytoLyt, Hologic Inc., or CytoRich Red, BD) if there will be a delay in processing.
  - If sample volume remains, an additional aliquot can be sent on ice for PCR or other testing. Alternatively, diluted specimens can be sent for the following:
    - Primary vitreoretinal lymphoma: Myd88 L265P mutation testing by PCR (seen in 80%), *IgH* gene rearrangement by PCR; interleukin 10/interleukin 6 ratio by ELISA (high if B-cell origin)
    - Infectious cause: Viral testing for HSV, VZV, EBV, or CMV by PCR; bacterial testing (16S universal PCR); fungal testing (28S universal PCR); toxoplasmosis by PCR; bacterial or fungal cultures
    - Unknown: Metagenomic deep sequencing
- Turn on the infusion line. Use vitrectomy to remove a diluted specimen in a second 10-mL syringe taking care to align the mouth of the vitrector to the residual vitreous to maximize obtaining vitreous.
  - Diluted samples can be sent for any of the tests above if undiluted sample volume needs to be preserved for flow cytometry and cytopathology.

Order of samples should be determined by the prioritized differential diagnosis.

- Additional residual sample can be saved at −80 degrees for add-on testing should ordered tests come back inconclusive.

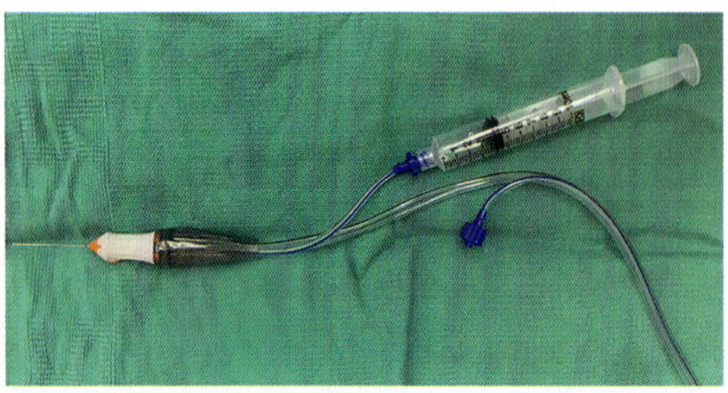

FIGURE 47.1. Use a 10-mL syringe connected to the aspiration tubing which is connected to the vitrectomy handpiece to manually aspirate about 2 mL of undiluted sample until the eye wall begins to collapse.

- Complete PPV after connecting the vitrectomy handpiece to the aspiration/vacuum tubing that is connected to the vitrectomy machine.
  - Fluid and vitreous obtained in the vitrectomy cassette can also be submitted for additional analysis including flow cytometry. Cortical vitreous may have a higher yield of lymphoma cells.

Alternative methods may be employed such as infusion of either PFCL or air to avoid collapse of eye while obtaining a larger undiluted sample, or use of in-line biopsy chamber with vitrector handpiece to avoid need for an assistant.

POSTOPERATIVE CONSIDERATIONS

- For suspected primary lymphoma, take into account overall cellular viability and look for a large monoclonal population of B cells when interpreting flow cytometry results; if viability is low, then a negative result may represent a false negative.
- For suspected primary lymphoma, take into account cell count and cellular viability when interpreting cytopathology. Large, atypical mononuclear cells with irregular nuclei are suspicious for large B-cell lymphoma and should be interpreted in context with concomitant flow cytometry results as well as Myd88 L265P mutation PCR testing if available.
- If preliminary analysis comes back negative or indeterminate, consider sending a residual sample for metagenomics deep sequencing.

CHAPTER 48

Retisert Placement

Ankur Mehra, MD • Andrew Pearson, MD

PREOPERATIVE CONSIDERATIONS

The only currently available scleral-fixated intravitreal implant is the 0.59-mg fluocinolone acetonide implant (Retisert, Bausch & Lomb, Irvine, CA). It is indicated for posterior segment chronic noninfectious uveitis and releases corticosteroid at 0.3-0.4 μg/day for ~36 months.

- Prior to implantation, confirm that there is no active infection and there are no choroidals present in the eye.
- Almost all phakic eyes in which the device is implanted will develop cataracts within 3 years.
- Consider an alternative treatment if the patient is a known steroid responder or at high risk of elevated IOP. If the resultant elevated IOP cannot be adequately controlled with medical management, glaucoma surgery may be needed.

Careful surgical positioning of the intravitreal implant is essential to avoid inadvertent placement in the suprachoroidal space or delayed extrusion of the implant strut.

SURGICAL PLANNING

- Educate the patient about the risks of cataract formation and elevated IOP.
- Plan to place the implant in one of the inferior quadrants to allow for future potential placement of a trabeculectomy or tube shunt.
- If the eye is vitrectomized, consider infusion line placement to avoid intraop hypotony.
- Prolene suture is recommended due to its longevity.

SURGICAL PROCEDURE: PLACEMENT OF THE RETISERT, A SCLERAL-FIXATED INTRAVITREAL IMPLANT (VIDEO 48.1)

- Place infusion line, if needed.
- Perform a partial conjunctival peritomy in the desired quadrant, exposing the sclera.
- Use wet-field cautery to obtain hemostasis and visualization of the sclera.

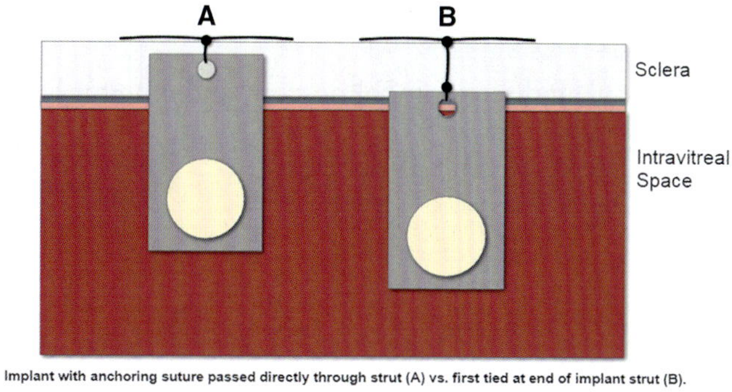

FIGURE 48.1. Intravitreal Retisert implant with anchoring suture passed directly through the strut **(A)** vs first tied at end of implant strut **(B),** which moves the anchoring spot for scleral fixation of the implant further back, allowing the implant to sit deeper within the wound once fixated to the sclera.

- In the selected quadrant, place two scleral marks using calipers and a marking pen, each 4 mm posterior to the limbus and 4 mm apart from each other.
- Enter the intravitreal space using a 20G MVR blade through a 4-mm full-thickness incision, parallel to the limbus and between the scleral marks.
- Elevate the lip of the incision using 0.3 forceps to inspect the wound.
  - The intravitreal space appears dark black and glistening as opposed to the suprachoroidal space that is gray or tan.
- Use Westcott scissors and Weck-Cel swabs to excise any prolapsed vitreous.
  - Alternatively, this can be achieved with the vitreous cutter.
- Thread a double-armed 8-0 or 9-0 Prolene suture through the hole in the implant strut, and tie a knot on top of the strut, leaving the needles on the suture.
  - This moves the anchoring spot for scleral fixation of the implant back, allowing the implant to sit deeper within the wound once fixated to the sclera (Fig. 48.1).
- Using each end of the Prolene, pass an anchoring suture through the sclera on each side of the wound at 90% depth.
  - Tie the knot such that the knot lies in the middle of the incision.
  - Leave the tails long and place to either side along the incision.
  - If the strut appears to extrude while tying the anchoring suture, release the knot tension and considering performing the below step before tying the anchoring suture.
- Place one or more interrupted 9-0 Prolene sutures along each side of the anchoring suture, taking care to ensure that the long tails of the anchoring suture are tied down under these (Fig. 48.2). Rotate to bury the knots.
  - Ensure that the anchoring suture knot and its tails lie flat underneath the conjunctiva to minimize the risk of suture extrusion.
- Confirm placement of the implant with indirect ophthalmoscopy.
- Tenon's and conjunctiva are then sutured back into place.

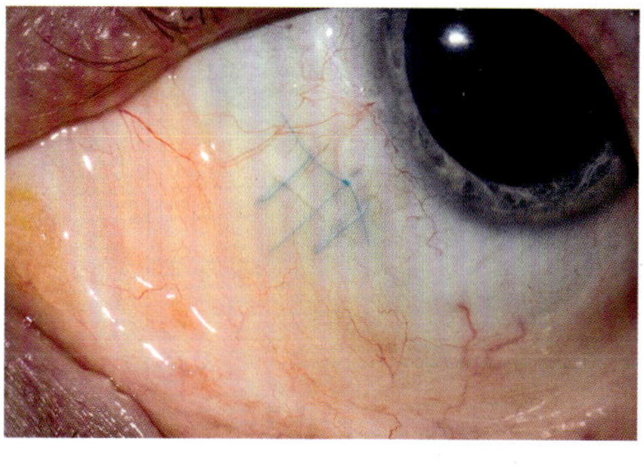

FIGURE 48.2. Postop appearance after scleral fixation of intravitreal Retisert implant. Position the Prolene suture tails underneath the two adjacent sutures as shown and bury the knot.

POSTOPERATIVE CONSIDERATIONS

- Confirm implant placement via indirect ophthalmoscopy and monitor for extrusion of implant strut.
- Monitor IOP and assess degree of cataract formation.

CHAPTER 49

RD Repair in Uveitis

Ananth Sastry, MD • Glenn J. Jaffe, MD

RD REPAIR ASSOCIATED WITH VIRAL OR TOXOPLASMA-RELATED RETINITIS

Preoperative Considerations

Viral retinitis of any etiology (HSV, CMV, VZV) or toxoplasma-related retinitis carries a high risk of RD with an increased risk of PVR and recurrent RD. When planning for surgical intervention, which often consists of PPV with silicone oil tamponade, consider the following:

- Determine the immunocompetence of the patient and ascertain etiology if compromised (eg, HIV/AIDS, immunosuppressive therapy).
- Medically manage any active retinitis or intraocular inflammation.
  - Antiviral medication such as intravenous acyclovir 10 mg/kg q8h for 7-10 days in any patient with active retinitis. Oral valacyclovir 1 g TID is an option for immunocompetent patients. Supplementation with intravitreal foscarnet (24 mg/mL, inject 0.1 mL) or ganciclovir (40 mg/mL, inject 0.1 mL) should be administered on presentation and weekly while there is active retinitis in the absence of a coexisting RD.
  - Toxoplasmosis: Systemic treatment options.
    - Double-strength trimethoprim/sulfamethoxazole (160 mg/800 mg) BID for 4 weeks
    - Azithromycin 500 mg daily for 4 weeks
    - Pyrimethamine 200 mg on day 1, followed by 50 mg daily for 4 weeks; sulfadiazine 2 g on day 1, followed by 1 g QID for 4 weeks, folinic acid 15 mg twice per week
    - Can be supplemented by intravitreal clindamycin (10 mg/mL, inject 0.1 mL) or used as an alternative in patients who cannot tolerate any of the above medications
  - Corticosteroids: Topical corticosteroids can be initiated on presentation for anterior inflammation. Dosage can be titrated according to the degree of inflammation. Systemic steroids can be started only after adequate antiviral/antiparasitic induction treatment has been initiated and there is evidence of response to treatment.
- Laser retinopexy for RD prophylaxis can be undertaken; however, there is currently conflicting evidence regarding its utility in infectious retinitis.

Surgical Planning

- Counsel patient on guarded visual prognosis.
- Take extra precautions with all sharps and surgical instruments during surgery, particularly in patients with HIV/AIDS. All OR team members should be notified regarding the presence of HIV prior to the start of the case. A metal side tray can be used as a safe zone to pass sharps off the field, back to the scrub tech. Double gloving may lower the probability of transmission from inadvertent needlestick injuries.
- Order intravitreal antiviral medication or clindamycin as above to inject at the end of the case.
- Place a SB is at your discretion depending on your comfort, number, and location of breaks, presence of PVR, etc. There is currently conflicting evidence regarding the utility of SB placement in addition to PPV with silicone oil tamponade in these cases.
- PFCL may also be utilized depending on the size of the retinal breaks and preference. See chapter titled *Perfluorocarbon Liquid.*

SURGICAL PROCEDURE: PPV WITH PLACEMENT OF SILICONE OIL

- Begin with a standard, 3-port, bimanual vitrectomy. A 23G, 25G, or 27G cannulas may be used.
- Insert iris hooks for mechanical pupillary dilation in cases of significant posterior synechiae precluding a view to the posterior segment. See chapter titled *Getting and Maintaining Your View.*
- Induce a PVD as gently as possible. Due to liquefactive necrosis of the retina, even minor vitreoretinal tractional forces can induce iatrogenic breaks. See chapter titled *PVD Induction.*
- Perform a core vitrectomy. See chapter titled *Vitrectomy Surgery Steps.*
- Consider use of PFCL depending on the number, size, and location of breaks. The presence of GRT may require the use of PFCL. Note that the presence of retinitis, retinal thinning, unrelieved traction, or breaks in a more posterior location may increase the risk of subretinal PFCL. See chapter titled *Subretinal Perfluorocarbon Liquid.*

The use of a side flow/dual-bore cannula (MedOne Surgical Inc) (Fig. 49.1) confers greater safety when injecting PFCL by minimizing excessive turbulent forces on the retina from the injection and thus reduces the chance of inadvertently creating a posterior break and forcing PFCL into the subretinal space.

- Complete a peripheral vitrectomy and meticulous shave of the vitreous base utilizing scleral depression.

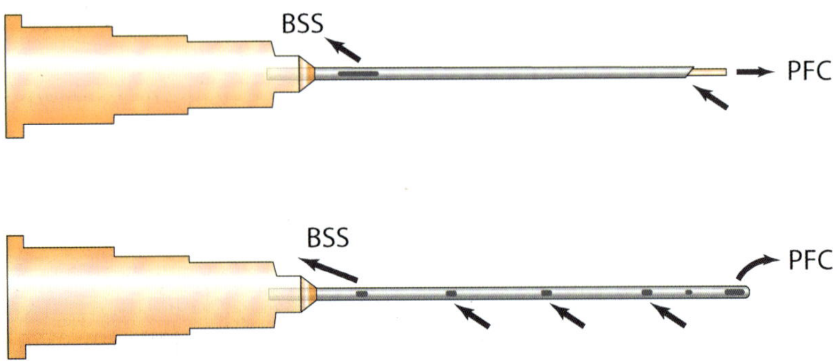

FIGURE 49.1. A side flow/dual-bore cannula (MedOne Surgical Inc) on bottom compared to a standard cannula on top.

- Shave all flaps and mark breaks with diathermy. See chapter titled *Retinal Break Localization*.
- Peel any inflammatory preretinal membranes using a bent MVR blade, Tano Diamond Dusted Membrane Scraper (Synergetics) or Finesse Flex Loop (Alcon) to create an edge and then MaxGrip (Alcon) or ILM forceps or equivalent to peel the membranes.
- Mark borders of necrotic or nonviable retinal tissue with diathermy. Perform retinectomy anterior to diathermy demarcation with the vitreous cutter by drawing the tissue into the port with aspiration and then cutting. Depending on the extent of retinal necrosis, some necrotic retina may be left in place. Avoid inadvertently cutting the RPE and choroid.
- Perform a FAX using a soft-tip cannula. If PFCL is in the eye, turn on the air infusion, aspirate the fluid between the PFCL bubble posteriorly and air bubble generated anteriorly, and then remove SRF through any breaks outside the PFCL bubble before aspirating the PFCL itself. Drain fluid over the optic disc. See chapter titled *Fluid Air Exchange*.

Some cases of toxoplasma-related RD have a tractional component to the RD. In such cases, segment around the inflammatory nidus, similar to segmenting in a diabetic TRD.

- Perform endolaser around all breaks and along all areas of retinitis or necrosis with at least three rows of barricade using 532-nm endolaser. See chapter titled *Endolaser Types and Settings*.
- Perform an air silicone oil exchange using a viscous fluid injector through the infusion port and using a vent or manually venting with a 0.12 forceps through another cannula. See chapter titled *Air Silicone Oil Exchange*.
- Remove all cannulas and suture all sclerotomy sites. Foscarnet (24 mg/mL, inject 0.1 mL), ganciclovir (40 mg/mL, inject 0.1 mL), or clindamycin (10 mg/mL, inject 0.1 mL) can be injected through the last valved cannula before it is removed to avoid significant elevation of IOP.

SURGICAL MANAGEMENT OF EXUDATIVE RD

Preoperative Considerations

While exudative RDs are often effectively managed with medical treatment alone, surgical management is appropriate when there is an insufficient response to medical treatment or if there is a suspicion for a possible rhegmatogenous component. See chapter titled *RRD vs Exudative RD vs Retinoschisis*.

- Confirm that the RD is exudative and not rhegmatogenous.
  - Perform a B-scan ultrasound and obtain images in all transverse quadrants with the patient's head lying to one side. SRF should pool in the dependent region. Then turn the patient's head to the other side and reimage. The SRF should now pool on the other side, which has now become dependent.
  - Obtain ultra-widefield fundus photography to examine the distribution of SRF.
  - Consider the presence of an occult retinal break if SRF does not shift on B-scan ultrasonography or there is asymmetric distribution of SRF following Lincoff's rules. See chapter titled *Retinal Break Localization*.
- Determine the etiology of the exudative RD (infectious, inflammatory, vascular, neoplastic, idiopathic, postsurgical). Many causes of exudative RD will respond to medical treatment or may resolve without any treatment at all (eg, serous RD after extensive retinal laser photocoagulation). Other mechanical causes such as optic nerve pit or compression of vortex veins from high circumferential SB may require a very specific and targeted surgical approach to correct the underlying cause.

Surgical Planning

- Counsel patient regarding expectations of surgery. Note that surgical management may not be definitive and exudative RDs can recur if the disease process cannot be adequately controlled. Additionally, discuss the risks of surgery including SRH, retinal incarceration (with external drainage), and RRD.
- Inform OR staff, microbiology, pathology, and/or cytology if you are planning to send vitreous or SRF for analysis. Order tubes and vials for fluid analysis ahead of time and properly label them.
- Use a 6-mm cannula, if available, and/or an infusion line with a 6-mm tip if there are concurrent choroidals. See chapter titled *Choroidals.*

SURGICAL PROCEDURE

Option 1: External Drainage of SRF. See chapter titled *External Subretinal Fluid Drainage.*

- Perform conjunctival peritomy in the quadrant of the SRF using Westcott scissors and 0.12 forceps.
- Hook the rectus muscles and loop the muscles with 2-0 silk ligatures to gain manual access to the more posterior sclera.
- Examine the RD either with indirect ophthalmoscopy or utilizing a 25G chandelier. The site of the most bullous RD can be marked with the indented edge of a scleral depressor as is performed in SB surgery. See chapter titled *Scleral Buckling Steps.*
- When selecting a drainage site, careful inspection should be performed both internally and externally to avoid areas of vortex veins or choroidal vessels.

Option 1A: Cutdown Drainage Method

- Make a 3-mm radial incision in the sclera with an MVR or no. 64 Beaver blade, down to the choroid. See chapter titled *External Subretinal Fluid Drainage.*
- In the center of this incision, cauterize through a focal point in the choroid using diathermy to gain access to the subretinal space. Egress of fluid should be seen if this step has been performed correctly.
- Confirm resolution of SRF by direct visualization under the microscope or indirect ophthalmoscopy.
- Upon drainage of the SRF, inject an equivalent volume of filtered air through the pars plana into the vitreous cavity with a 30G needle. Alternately, place an AC infusion at the start of surgery. See chapter titled *Choroidals.*
- Consider leaving the scleral drainage site open unless there is concern for hypotony or retinal incarceration. Alternatively, suture the wound with 7-0 Vicryl.
- Remove the silk ligatures, and close the peritomy with 6-0 plain gut.

Option 1B: Needle Drainage Method

- Fashion a guarded needle by placing a 270 sleeve over a 3/8 inch 26G needle. Trim the sleeve to allow 2-3 mm of needle to remain exposed (Fig. 49.2). Affix the needle to a 3-mL syringe with the plunger removed. Alternatively, you can use a commercially available 25G needle connected via tubing to the aspiration port of the vitrectomy machine. See chapter titled *External Subretinal Fluid Drainage.*
- Place the needle through the sclera tangentially (not perpendicular to the sclera) with the bevel away from the retina. Under direct visualization with indirect ophthalmoscopy or under a widefield microscopic viewing system with chandelier illumination, observe the needle tip entering the subretinal space. See chapters titled *Lenses and Viewing Systems* and *The Chandelier Buckle.*
- Apply tension on the silk ligatures or gently modulate the foot pedal if using a 25G needle connected to the aspiration port of the machine to promote passive egress of

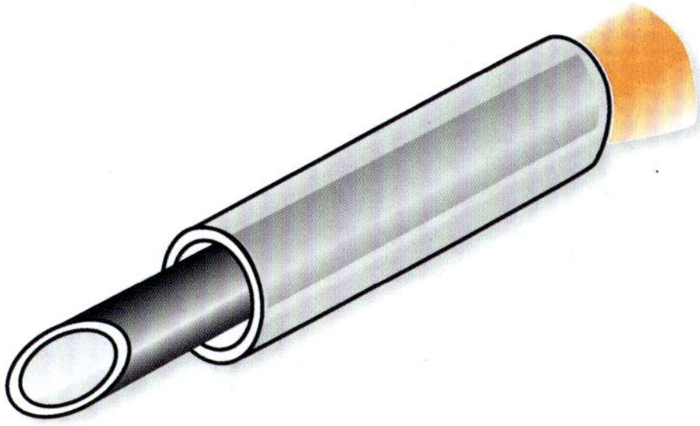

FIGURE 49.2. Needle drainage method. Fashion a guarded needle by placing a 270 sleeve over a 3/8 inch 26G needle. Trim the sleeve to allow 2-3 mm of needle to remain exposed.

SRF. Fluid can also be manually aspirated by an assistant using attached tubing. This method may be preferable if sending fluid for laboratory studies.

- Upon drainage of the SRF, inject an equivalent volume of filtered air through the pars plana into the vitreous cavity with a 30G needle. Alternatively, place an AC infusion at the start of surgery. See chapter titled *Choroidals.*
- Remove silk ligatures, and close the peritomy with 6-0 plain gut.

Option 2: PPV With Internal Drainage of SRF. See chapter titled *Posterior SRF During Vitrectomy for RRD.*

- Set up a standard 3-port vitrectomy using 23G, 25G, or 27G cannulas. See chapter titled *Gauge Selection and Cannula Placement.*
- Perform a core and peripheral vitrectomy with induction of PVD if necessary. Close shaving of vitreous base is usually not necessary. See chapter titled *Vitrectomy Surgery Steps.*
- Using diathermy, create a retinotomy in the most posterior aspect of the RD, preferably nasal to the optic disc. See chapter titled *Posterior SRF During Vitrectomy for RRD.*
- The aspiration port of the vitrector tubing can be connected to a 10-mL syringe. An assistant can gently aspirate, while you place the port over the drainage retinotomy site to extract the SRF for laboratory studies. This may have a higher yield than sending the entire vitrectomy cassette for analysis. See chapter titled *Diagnostic Vitrectomy.*
- Perform a FAX using a soft-tip cannula over the drainage retinotomy site. See chapter titled *Fluid Air Exchange.*
- Apply three rows of endolaser barricade around the drainage retinotomy site using 532-nm endolaser. See chapter titled *Endolaser Types and Settings.*
- Perform an air gas exchange with the desired concentration of SF_6 or C_3F_8 gas. See chapters titled *Air Gas Exchange* and *Gas Tamponade.*
- Remove all cannulas. Suturing is not necessary if appropriate conjunctival displacement had been performed and self-sealing wounds are observed.

CHAPTER 51

Transscleral Choroidal Biopsy

Michael Seider, MD

PREOPERATIVE CONSIDERATIONS

- Diagnostic transscleral biopsy
  - Perform B-scan ultrasonography in clinic to determine the tumor thickness. The transscleral biopsy technique is most preferred for anterior uveal tumors (ciliary body, anterior/equatorial choroid) with thickness of 2-3 mm or greater. Transvitreal biopsy may be safer for thinner and/or more posterior tumors because of direct visualization.
  - Consider coordinating with pathology (specializing in cytology, if possible) to have staff present in the OR to confirm diagnostic transscleral specimen adequacy. Note, this may result in a destruction of your initial biopsy "pass," and others may need to be taken for cytologic analysis after adequacy is established. If immediate surgical decision-making depends on the biopsy results, pathology may be able to provide a "wet read" in the OR as well.
  - When diagnostic biopsy is performed in conjunction with prognostic biopsy, it may help confirm that the tissue being sampled is the intended tissue, as prognostic biopsy results may be provided even if nontumor tissue is submitted.

Never perform a biopsy for possible retinoblastoma as this may result in tumor spread. Biopsy for medulloepithelioma is also not recommended as spread and metastatic disease has been reported, especially with larger "open" biopsies.

- Prognostic transscleral biopsy
  - Performed for uveal melanoma tumors to characterize the cytogenetic abnormalities and/or gene expression profile to determine the likelihood of eventual metastasis
- Concomitant radiotherapy
  - Transscleral tumor biopsy is likely most safe when combined with tumor radiotherapy (either radioactive brachytherapy plaque at the time of biopsy or external beam radiotherapy soon afterward) to sterilize the needle tract from possible migrating malignant cells.

SURGICAL PROCEDURE: TRANSSCLERAL FINE NEEDLE ASPIRATION TUMOR BIOPSY (VIDEO 51.1)

- Use transillumination (transpupillary and transscleral) to mark the borders of the tumor base on the sclera with a surgical pen (Fig. 51.1). Beware of "penumbra" or shadowing, in which a tall tumor may result in a transillumination shadow on the sclera adjacent to the tumor even though no tumor is present there. To avoid this, make sure to transilluminate thick tumors from multiple angles and do not mark any area of sclera unless a shadow persists during this entire process.

> **Nonuveal melanoma tumors (such as uveal metastasis) may not cause a tumor shadow. Indirect ophthalmoscopy with a scleral marker may be used in such cases to identify a suitable biopsy site.**

- Use a 25G-27G hollow bore needle for your biopsy (1/2 or 5/8 inches in length). We have developed a novel technique for transscleral tumor biopsy that uses the 25G Hanscom SRF drainage needle (Beaver-Visitec), which has a silicone guard that prevents inadvertently passing the needle "too deep" and engaging retina or vitreous. This technique is simple, effective, and safe.
- Attach your needle to IV extension tubing to uncouple the syringe and needle—ideally, a short amount (12 inches or less) of fine "IV extension" (pediatric) tubing is best. Connect the tubing to a 10-mL syringe.
- Ensure that the biopsy site is well exposed (peritomy, Tenon dissection, looping extraocular muscles for retraction as needed) and dry with decent hemostasis (cautery is usually not necessary unless the biopsy site is anterior to the extraocular muscle insertions).
  - Optional step: create a partial-thickness scleral flap in the area of intended biopsy, which is intended to reduce the risk of tumor cell escape from the biopsy site (although this is rare). This flap may be closed with suture after biopsy.
- Identify an area of sclera corresponding to the center of the tumor, which is usually the thickest portion of the tumor. Begin your needle pass just proximal to this area—ideally the tumor is entered (sclera is perforated) at the tumor's thickest point to avoid perforating the tumor.
- Enter the sclera with the needle with the bevel facing you, so you can visualize the bevel entering sclera (unless the Hanscom needle is used, in which case the face the bevel should face the sclera) and only advance the needle 1-2 mm beyond where the view of the bevel is lost.
- Pass your needle at a steep angle to create a longer scleral tunnel, which will impede unintended outflow of potentially malignant cells after biopsy. Just before perforating sclera (entering the uveal tumor), reorient your needle perpendicular to sclera so that the tumor is not entered at an extreme angle (which reduces the risk of tumor perforation/entering the vitreous cavity).

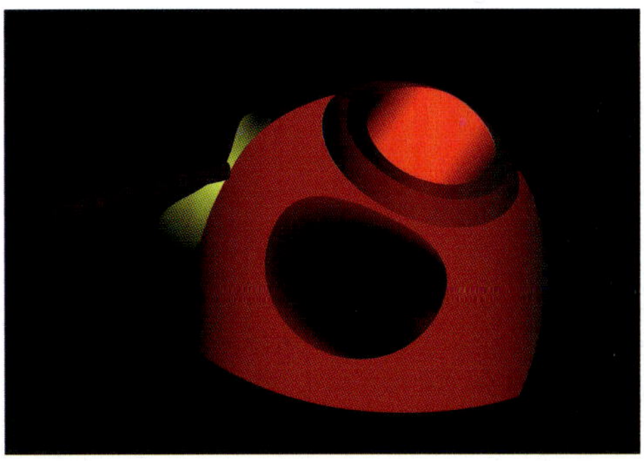

FIGURE 51.1. Use transpupillary and transscleral transillumination to mark the borders of the tumor base on the sclera with a surgical pen. Beware of "penumbra" or shadowing, in which a tall tumor may result in a transillumination shadow on the sclera adjacent to the tumor even though no tumor is present there. To avoid this, make sure to transilluminate thick tumors from multiple angles and do not mark any area of sclera unless a shadow persists during this entire process.

- Once the needle is believed to be in the area of the tumor, ask an assistant to pull on the syringe plunger. It is normal to develop a vacuum in the syringe and for the assistant to feel significant resistance. If the assistant notices a loss of vacuum and/or aspiration of clear fluid into the tubing/syringe, tell your assistant to immediately release aspirating force—this may indicate that your needle has perforated the tumor/retina and inadvertently entered the vitreous cavity.
- Once the assistant has applied aspiration force, initiate low-amplitude/frequency in-and-out and 90-180 degree rotational movements with the needle to improve biopsy yield.
- Ask your assistant to stop aspirating before the needle is removed from the sclera to avoid aspirating room air and moving your specimen to the needle hub where expulsion into transport media may be more difficult.
- Immediately after needle removal from the sclera, apply cautery to the scleral tunnel to destroy potentially malignant cells. If significant outflow of liquid from your scleral pass is noted, dry this area to ensure malignant cells are removed.
- Consider rinsing the area afterwards with saline/BSS to remove any invisible liberated malignant cells.
- Transfer your biopsy specimen to transport media (use the smallest collection vial available to avoid specimen loss). Flush the needle with room air to expel contents into the transport media. Disconnect the syringe and repeat this procedure if necessary. Consider aspirating some transport media into the needle and flushing it similarly into the transport media to improve yield. Especially if your retrieved specimen is small (or invisible!), communicate with pathology to centrifuge your transport media (similar to creating a "cell block") and not attempt to pass it through filter paper to "catch" the specimen, as this may result in specimen loss.
- Repeat the biopsy procedure as needed for additional passes (use a fresh needle/tubing/syringe for each pass).
- Perform indirect ophthalmoscopy to confirm no retinal perforation, VH, or RRD. Significant intratumoral/subretinal hemorrhage is not uncommon.
- Close conjunctiva.
- Alternatively, if a larger tumor biopsy specimen is desired (only recommended in select cases):
  - Moderate sized biopsy: fashion a tunneled incision with a small blade instead of a needle (Super Sharp or MVR) and enter the tumor substance with biopsy forceps.
  - Large biopsy (when definitive histopathology desired or tumor identity quite uncertain): create a rectangular-shaped partial-thickness scleral flap (3-4 mm in length) hinged on one side, reflect it, and within the bed, create a rectangular-shaped area of scleral excision with your blade (Fig. 51.2). Withdraw this inner scleral flap from the eye and incise the exposed intraocular tumor (1-3 mm thickness) to create a biopsy specimen with partial-thickness scleral bed attached. After specimen removal, close the outer scleral flap securely with suture.

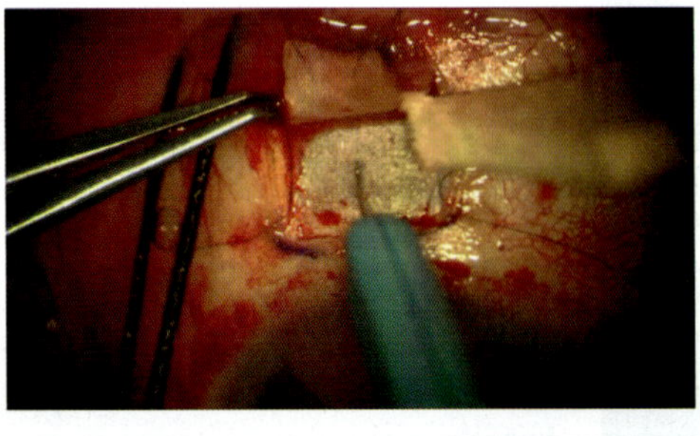

FIGURE 51.2. Create a rectangular-shaped partial-thickness scleral flap (3-4 mm in length) hinged on one side, reflect it, and within the bed, create a rectangular-shaped area of scleral excision with your blade.

POSTOPERATIVE CONSIDERATIONS

If the biopsy site is anterior, check it at the slit lamp at subsequent postop exams to ensure no extraocular tumor growth in the biopsied area. If biopsy site is not visible at the slit lamp (most common), use B-scan during follow-up to ensure no extrascleral tumor extension occurred in this area.

- Cut out the chorioretinal specimen.
  - This can be achieved unimanually with vertical scissors if PFCL is used.
    - Make your initial incision only through retina to expose the underlying choroid and then make an incision through the choroid. Then additional cuts can be made to incorporate both retina and choroid in a single bite.
  - Alternatively, a bimanual technique using forceps and intraocular scissors can be used.
    - This is helpful when PFCL is not used. The forceps help reflect the tissue to identify the appropriate surgical plane.
  - Leave the chorioretinal biopsy hinged at one corner if PFCL is not used.
    - This prevents the sample from floating away while the sclerotomy is being widened for its removal.
    - If PFCL was used, the entire specimen can be freed as the PFCL will stabilize the tissue in place.
- Remove the cannula in the region of the peritomy.
- Lower the infusion pressure to 25-30 mm Hg.
  - Presence of a high infusion pressure in the presence of a large sclerotomy can create significant turbulence that can disturb the PFCL and/or sweep the chorioretinal biopsy away into the vitreous cavity.
- Widen the sclerotomy with an MVR blade.
- Cut the final hinge of the chorioretinal specimen if needed.
- Remove the chorioretinal biopsy with intraocular forceps, *en bloc* if possible, and transfer to a piece of filter paper. Avoid extensive crush artifact if possible.
  - Sometimes the retina and choroid may come out as separate pieces.
  - Have your assistant gape the edges of the sclerotomy with 0.12 forceps so that your specimen can be more easily delivered.
- Preplace an 8-0 Vicryl suture in the enlarged sclerotomy and replace the cannula in the sclerotomy.
- Examine the retinal periphery for any retinal breaks with scleral depression.
- If an exudative RD is present, inject additional PFCL to displace SRF further anteriorly.
  - In this scenario, create an anterior drainage retinotomy in an area that can be well tamponaded (not inferior periphery), drain SRF through the retinotomy, and apply endolaser around the retinotomy.
- Remove all PFCL via FAX. See chapter titled *Fluid Air Exchange.*
- Inject your tamponade agent of choice.
  - Silicone oil is commonly used, but C_3F_8 tamponade may be appropriate in cases without an exudative RD. See chapters titled *Gas Tamponade* and *Silicone Oil Tamponade.*
- Remove the remaining cannulas and suture the sclerotomies with 8-0 Vicryl suture.
- Position your patient such that the chorioretinal biopsy site is well tamponaded for the first 3-5 days.

Modifications to the chorioretinal biopsy technique in the presence of an exudative RD include injection of PFCL to flatten the retina at the planned biopsy site, creation of an anterior drainage retinotomy through which SRF is drained, and uniform use of silicone oil tamponade at the end of the case. See chapter titled *Silicone Oil Tamponade.*

Section XI

Challenging Vitreoretinal Surgical Scenarios

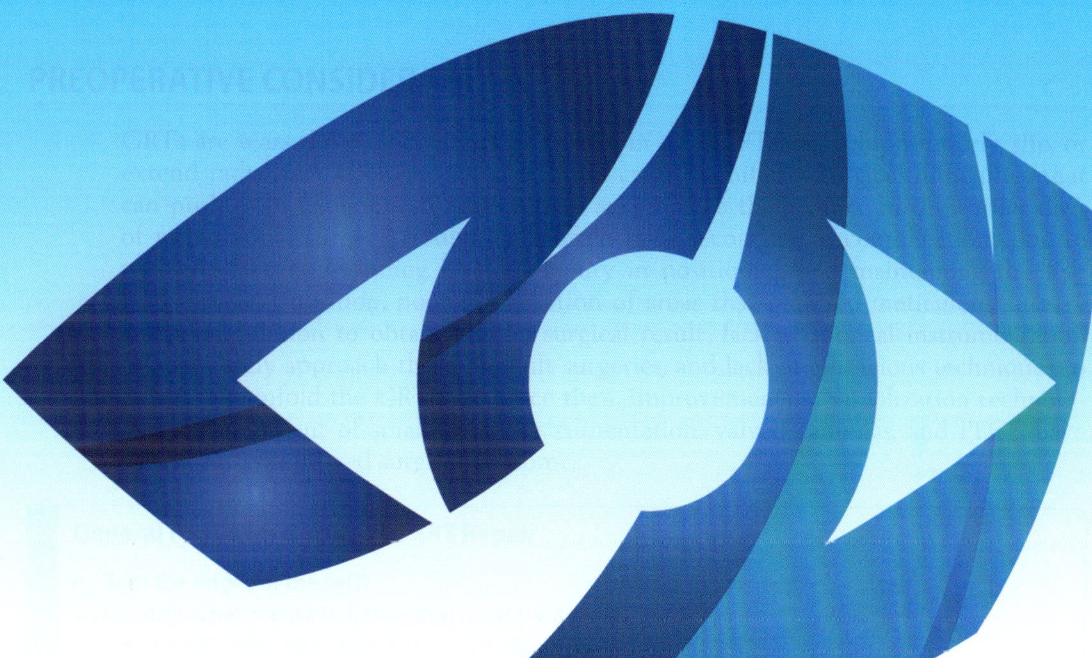

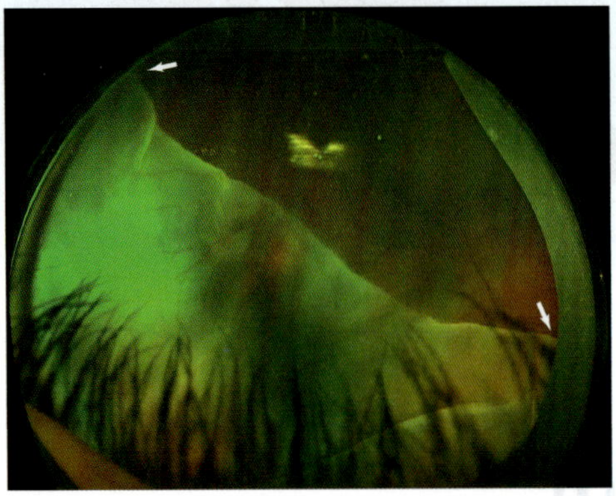

FIGURE 53.1. Pay attention to the horns (*arrows*) of the GRT where it is most prone to opening postop if not well treated.

- There is often a strong vitreous adhesion to the anterior margin of the GRT. But, the vitreous is usually free from the posterior margin, allowing the retina to fall back.
- Pay attention to the horns of the GRT where it is prone to open postop if not well treated (Fig. 53.1).

Consider a SB in cases with preexisting PVR. If a SB is placed, use a low-lying SB (41, 42, or 4050 band) to decrease risk of retinal slippage or radial folds.

- Mark the posterior edge of the GRT and any other breaks. Diathermy helps with hemostasis and aids in visualization of the GRT, as the case progresses.
- Lensectomy is typically not necessary unless visualization precludes achieving vitreous base surgical goals. See chapter titled *Pars Plana Lensectomy*.
  - Optimal visualization can be obtained by pharmacological dilation, iris retractors, wide-angle viewing systems, and scleral depression. Advanced lighting systems such as chandeliers may be helpful. See chapter titled *Getting and Maintaining Your View*.
- Truncate the anterior flap of devitalized retina to reduce the chance of developing anterior loop PVR (Fig. 53.2).
- Inject PFCL over the optic disc to unfold the GRT out to the periphery. If the GRT flap has flipped over, tilt the eye as the flap unrolls and use a soft-tip cannula or Tano Diamond Dusted Membrane Scraper (Synergetics) to unroll the edge of the GRT.
- Apply three rows of laser retinopexy with multiple confluent or nearly confluent laser burns along the posterior edge of the GRT. Laser the GRT out to the ora. Laser other breaks and lattice as well. White-without-pressure is associated with

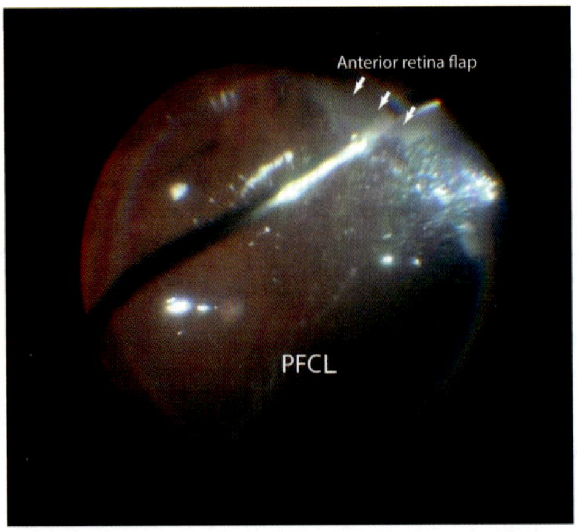

FIGURE 53.2. Truncate the anterior flap of devitalized retina to reduce the chance of developing anterior loop PVR.

development of a GRT in the fellow eye, so treat WWP in both eyes as well. There is no clinical evidence that routine 360-degree treatment is beneficial without concomitant pathology. See chapter titled *Endolaser Types and Settings.*

- Perform FAX while preventing slippage of the flap of the GRT, the development of folds, or residual SRF pockets. Carefully and meticulously "milk" the SRF along the edge of the GRT following PFCL administration for adequate "seating" of the flap.
  - Rotate the eye to place the GRT in the most dependent position, maintain suction, meticulously dry at the air/PFCL interface and edges of the GRT. Drain for a longer duration than in RRD without a GRT to avoid slippage.
- Exchange the PFCL or air for gas or silicone oil. Factors determining the use of a specific tamponade agent include the presence of PVR, location of the GRT (inferior or superior), the need for postop travel, and/or compliance issues. The presence of a superior break would allow for extended gas tamponade (ie, C_3F_8 gas). The presence of an inferior GRT, the need for travel, PVR, or potential poor compliance may make silicone oil a better tamponade agent. See chapters titled *Gas Tamponade* and *Silicone Oil Tamponade.*
- Treatment of the fellow eye is generally indicated for lattice, retinal break(s), or WWP. The fellow eye of those with Marfan or Stickler syndrome or a history of trauma should be considered for prophylactic treatment such as 360 laser or SB.

CHAPTER 54

Proliferative Vitreoretinopathy Surgery

Mohammad Dahrouj, MD, PhD • Dean Eliott, MD

Grade the PVR according to the Updated PVR Grade Classification (1991):

Grade A	**Vitreous haze, pigment clumps in vitreous or on inferior retina**
Grade B	**Inner retinal surface wrinkling, retinal stiffness, vessel tortuosity, rolled and irregular edge of retinal break(s), decreased vitreous mobility**
Grade C	**Focal, diffuse or circumferential full-thickness folds, subretinal strands Stratified based on clock hour extension and anatomic location: posterior vs anterior**

MEMBRANE PEELING

- Take advantage of various stains to help with visualization of vitreous (triamcinolone), membranes (triamcinolone), and ILM (ICG). See chapter titled *Intraoperative Visualization Agents.*
- Fine pigment deposits often indicate the presence of preretinal membranes.
- Begin preretinal membrane peeling at the disc and proceed outward. Peel membranes in one large sheet, although not always possible especially for immature membranes.
- If a membrane cannot be grasped with forceps, use a Tano Diamond Dusted Membrane Scraper (Synergetics) or Finesse Flex Loop (Alcon).
- Remove subretinal bands if they are causing significant traction. In pediatric cases or in young adults with an attached hyaloid, subretinal bands can often be left in place.
- Remove the subretinal bands via an access retinotomy (Fig. 54.1). Grasp the membranes and pull gently or roll the membranes around the forceps or light pipe to mobilize the band without breaking it.
- Remove the subretinal bands and membranes via a retinectomy, most commonly an inferior 180-degree retinectomy.
- In anterior PVR, there may be a fibrous circumferential membrane adherent to the pars plana and ciliary process (and occasionally even the iris) that results in anterior displacement of the retina. Use an MVR blade or vitreous cutter to create an

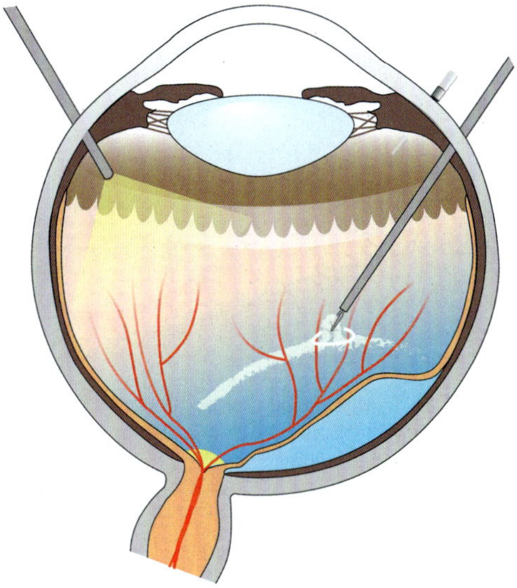

FIGURE 54.1. Remove subretinal bands via an access retinotomy. Grasp the membranes and pull gently or roll the bands around the forceps or light pipe to mobilize the band without breaking it.

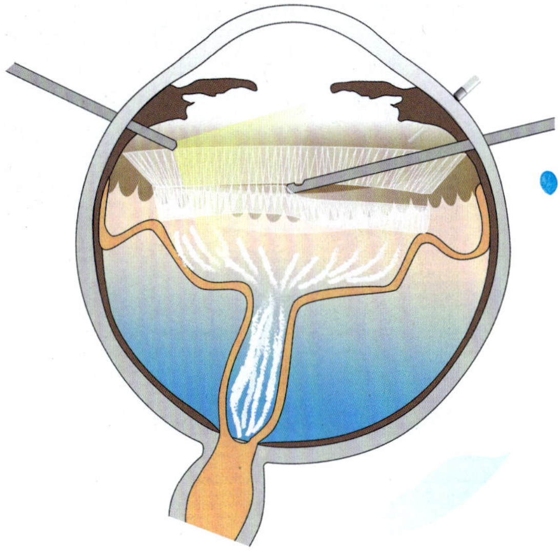

FIGURE 54.2. Use an MVR blade or vitreous cutter to create an opening in the membrane. Then use the vitreous cutter or scissors to extend the opening circumferentially and relieve the traction.

opening in the membrane. Use the vitreous cutter or scissors to extend the opening circumferentially and relieve the traction (Fig. 54.2).

- After membrane peeling, perform a careful peripheral retinal exam to identify all retinal breaks. See chapter titled *Retinal Break Localization*.

RETINECTOMY (VIDEO 54.1)

The frequency of relaxing retinectomy in PVR repair has increased and may be performed in up to ⅔ of cases. Three types of retinectomies are performed: inferior 180 degrees (most common), 360 degrees, and small posterior focal.

- Consider performing a retinectomy after membrane peeling if there is unrelieved traction due to retinal foreshortening. In some cases, place a SB to relieve the residual traction and obviate the need for retinectomy.
- Create the retinectomy posterior to the vitreous base.
- A 180-degree inferior retinectomy is the preferred retinectomy in most eyes with several clock hours of inferior PVR.
- When performing a 180-degree inferior retinectomy, make the edges at 3 and 9 o'clock since reproliferation typically occurs inferiorly (Fig. 54.3).
- In cases where a 180-degree retinectomy is insufficient, consider enlarging it up to 270 degrees. If a retinectomy larger than 270 degrees is required, then consider a 360-degree retinectomy.
- Use PFCL to stabilize the posterior retina while performing a peripheral retinectomy.
- Maintain hemostasis at the retinectomy edge to decrease recurrent PVR. Use endodiathermy to delineate the intended retinectomy edge before starting the retinectomy and/or raise the infusion pressure to prevent bleeding during the retinectomy.
- Endolaser along the retinectomy edge promotes long-term retina-RPE adhesion at the retinectomy margin.
- Completely excise the anterior retina to prevent postop proliferation, traction, VEGF production, and hypotony.
- Use the vitreous cutter (or vertical scissors in low-lying RD) to cut the retina.
- Use either silicone oil or C_3F_8 gas as tamponade. Air and SF_6 gas have worse outcomes in PVR cases. See chapters titled *Gas Tamponade* and *Silicone Oil Tamponade*.

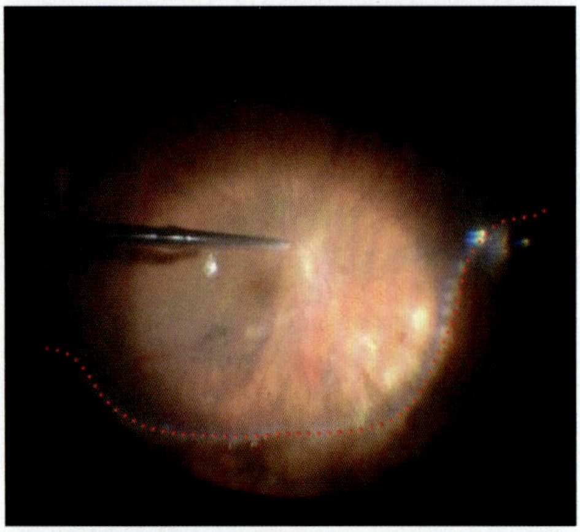

FIGURE 54.3. Make a 180-degree inferior retinectomy with the edges at 3 and 9 o'clock since reproliferation typically occurs inferiorly.

LENSECTOMY

Pars plana lensectomy should be performed on a case-by-case basis. In advanced PVR cases with anterior PVR, however, have a low threshold to perform lensectomy including removing the entire capsular bag since secondary IOL implantation at a later date is rarely performed. See chapter titled *Pars Plana Lensectomy.*

Advantage of lensectomy in PVR cases:

- More complete anterior vitrectomy
- Access to anterior membranes
- Release of anterior retinal and ciliary body traction
- Aphakia correlates with normal postop IOP.

SB FOR PVR

- A SB is recommended for most PVR cases, especially if there are multiple breaks or extensive inferior pathology. See chapter titled *Scleral Buckling Steps.*
- With 360-degree retinectomy or extensive 360-degree anterior laser, a SB may not be necessary.
- A SB helps relieve potential future traction at the retinectomy edges (such as at the 3 and 9 o'clock sites).

AVOID SLIPPAGE

Retinal slippage can occur during FAX and PFCL removal, especially in cases with a large retinectomy. This occurs when a thin film of SRF is trapped posteriorly by the enlarging air bubble, causing the retina to slide posteriorly.

- Exchange the fluid anterior to the PFCL for air, and then aspirate any remaining fluid along the edge of the retinectomy with a soft-tip cannula. Then remove the PFCL. See chapter titled *Giant Retinal Tear.*
- Consider a direct PFCL silicone oil exchange. See chapter titled *Perfluorocarbon Silicone Oil Exchange.*

AVOIDING RETENTION OF PFCL

- Use a lower infusion pressure to decrease turbulence.
- Use valved cannulas.
- To avoid PFCL entering the subretinal space, all traction should be relieved before injecting PFCL.
- Perform a saline rinse after the FAX. See chapters titled *Perfluorocarbon Liquid* and *Fluid Air Exchange.*

CHAPTER 55

Choroidals

Xi Chen, MD, PhD

PREOPERATIVE CONSIDERATIONS

In an eye with a choroidal detachment, perform B-scan ultrasonography to exclude masquerades (tumor), determine type of choroidal (serous, hemorrhagic, serosanguineous), and whether there is apposition and if not, which quadrant has the highest choroidal.

Serous Choroidals

- Find the underlying cause and fix it.
  - Is there a wound leak or open globe?
  - Is there overfiltration from a trabeculectomy/tube?
  - Is the eye hypotonous from another reason such as RD or inflammation?
- Usually correction of the underlying cause leads to resolution of serous choroidals.
- If nonappositional, observe unless associated with RRD.
- If appositional and persistent despite resolution of the underlying cause, consider surgical drainage to relieve apposition.

Hemorrhagic Choroidals

- Consider discontinuation of antiplatelet or anticoagulant agents in consultation with internist.
- Discourage Valsalva or eye rubbing.
- If nonappositional, observe.
- If appositional, consider oral steroids to promote clot liquefaction to facilitate more complete surgical drainage.
- If appositional for 7-10 days, consider surgical drainage, even if incomplete drainage, to relieve central apposition.
- If the AC is flat, IOP high despite medical management, or corneal decompensation occurs, earlier surgical intervention may be warranted.

SURGICAL PLANNING

- Manage patient expectations about guarded visual prognosis.
- Let the OR team know what you need.

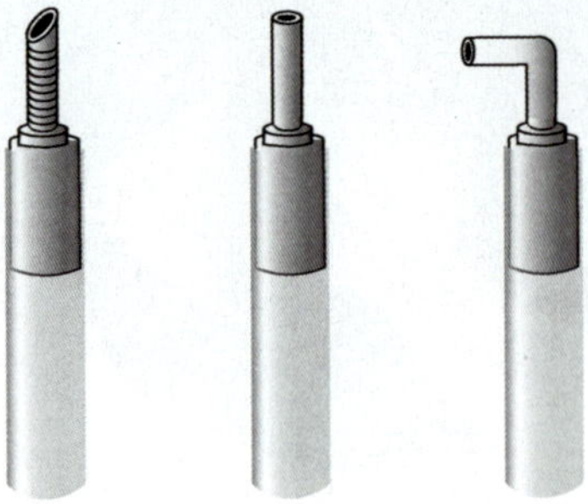

FIGURE 55.1. AC maintainers: straight corrugated AC maintainer vs straight, smooth AC maintainer vs 90-degree AC maintainer.

- AC maintainer (straight corrugated AC maintainer vs straight, smooth AC maintainer vs 90-degree AC maintainer) (Fig. 55.1)
- Infusion line with 6-mm tip or 6-mm cannula if planning vitrectomy

SURGICAL PROCEDURE: DRAINAGE OF CHOROIDALS (VIDEO 55.1)

- Perform B-scan ultrasonography and/or re-examine patient to ensure the size and location of the choroidals have not significantly changed.
- Reform AC if flat or shallow. Can use BSS, infusion fluid, or viscoelastic that may help maintain AC depth.
- If using a straight AC maintainer, place it around 3 or 9 o'clock at the limbus after creating an entry paracentesis with Zeigler knife or paracentesis blade. May not need 7-0 Vicryl suture to secure into place.
- If using a 90-degree AC maintainer, place at 6 o'clock limbus and secure with 7-0 Vicryl (Fig. 55.2).
- If choroidals are appositional, take down conjunctiva in quadrant of planned pars plana drainage site (often superonasal but where choroidal appears particularly liquefied or highest on ultrasonography) using toothed 0.12 forceps and Wescott scissors.
- Use wet-field cautery to obtain hemostasis and visualization of the sclera.

The suprachoroidal space is continuous, so one or two external drainage sites may be enough for sufficient drainage of nonloculated choroidals.

- Use an MVR blade to pass through sclera and *just* enter the suprachoroidal space 3-4 mm posterior to the limbus in the quadrant of highest choroidal detachment or superonasally in appositional choroidals with incision parallel to limbus. Hemorrhage drains quite slowly. A more posterior site for drainage of choroidals may be chosen. A No. 64 Beaver blade can also be used instead of an MVR blade.

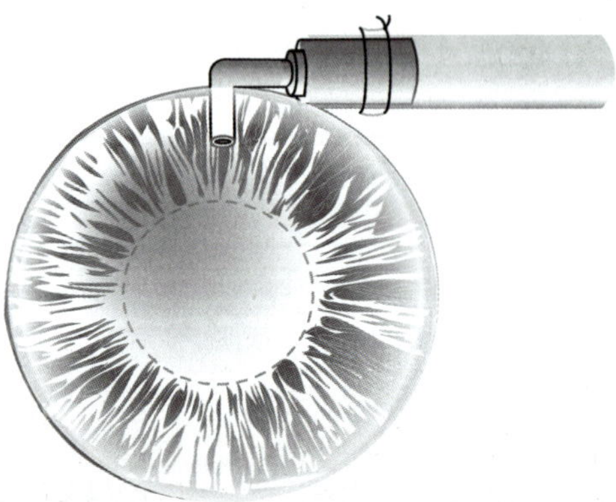

FIGURE 55.2. If using a 90-degree AC maintainer, place in the AC at 6 o'clock at the limbus and secure with a 7-0 Vicryl as shown.

- To promote drainage and access loculated pockets of liquefaction, insert a blunt cyclodialysis spatula into the suprachoroidal space and snake it along the inner sclera. External scleral massage with a cotton tip toward the drainage sclerotomy can help squeeze pockets of liquefied blood toward the external drainage site.
- Monitor progress with intraop B-scan ultrasonography or indirect ophthalmoscopy.
- Sometimes, you may need to create a second, or rarely a third, drainage site at the level of the pars plana in the superotemporal or one of the inferior quadrants to relieve choroidal apposition and promote additional drainage.
- You can leave open one but not all of the scleral drainage sites without suture, unless there is concern for retinal or vitreous incarceration or postop hypotony.
- Remove the AC maintainer and suture the corneal entry site with 10-0 nylon. Bury the knot.
- Consider simultaneous vitrectomy if absolutely necessary with attention to maintain intraop IOP to decrease the risk of recurrent choroidals.

No need to drain a limited hemorrhagic choroidal that develops intraop. If repairing a concurrent RD, place slightly expansile gas for any necessary retinal tamponade. If you use silicone oil, there will be an underfill as the choroidal resolves.

POSTOPERATIVE CONSIDERATIONS

After successful drainage, any residual nonappositional hemorrhagic choroidals may take months to fully resolve. Secondary nonrhegmatogenous SRF may also be slow to resolve.

CHAPTER 56

Submacular Hemorrhage

Kenneth Taubenslag, MD • Joseph Martel, MD

PREOPERATIVE CONSIDERATIONS

- Determine the duration and etiology of the hemorrhage. Any condition causing CNV can lead to massive submacular hemorrhage. Trauma or RAM rupture can also cause a submacular hemorrhage.
- Get OCT to quantify thickness of the blood and determine whether the majority is subretinal or subRPE. SRH is more amenable to displacement than subRPE blood.
- Consider surgical intervention for thick hemorrhages of limited duration (preferably ≤7 days).
- Consider observation for limited or mostly extrafoveal hemorrhage, which may reabsorb spontaneously with less significant visual sequelae compared to massive fovea-involving hemorrhage.
- Discuss with anticoagulation prescriber the possibility of holding anticoagulation for a short time if considering surgical intervention.
- There is no consensus on preferred management. Management will depend on surgical candidacy, preference, status of the contralateral eye, and resource availability.

Surgical Planning

- Manage patient expectations. Eyes with advanced AMD or long-standing hemorrhage have a poorer visual prognosis.
- Consider subretinal therapeutic options.
- Communicate with the OR any special vitreoretinal surgical needs.
  - Recombinant rtPA
  - Anti-VEGF agent
  - Syringe that connects to fluid injection tubing
  - 41G subretinal needle (DORC) or 38G Subretinal Polytip Cannula (MedOne Surgical Inc)
  - Intraop OCT

SURGICAL PROCEDURE: SUBRETINAL DISPLACEMENT OF MASSIVE SUBMACULAR HEMORRHAGE (VIDEO 56.1)

- Perform a complete PPV with posterior hyaloid separation. See chapter titled *PVD Induction*.
- Prepare 50 ug rtPA (12.5 mcg/0.1 mL) in a 1-mL syringe.

For a controlled subretinal injection without the need for a skilled assistant, connect injection syringe to the viscous fluid injection tubing connected to the vitrectomy platform. See chapters titled *Vitrectomy Machine Settings* and *Silicone Oil Tamponade*.

- Attach a subretinal needle (such as DORC 23G 41G needle or MedOne Surgical 38G Subretinal Polytip Cannula) to the syringe and engage the hemorrhage close to the arcade within the hemorrhagic neurosensory macular detachment to enter the subretinal space (Fig. 56.1A).
- Inject the recombinant tPA (about 0.4 mL) either with the aid of an assistant or, if using the viscous fluid injection system, by slowly uptitrating the injection pressure. Slow and controlled injection is necessary to reduce the risk of an FTMH.
- In addition to subretinal rtPA, concurrent injection of a small subretinal air bubble may enhance inferior displacement by reducing the buoyancy of the liquefied blood (Fig. 56.1B).

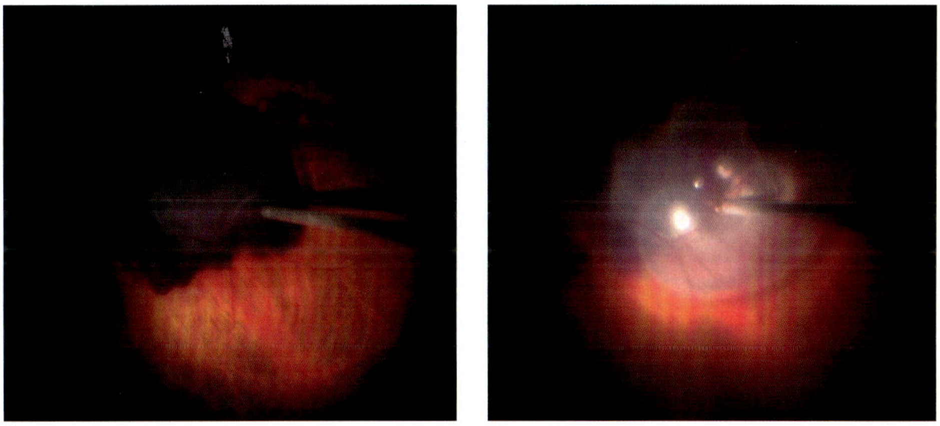

A B

FIGURE 56.1. **A.** The subretinal needle is placed into an area closest to the arcade where the submacular hemorrhage is thickest. **B.** In addition to rtPA, sometimes a small air bubble (~0.2 mL) is also injected into the subretinal space.

If opting for subretinal pneumatic displacement, the vitreous cavity gas fill is important in preventing subretinal migration of the air superiorly. After a partial FAX, an air gas exchange with 20% SF_6 to achieve a 50% vitreous cavity fill is recommended (Fig. 56.2).

- FAX with 20% SF_6 gas bubble. See chapter titled *Fluid Air Exchange*.
- If not using subretinal bevacizumab, intravitreal anti-VEGF injection should be considered.

Anti-VEGF may be injected intravitreally or may be mixed with the recombinant tPA. If injecting into the subretinal space, 0.1 mL of bevacizumab (2.5 mg) may be used in combination with the 0.4 mL of rtPA.

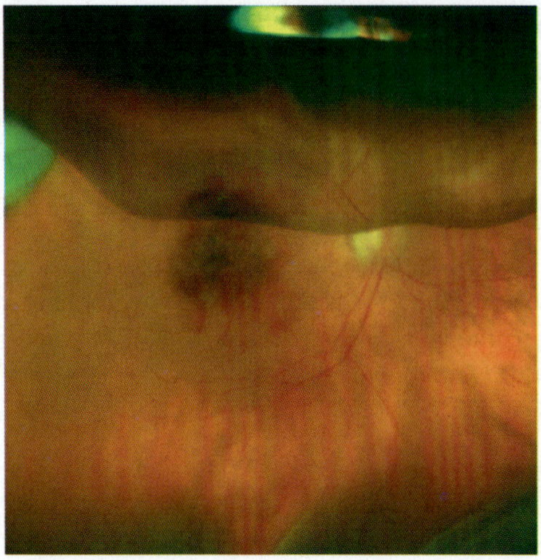

FIGURE 56.2. A partial FAX followed by an air gas exchange is performed to achieve a gas fill of close to 50%.

- Instruct the patient on partial facedown positioning (or upright positioning with downgaze) so that the bottom meniscus of the intravitreal gas bubble is on the superior 1/3 of the submacular hemorrhage. The goal is for the bubble to displace the hemorrhage inferior to the macular region. This positioning can be maintained for at least 72 hours. See chapter titled *Postop Positioning*.

POSTOPERATIVE CONSIDERATIONS

- Even after successful displacement, residual hemorrhage may take weeks to reabsorb.
- Displacement of the hemorrhage should occur within the first 24 hours postop. Additional displacement beyond the first 24 hours is typically minimal.
- Continue anti-VEGF therapy if clinically indicated.
- Restart anticoagulation, if appropriate.

CHAPTER 57

Subretinal Perfluorocarbon Liquid

Glenn C. Yiu, MD, PhD

PREOPERATIVE CONSIDERATIONS

PFCLs such as perfluoro-n-octane are widely used in vitreoretinal surgery, but inadvertent subretinal PFCL retained after surgery may be associated with retinal toxicity and visual scotomas. See chapter titled *Perfluorocarbon Liquid*. Preop considerations must take various clinical and surgical factors into account when deciding how to manage the subretinal PFCL.

- Determine if patient is a surgical candidate based on the location, amount, and duration of subretinal PFCL.
    - *Location:* Smaller amounts of extramacular or peripheral PFCL may be observed or delineated with barricade laser to prevent its migration. Spontaneous posterior migration may occur, especially if the subretinal PFCL is located in the superior periphery.
    - *Amount:* Larger number or size of subretinal PFCL bubble(s) are associated with larger areas of retinal toxicity and/or scotomas and may have a higher propensity for spontaneous migration.
    - *Duration:* Longer duration of subretinal PFCL may be associated with irreversible retinal toxicity; manage patient expectations of possible permanent scotomas even after removal of subretinal PFCL.

Surgical Planning

- Obtain details of previous vitreoretinal surgeries to confirm prior use of PFCL and likely duration of subretinal PFCL retention.
- Perform detailed dilated funduscopic exam to determine if any additional retinal pathology is present, such as ERM, PVR, or recurrent RD.
- Obtain retinal imaging including OCT to confirm diagnosis of subretinal PFCL based on "omega sign" to distinguish it from residual subretinal or intraretinal fluid (Fig. 57.1) and to determine the visual prognosis based on loss, disruption, or disorganization of outer retinal layers.

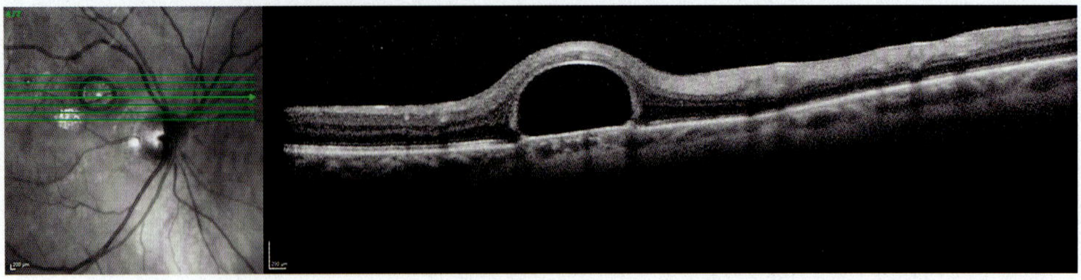

FIGURE 57.1. OCT image of a retained subretinal PFCL bubble in the superonasal macula 1 month after PPV with laser and gas for a RD in an 80-year-old man, demonstrating the "omega" sign.

SURGICAL PROCEDURE: REMOVAL OF RETAINED SUBRETINAL PFCL

Surgical removal of subretinal PFCL may be achieved by aspiration or displacement. VIDEO Video 57.1.

- Aspiration of subretinal PFCL
  - Use a 38G or 41G subretinal cannula (Fig. 57.2) to enter the subretinal PFCL bubble and then gently aspirate.
  - If such a cannula is unavailable, depending on the size and location of subretinal PFCL, make a retinotomy at the top or edge of the PFCL bubble. Perform endodiathermy and use a soft-tip cannula connected to aspiration on the vitrectomy machine to directly aspirate the PFCL, if not located precisely in the fovea.
  - You can directly aspirate the subretinal PFCL with a soft-tip cannula placed close to the overlying retina without the creation of a retinotomy and without the use of a subretinal cannula in some cases.
  - Injecting additional PFCL over the macula, before subfoveal PFCL aspiration, may reduce the size of the therapeutic FTMH.
  - Adjunctive ILM removal before or after PFCL removal may facilitate closure of the drainage site and minimize risk of postop FTMH formation.
- Displacement of subretinal subfoveal PFCL
  - For subfoveal PFCL, direct aspiration may risk FTMH and central scotoma formation. Instead, displacement should be considered.
  - Induce a macular RD by injecting infusion fluid into the subretinal space through an extrafoveal or extramacular location using a 38G or 41G subretinal cannula or via a retinotomy created by diathermy and soft-tip cannula.
  - Aspirate the subretinal PFCL through the retinotomy using either a subretinal or soft-tip cannula.
  - Injection of additional PFCL over the macula may help displace the subfoveal PFCL to the retinotomy site.
  - Use a Tano Diamond Dusted Membrane Scraper (Synergetics) of Finesse Flex Loop (Alcon) to gently displace the PFCL to the retinotomy site.

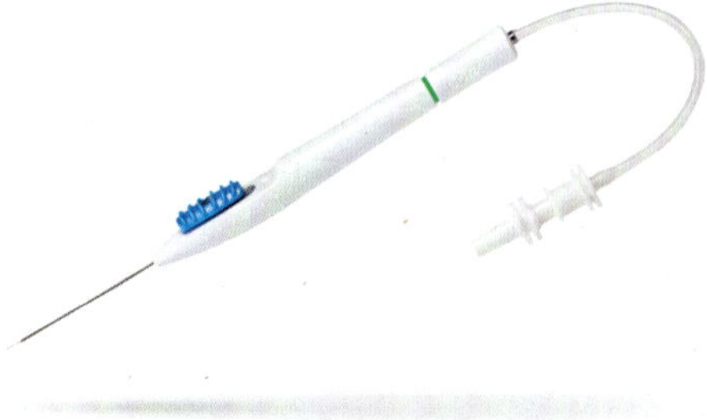

FIGURE 57.2. 41G subretinal cannula.

- Alternatively, after creating a macular RD with an inferior peripheral retinotomy, perform a FAX followed by postop positioning in an upright position to allow the subretinal PFCL to displace toward the inferior periphery. See chapters titled *Fluid Air Exchange* and *Postop Positioning*.

> **Intraop OCT may permit dynamic, real-time guidance to facilitate subretinal PFCL aspiration (Video 57.2).**

POSTOPERATIVE CONSIDERATIONS

- Incomplete removal of small, residual subretinal PFCL bubbles may occur, especially if extrafoveal or if visual prognosis is unlikely to change with further intervention.
- Patients should understand that visual scotomas and vision may not immediately recover, or improve at all, depending on the duration of subretinal PFCL retention.
- Use postop OCT to monitor anatomic restoration of outer retinal layers and guide visual prognosis.

CHAPTER 58

Subretinal Silicone Oil

Jeremy Lavine, MD, PhD • Sumit Sharma, MD

PREOPERATIVE CONSIDERATIONS

- The underlying mechanism for subretinal silicone oil is traction on a retinal break either due to traction from residual vitreous or PDR or PVR membranes.
- To address subretinal silicone oil, identify
  - Undetected posterior hyaloid
  - Vitreous traction
  - Preretinal membranes
  - Subretinal membranes

Surgical Planning

- Manage patient expectations.
  - Subretinal silicone oil suggests that one or more prior surgeries have been performed.
  - Visual outcomes are guarded particularly in the setting of PVR or PDR.
- Anticipate instrumentation.
  - SB. See chapter titled *Scleral Buckling Basics*.
  - Viscous fluid extractor. See chapter titled *Silicone Oil Tamponade*.
  - Maxgrip (Alcon) or similar style forceps.
  - Retinal pick with or without endoillumination
  - Chandelier illumination
  - Diathermy
  - PFCL. See chapter titled *Perfluorocarbon Liquid*.
  - Soft-tip cannula
  - Endolaser. See chapter titled *Endolaser Types and Settings*.
  - Longer tamponade agent: C_3F_8 gas vs silicone oil.

SURGICAL PROCEDURE: SUBRETINAL SILICONE OIL REMOVAL (VIDEO 58.1)

- Consider placing a SB in cases of PVR with subretinal silicone oil.
  - Even if a 180-degree retinectomy is anticipated, the SB can alleviate traction from the vitreous base on the retinectomy edges.
  - SB is not necessary in eyes with 360-degree retinectomy.

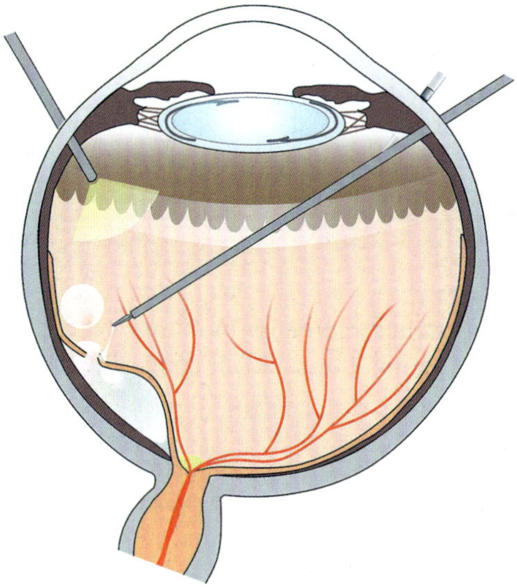

FIGURE 58.1. Remove traction around an existing break, enlarge the preexisting break, and watch silicone oil exit the subretinal space into the vitreous cavity.

- Remove intravitreal silicone oil using the viscous fluid extractor. See chapter titled *Silicone Oil Tamponade*.
- Identify the problematic retinal traction.
  - Segment or delaminate PDR membranes.
  - Peel surface PVR membranes. See chapter titled *Proliferative Vitreoretinopathy Surgery*.
    - Use a pick to identify edges.
    - Stain PVR membranes with triamcinolone when needed. See chapter titled *Intraoperative Visualization Agents*.
    - Use forceps to strip membranes working from posterior to anterior.
- Removal of subretinal silicone oil
  - Remove traction around an existing break, enlarge the preexisting break, and watch silicone oil exit the subretinal space into the vitreous cavity (Fig. 58.1).
  - If there is intrinsic contraction and foreshortening of the retina leading to persistent traction despite membrane peeling, perform a retinectomy (this is the more common scenario in these cases).
    - Use endodiathermy to mark the retinectomy edge and provide hemostasis.
    - Use the vitrector to remove the retina anterior to the diathermy.
    - Then silicone oil will easily exit the subretinal space or flip the retina to allow easier egress of the subretinal silicone oil.
    - Excise or photocoagulate retina anterior to the retinectomy edge to reduce risk of NVI or NVA.

Subretinal Silicone Oil that does not Escape the Subretinal Space

- If silicone oil does not retain its greater buoyancy than BSS, suspect that the retained silicone oil is mixed with PFCL making it heavier.
- In this case, relieve the retinal traction and aspirate the fluid with the vitrector or soft-tip cannula.
- Use the viscous fluid extractor to remove anterior silicone oil that has escaped from the subretinal space.
- Complete the RD repair.
  - Relieve all traction by peeling all preretinal and subretinal membranes and by performing a retinectomy if necessary.
  - Flatten the retina with PFCL.

- Apply endolaser to the retinal breaks and retinectomy edge. See chapter titled *Endolaser Types and Settings.*
- Perform FAX. See chapter titled *Fluid Air Exchange.*
- Use a longer-lasting tamponade agent such as C_3F_8 gas or silicone oil.
  - Do not be afraid to use silicone oil again once all retinal traction has been removed.

SUBRETINAL MEMBRANES

- Subretinal silicone oil changes the subretinal microenvironment.
  - Subretinal membranes in the presence of subretinal silicone oil can behave like preretinal membranes.
    - Suspect sheets of membrane.
    - Subretinal membranes without subretinal silicone oil are typically in cords.
  - Use a lighted pick with blunt edge toward the subretinal space or Tano Diamond Dusted Membrane Scraper (Synergetics) to flip the retina.
  - Use forceps and potentially bimanual technique to peel subretinal membranes.
  - A chandelier can be placed. See chapter titled *The Chandelier Buckle*.
    - Use two forceps or forceps with pick or lighted pick to remove the membranes.

CHAPTER 59

Uveal Effusion Syndrome

Francisco A. Folgar, MD

PREOPERATIVE CONSIDERATIONS

Nonsurgical options include:

- High-dose oral, periocular, or topical corticosteroids. These may have a greater effect in eyes without nanophthalmos and without abnormal scleral thickening.
- Topical prostaglandin analogues
- Oral carbonic anhydrase inhibitors

SURGICAL PROCEDURE: SCLERAL WINDOW SURGERY (VIDEO 59.1)

- Goal: To allow uveal effusions to resolve by reducing scleral resistance and increasing fluid outflow from the uveal tract and suprachoroidal space.
- Perform a 360-degree conjunctival peritomy and blunt dissection of Tenon capsule.
- Isolate each of the four rectus muscles with a muscle hook and 2-0 silk tie loop to expose each oblique quadrant.
- Maintain hemostasis of the sclera with wet-field diathermy.
- Mark the corners of a 5-mm × 5-mm square in each oblique quadrant, with the anterior margin located 3 mm posterior to the rectus muscle insertions.
- Use a No. 57 scleral blade (or similar) to create a 5-mm × 5-mm lamellar scleral flap of about 50%-75% thickness. Start at the anterior margin and retract the flap posteriorly.
- Use a 30-degree corneal blade (or similar) to create a 2.5-mm incision (parallel to the limbus) through the scleral bed, down to the choroid.
- Use a Kelly trabeculectomy punch to widen the incision into an oval scleral window (Fig. 59.1).
- After opening the scleral window, excise the scleral flap with scissors.
- Repeat the procedure in each of the four oblique quadrants.
- Reappose the conjunctiva at the limbus with 7-0 Vicryl or 8-0 plain gut suture.

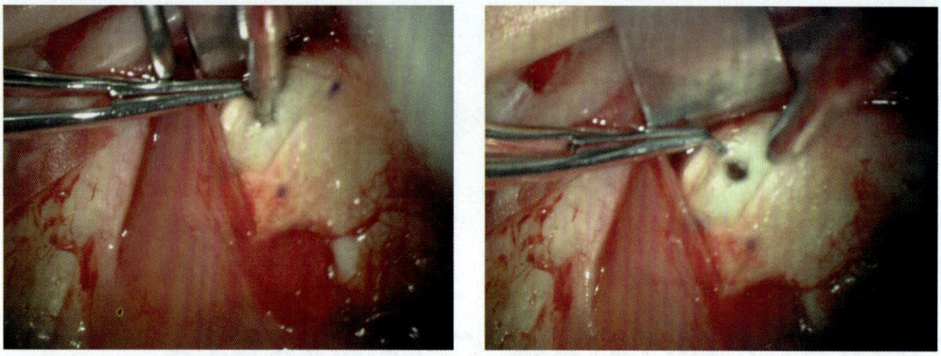

FIGURE 59.1. Use a Kelly trabeculectomy punch to widen the incision into an oval scleral window.

Additional Surgical Considerations

- Create scleral windows in all four oblique quadrants or just the inferotemporal and inferonasal quadrants in cases of inferior uveal effusion.
- Place the excised scleral flaps in formalin for surgical pathology.
- If choroidal perforation occurs intraop, close the scleral window with the scleral flap and Vicryl suture.
- If the globe softens intraop, reform the globe with a 30G intravitreal injection of infusion fluid through the pars plana.
- Use mitomycin C to treat the scleral bed to prevent fibrosis of the scleral window. This may be particularly beneficial in pediatric or repeat surgeries.

POSTOPERATIVE CONSIDERATIONS

Residual nonappositional uveal effusions can take several months to resolve.

CHAPTER 60

Endophthalmitis

Andrew N. Antoszyk, MD

PREOPERATIVE CONSIDERATIONS

An eye with clinical findings consistent with endophthalmitis should be considered infectious until proven otherwise. This is a true ocular emergency.

- Conduct a thorough history to determine if this is postsurgical or posttrauma.
- Consider an endogenous source if not postop or posttrauma.
- Assess anterior segment for defects in sclera and cornea.
- Perform ultrasonography to exclude masquerades (tumor) and determine if there is a concomitant RD, IOFB, and/or choroidal. See chapter titled *Intraocular Foreign Body*.
- Eyes with HM or better vision due to endophthalmitis following intraocular surgery or intravitreal injection may be managed with a vitreous or AC tap and intravitreal antimicrobials. If LP only vision or a concomitant penetrating injury with a retained IOFB, plan PPV and intravitreal antibiotics.
- If an IOFB is suspected, perform B-scan ultrasonography lightly through the eyelids to look for one or more IOFBs. If none are found on B-scan, promptly obtain an orbital CT scan with 1.5 mm cuts to look for IOFBs. An MRI is contraindicated in an eye with a metallic IOFB.
- Order a tetanus shot if not up-to-date.
- Consider systemic antibiotics.

Take a detailed history to narrow down your diagnostic testing and planned treatment. If source unclear, use a "shotgun approach" to treat multiple potential infectious sources with intravitreal antibiotics, antifungals, and antivirals.

Surgical Planning

- Determine what specialized diagnostic testing will be required.
  - If you suspect a postop infection or postinjection infection, obtain cultures from the AC and/or vitreous cavity and send for Gram and fungal stains and anaerobic, aerobic, and fungal cultures. For fastidious organisms, consider PCR testing.

- If a viral (HSV, VZV, CMV) or protozoic (toxoplasmosis) etiology is suspected, then PCR confirmatory testing will be needed.
- Let the OR know what you need, for example, graft material, sutures for corneal and scleral wounds, viscoelastic material to reform the AC or to help reposit exposed uvea, specialized instrumentation for lensectomy, or IOFB removal.
- Let the pharmacy know what you need. Order 0.5 mL of intravitreal ceftazidime 2.25 mg per 0.1 mL and 0.5 mL of vancomycin 1 mg per 0.1 mL. If a fungal etiology is suspected, order 0.5 mL intravitreal amphotericin 5 µg per 0.1 mL or voriconazole 50 µg per 0.1 mL. Use 0.1 mL of each.
- Some surgeons may also choose to inject subconjunctival antibiotics and steroid such as vancomycin 25 mg per 0.5 mL and dexamethasone 4 mg per 1 mL.
- If topical fortified medications are needed, the following formulations may be used:
  - Topical amphotericin B 0.15%
  - Topical voriconazole 1%
  - Topical tobramycin or gentamicin 1.4%
  - Topical vancomycin 5%
  - Topical amikacin 2.5%
  - Topical cefazolin 5%
  - Topical ceftazidime 5%

If PPV cannot be started within about an hour of patient presentation, a vitreous and/or AC tap and intravitreal injection of selected antimicrobials can be performed while waiting.

SURGICAL PROCEDURE (VIDEO 60.1)

- Administer a retrobulbar block of 50:50 mixture of 4% lidocaine and 0.75% bupivacaine. If there is an open globe, then general anesthesia is preferred.
- Prep the eyelashes, eyelids, and periorbital skin using 5% Betadine. Place a lid speculum. For open globes, use a Jaffe lid speculum (Fig. 60.1) that does not place pressure on the globe.
- Insert a 25G valved cannula inferotemporally and place the infusion line but keep the infusion off. See chapter titled *Vitrectomy Surgery Steps*.
- Place superotemporal and superonasal valved cannulas. See chapter titled *Gauge Selection and Cannula Placement*.
- Consider performing an AC tap with 30G needle on a TB syringe. Aspirate 0.1 mL and send for anaerobic, aerobic, and fungal cultures as well as Gram and fungal stains.

If significant fibrin in the AC is obscuring the view of the tip of the infusion in the vitreous cavity, inject viscoelastic into the AC. Insert one of the 25G cannulas temporally into the AC and move the infusion to this cannula. Create an AC paracentesis with a #57 blade and use the vitrector to aspirate and cut the fibrin membrane in the AC to clear the visual axis.

Insert either a 6-mm cannula into the vitreous cavity for the infusion line that is easier to visualize or an infusion line that has a 6-mm tip.

- Prime the infusion line and connect it to the inferotemporal cannula but do not turn the infusion on. Make sure the tip of the infusion line is visualized in the vitreous cavity. Disconnect the tubing at the connection located about 6 inches away

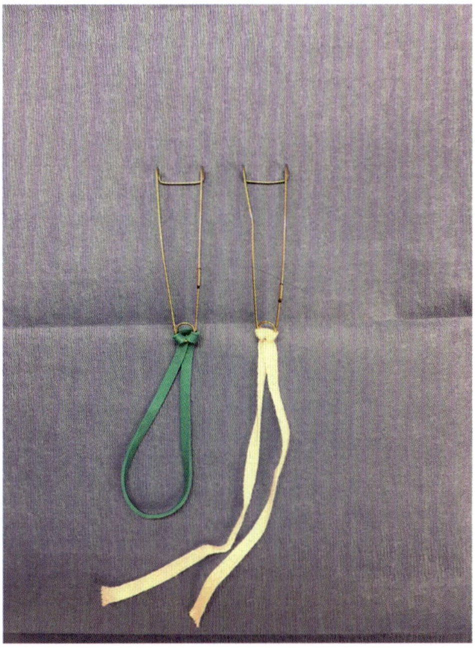

FIGURE 60.1. Jaffe lid speculum does not exert pressure on an open globe.

from the vitreous cutter handpiece. Attach a 10-mL syringe to sterile tubing that is connected to the vitreous cutter handpiece (Fig. 60.2). While cutting with the vitrector, have your assistant manually and slowly aspirate using the 10-mL syringe. Once an adequate undiluted vitreous sample of about 1 mL has been obtained or the eye gets soft, turn on the infusion. Push this undiluted sample through the vitreous cutter handpiece into an Eppendorf tube and send for microbial testing. See chapter titled *Diagnostic Vitrectomy*. Alternatively, aspirate the undiluted sample into the 10-mL syringe that is then capped and send the sample in the syringe to microbiology for Gram stain and culture.

- Once the infusion is turned on and the eye is re-pressurized, obtain an additional diluted vitreous sample again in the same manner with simultaneous cutting and manual aspiration.
- Once the two vitreous samples, diluted and undiluted, are obtained, reattach the sterile tubing so that the vitrectomy can be performed with automated aspiration.
- The view will dictate the degree of vitrectomy that can be completed.
  - Perform only whatever can be safely accomplished.
  - Start with a core vitrectomy and then proceed peripherally as able.
  - Thick plaques of posterior cortical vitreous may be lifted to induce a PVD; however, there is a higher than normal risk of creating iatrogenic breaks.
- Send the cassette from the vitrectomy machine for testing if you did not get sufficient sample.
- Inject the selected intravitreal antimicrobials. Is there a wound leak or open globe?

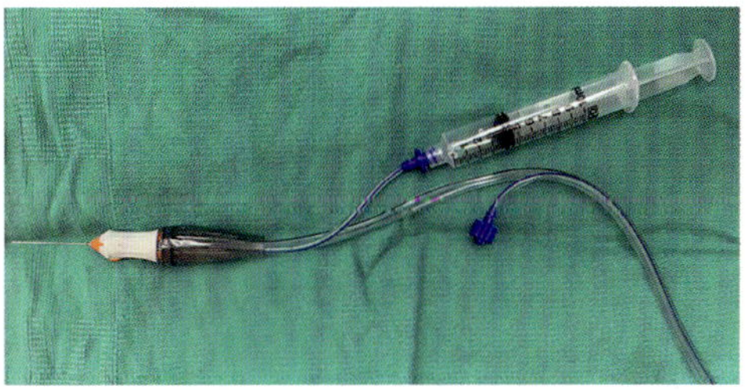

FIGURE 60.2. A 10-mL syringe is attached to sterile tubing that is then connected to the vitreous cutter handpiece to obtain an undiluted vitreous specimen.

- Repair corneal wounds with 10-0 nylon sutures (bury knots) and 7-0 Vicryl or 8-0 nylon sutures for scleral wounds. Corneal melts with perforations may need a corneal graft and scleral defects can be repaired with Tutoplast pericardium or a scleral patch.

Repair wounds and remove IOFBs

- If there is a retained IOFB, remove it promptly at the time of vitrectomy. If the view is poor due to crystalline lens opacification, then perform a lensectomy and as complete a vitrectomy as the view permits. Remove the IOFB. See chapter titled *Pars Plana Lensectomy*.

POSTOPERATIVE CONSIDERATIONS

- The effectiveness of postop systemic antimicrobials is debatable unless the patient has an endogenous source. In this latter scenario, obtain an infectious disease consult to aid in performing a systemic workup to determine the infectious source and to recommend an intravenous antimicrobial regimen. Can consider oral 4th generation fluoroquinolone for 5 days as well.
- Begin oral prednisone 1 mg/kg 24 hours post intravitreal antimicrobials if the eye is otherwise improving. Do not use in cases of endogenous endophthalmitis. Use cautiously in patients with diabetes and in conjunction with the physician managing their diabetes.
- Start topical prednisolone acetate 1% every hour while awake or difluprednate 0.05% every 2 hours while awake on postop day 1.
- Start a topical cycloplegic with homatropine 5% or atropine 1% one drop BID.
- First sign of improvement is often resolution of pain. Repeat intravitreal antibiotics after 48 hours if pain has not resolved or substantially improved and/or if clinical appearance worsens. It is not unusual for any hypopyon to worsen in the initial 24 hours following treatment, even though the eye is improving.
- Base antimicrobial choices on cultures results and sensitivities when available.

CHAPTER 61

Intraocular Foreign Body

Johnathan Warminski, MD • Jawad Qureshi, MD, MBA

PREOPERATIVE CONSIDERATIONS

Up to 41% of open globes can have an IOFB. Remember that there could be more than one IOFB. Ascertain the mechanism of injury and material composition of the IOFB and obtain radiologic imaging with orbital CT scan, in consultation with a radiologist, to allow for analysis of the location and size of the IOFB.

CT imaging of the orbits with thin cuts of 1-1.5 mm is usually the modality of choice to rule out IOFB. CT can detect glass, stone, metal but may not always detect plastic, wood, ceramic, or metal IOFBs smaller than 0.5 mm. Wood may resemble air on CT.

Do not do an MRI if the IOFB may be magnetic. MRI can detect nonmagnetic metallic IOFBs smaller than 0.5 mm as well as wood, glass, ceramic, and plastic.

Evaluate the integrity of the globe, locate the entry site, and identify other findings that may need to be addressed intraop such as hyphema, traumatic cataract, retinal break, choroidal hemorrhage, and RD. Shield the eye if the globe is open. Consider systemic antibiotics prior to surgery. Systemic fluoroquinolones have good intraocular penetrance and a broad profile; vancomycin and a cephalosporin (eg, ceftazidime) are other options. See chapter titled *Endophthalmitis*.

Surgical Timing

When possible, remove the IOFB at the same time as open globe repair. When this is not feasible, remove the IOFB as soon as possible to reduce the risk of infectious endophthalmitis and an inflammatory reaction. It is less than ideal to proceed without appropriate imaging to identify any IOFBs; however, open globe repair should not be delayed if imaging cannot be promptly obtained.

Materials and OR Equipment Often Needed

- Suture
  - Repair the open globe prior to removing the IOFB. Use 8-0 nylon for scleral wounds, 9-0 nylon for the limbal wounds, and 10-0 nylon for corneal wounds.

- Use larger gauge vitrectomy such as 20G or 23G.
- Endolaser
- Endocautery
- Based on the size/shape/composition of the IOFB, consider intraocular forceps, 20G foreign body forceps, 20G intraocular magnet, 20G IOFB snare (eg, commercially available) or Finesse Flex Loop (Alcon), or Prolene suture fashioned as a loop, or external magnet.
- Chandelier illumination, if bimanual approach planned. See chapter titled *The Chandelier Buckle*.
- Use PFCL to protect the macula from IOFB manipulation.
- Silicone oil. See chapter titled *Silicone Oil Tamponade*.
- Viscoelastic, if anterior segment approach is needed.
- Fragmatome, if lensectomy necessary. See chapter titled *Pars Plana Lensectomy*.
- SB, if RD present or if a scleral laceration is present. See chapters titled *Scleral Buckle Basics* and *Retinal Detachment in Open Globe Injury*.

Check that the patient is up-to-date on their tetanus shot.

SURGICAL PROCEDURE (VIDEO 61.1)

No two cases will be alike.

- Close the entry wound.
  - Use 10-0 nylon suture for corneal wounds.
  - Use 9-0 nylon for limbal wounds.
  - Scleral wounds
    - Perform peritomy around limbus and reflect Tenon's with Westcott or Stevens scissors. Caution in the quadrant of the suspected wound.
    - Place 2-0 silk bridle sutures around the rectus muscles with muscle hook.
    - Expose scleral wound, perform Weck-Cel vitrectomy if vitreous present.
    - Close scleral wound with 8-0 nylon suture and evert scleral edges.
    - Consider placing encircling SB for coexisting RD or prophylaxis of RD.
- Repair associated ocular injury and improve intraop view.
  - Hyphema
    - Create paracentesis and wash out AC using BSS.
  - Traumatic cataract
    - Place cannulas as described below.
    - Using a MVR blade, pierce the capsule of the lens at its equator.
    - Insert light pipe and vitrectomy probe into the lens and attempt to vitrectomize the cataract in place.
      - Slow cut rate significantly. See chapter titled *Vitrectomy Machine Settings*.
      - The lens is soft enough to be removed with vitrectomy alone in most IOFB patients.
    - If the 23G vitrectomy probe is insufficient, use the fragmatome before addressing the IOFB. See chapter titled *Pars Plana Lensectomy*.
    - Mark retinal breaks with diathermy and laser after IOFB removal. See chapter titled *Retinal Break Localization*.
    - Consider long-lasting tamponade agent.
  - Concurrent RD
    - If scleral wound is present, then place encircling SB after repair of wound.
    - After IOFB is removed, reattach retina. See chapter titled *Retinal Detachment in Open Globe Injury*.
    - Consider silicone oil for tamponade.

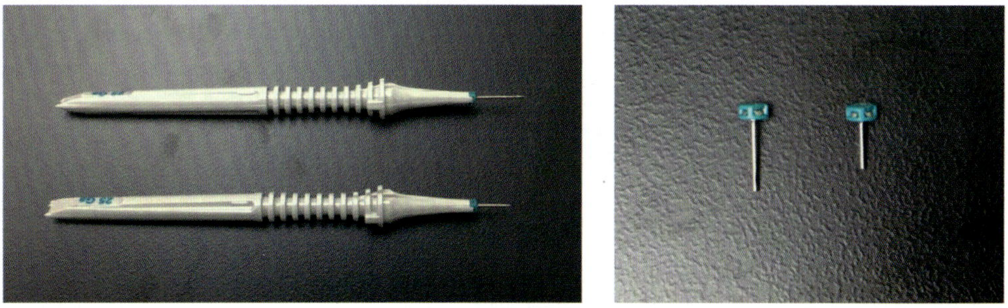

FIGURE 61.1. If poor visualization, use a cannula that is 6 mm long for the infusion line.

- Removal of IOFB
  - Place infusion cannula for PPV. See chapter titled *Gauge Selection and Cannula Placement*.
    - Use a straight/nonbeveled entry to reduce chance of suprachoroidal infusion.
    - If poor visualization, use a 6-mm cannula for infusion line (Fig. 61.1). See chapter titled *Getting and Maintaining Your View*.
  - Place additional cannulas.
    - Use a similar nonbeveled entry.
    - Orient the incision parallel to the limbus to allow for enlargement to remove IOFB if necessary.
  - Perform PPV. See chapter titled *Vitrectomy Surgery Steps*.
    - Create PVD if not already present: stain vitreous with triamcinolone. See chapter titled *PVD Induction*.
    - Carefully shave vitreous base to visualize possible additional foreign material and decrease vitreous snag when removing IOFB.
  - Remove IOFB.
    - Consider placing PFCL to protect macula from inadvertent contact with IOFB.
    - Try not to remove IOFB through the entry wound. Remove IOFB through an enlarged, strategically placed sclerotomy instead. The larger the wound, the easier the removal. Preop CT measurements may guide wound size.
      - Remove one cannula and enlarge the wound with MVR blade.
      - If RD repair needed after IOFB removal, make sclerotomy for IOFB removal at the 12 o'clock position if possible.
      - Consider a limbal wound to remove IOFB in an aphakic eye.
        - Ensure the corneal endothelium is coated with viscoelastic prior to removal.

Sutures placed in limbal wound may cause corneal striae that may make intraop visualization challenging.

- Forceps
  - If IOFB is small, then grasp with intraocular forceps of choice.
  - Consider larger IOFB forceps if available (Fig. 61.2).
  - Grasp oblong IOFB at the smallest end.
- Intraocular magnet
  - Will not hold IOFB strongly enough for removal through a sclerotomy. A bimanual approach is necessary.
  - Place chandelier for illumination.
  - Enlarge sclerotomy to adequate size.
  - Lift IOFB off retina and transfer to forceps for removal (Fig. 61.3).

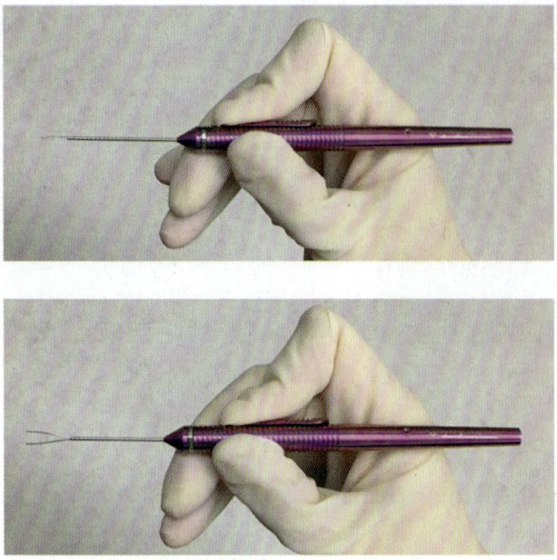

FIGURE 61.2. Consider larger IOFB forceps to remove the IOFB.

- Snare
  - Unusually shaped, round, large foreign bodies often cannot be grasped with forceps and will require a snare. Commercially available snares can be purchased or the Finesse Flex Loop (Alcon) can be used or a snare can be fashioned from Prolene suture (Fig. 61.4).
    - Straight cannula, 25G or 27G anterior segment cannula.
    - 9-0 Prolene suture looped through the cannula.
    - Suture can be retracted by assistant or by capturing in the plunger of BSS-filled syringe.
    - Suture can also be tied at apex with 2 or more loops to create a basket effect.

If not possible to fashion a snare from Prolene suture for an unusually shaped IOFB, insert a 1.5 French NCircle Nitinol Tipless Stone Extractor (Cook Medical) through an enlarged sclerotomy. Once in the vitreous cavity, carefully extend the 1 cm basket out of the instrument shaft. Place the IOFB in the center of the basket and then use the external handpiece knob to tighten the basket around the IOFB. Remove the IOFB from the eye.

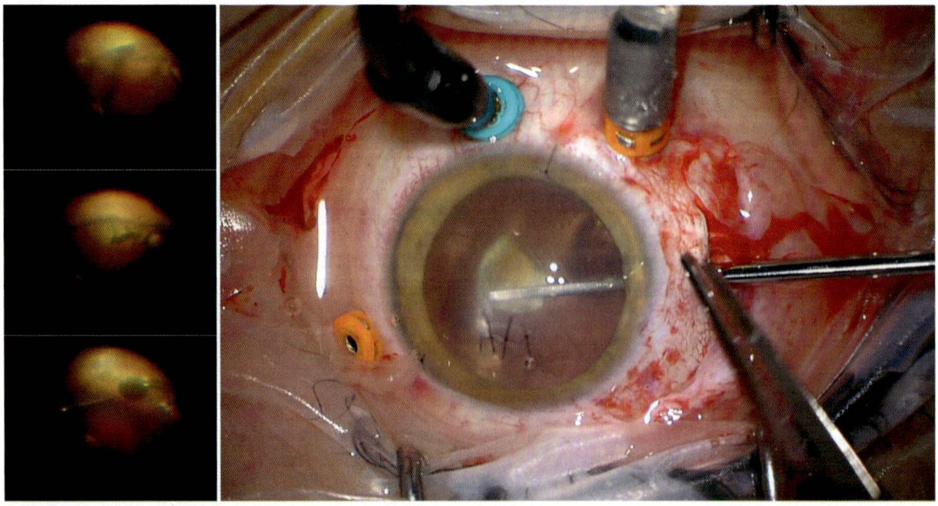

FIGURE 61.3. Lift IOFB off retinal surface and transfer to forceps for removal.

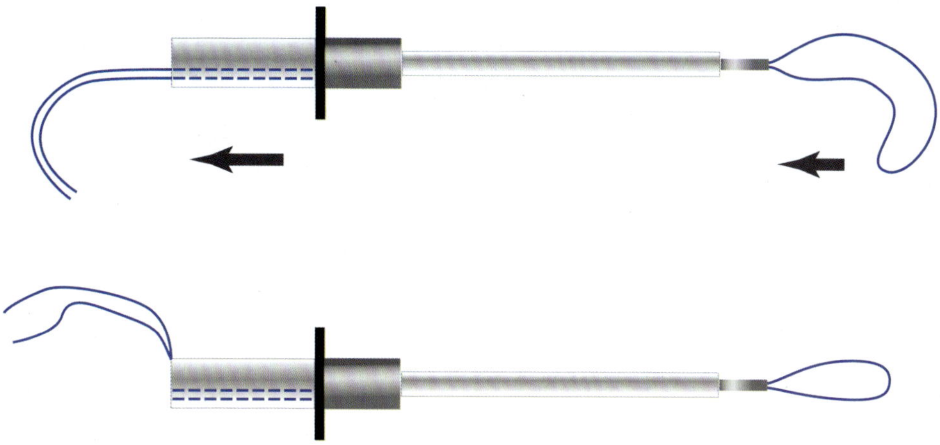

FIGURE 61.4. A Prolene suture snare can be fashioned to assist with IOFB removal.

        - Remove cannula and enlarge sclerotomy to appropriate size.
        - Ensnare the IOFB, tighten, and remove.
        - If IOFB is oblong, then grasp it nearest to the end as possible to ease removal through sclerotomy.
    - Consider external magnet (this approach carries risk of choroidal hemorrhage) if metallic IOFB is embedded in sclera. See chapter titled *Choroidals*.
        - Use transillumination through external sclera to identify IOFB location.
        - Create sclerotomy at site of IOFB to expose embedded IOFB.
        - Use external magnet to remove.
        - Consider repositing or excising any expulsed tissue.
        - Close sclerotomy with 8-0 nylon suture.
- After IOFB removal:
    - Reattach retina if RD present. See chapter titled *Vitrectomy for RRD*.
    - Endolaser to retinal break(s) and possibly endolaser 360 degrees peripherally.
    - Consider silicone oil tamponade vs gas. See chapters titled *Gas Tamponade* and *Silicone Oil Tamponade*.
    - Administer 0.1 mL of intravitreal vancomycin 1 mg/mL and 0.1 mL of ceftazidime 2.25 mg/mL after eye watertight. Check allergies.
- Inject 0.3 mL of subconjunctival vancomycin (50 mg/1 mL) and 0.3 mL of dexamethasone 4 mg/1 mL.

Intravitreal antibiotics are immiscible with silicone oil and thus are concentrated in the fluid surrounding the silicone oil bubble. Because standard antibiotic dosing in an oil- or gas-filled eye can result in retinal toxicity, only 1/10th to 1/4th of the usual dose of intravitreal antibiotics should be used in such cases. Alternatively, consider using standard dosing of intravitreal antibiotics to irrigate the retinal surface prior to FAX. See chapter titled *Endophthalmitis*.

POSTOPERATIVE CONSIDERATIONS

- Have a high index of suspicion for endophthalmitis.
- With that in mind, control postop inflammation with topical steroid. Consider course of systemic steroids in nondiabetics.
- Use topical antibiotic and cycloplegic drops.
- Oral fluoroquinolone for 10 days. Check allergies.
- Monitor closely in the postop period.

CHAPTER 62

Retinal Detachment in Open Globe Injury

Durga S. Borkar, MD • Carl H. Park, MD

PREOPERATIVE CONSIDERATIONS

- Ask whether your patient has had a recent tetanus shot.
- Exclude an IOFB with CT scan and/or B-scan ultrasonography. If the globe is open, perform the B-scan gently through the eyelids. MRI is contraindicated if a metallic IOFB may be present. Remove any IOFB promptly. See chapter titled *Intraocular Foreign Body*.
- Is there a view posteriorly? If not, perform B-scan ultrasonography through the lids to provide information about the status of the posterior segment.
- In general, RDs are not repaired at the time of primary globe repair. An exception may be in cases of localized RD in the setting of a limited globe injury where a retinal break or incarceration site may be seen on direct visualization. Sufficient posterior view in such an instance may allow for repair of the RD at the time of the primary globe repair.
- Repair a localized RD with focal pathology at the time of the primary globe repair and IOFB removal if the view permits. In most cases of significant trauma with IOFB, however, the posterior view is suboptimal and thus closure of the rupture and removal of the IOFB may be the most that can be accomplished during the first surgery.
- If there is an associated VH or RD, perform PPV within 10-14 days after primary closure. If an RD is detected on ultrasonography but there is cataract or corneal opacity, cataract extraction (with or without IOL implantation) and/or temporary keratoprosthesis with penetrating keratoplasty may be needed.
- Is a choroidal detachment present? Is it serous or hemorrhagic? Will it be necessary to drain the hemorrhagic choroidal detachment?
- For very posterior ruptures that could not be completely closed during primary repair, waiting at least 2 weeks may allow for secondary closure of the posterior rupture site.

Surgical Planning

- A detailed, well-documented conversation with the patient will manage expectations about the visual outcome.
  - VA at the time of injury, the configuration of the globe injury/RD, and the presence or absence of an APD can help guide the discussion about visual outcome.
  - Discuss the possibility of a poor visual outcome, loss of the globe, and sympathetic ophthalmia.
- Let the OR team know if you will need any additional instruments that may not otherwise be readily available.
- General anesthesia may be needed since it may not be advisable to perform a retrobulbar block if the globe is open. Also, the length of the procedure and the younger demographic of the open globe injury patient may warrant general anesthesia.
- A 23G surgical platform is often chosen given the diverse instrumentation available and the expected confrontation of fibrous/scar type, tissues which may not engage well with a 25G or 27G vitrector. See chapter titled *Gauge Selection and Cannula Placement*.
- An SB is often placed (if a prophylactic SB was not placed at the time of primary repair) in eyes with posterior segment pathology in addition to performing a PPV.

VIDEO

SURGICAL PROCEDURE: REPAIR OF RD IN EYE WITH OPEN GLOBE INJURY

- Use a sterile drape with an opening for the globe.
- Place a Jaffe lid retractor (Fig. 62.1) and secure with clamps.
- Reform the AC if flat or shallow, using BSS, infusion fluid, or viscoelastic. If a hyphema is present, perform an AC washout. Leaving some viscoelastic as tamponade in the AC during surgery may keep blood out of the AC.
- If hemorrhagic choroidals are present, drain the blood externally through a scleral incision, typically at least 3-4 mm from the limbus. Multiple drainage incisions in different quadrants may be needed. See chapter titled *Choroidals*.

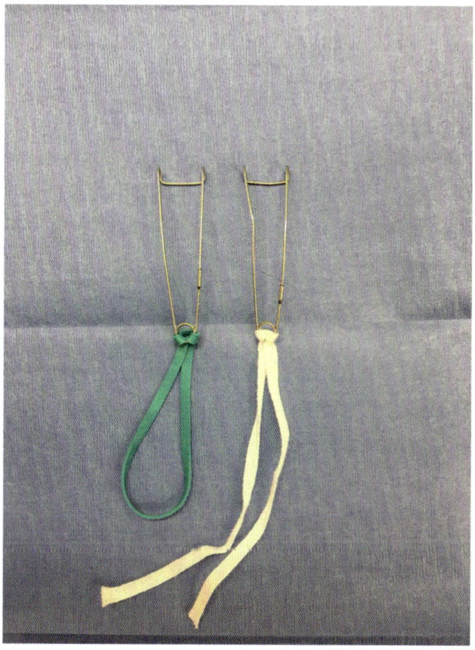

FIGURE 62.1. Jaffe lid retractor.

- Evaluate the location of the scleral laceration and sutures and adjust the placement of the three cannulas. Placement of the cannula into the choroidal space and/or subretinal space may result in iatrogenic damage and complications. See chapter titled *Gauge Selection and Cannula Placement*.
  - In cases where the view is poor and/or an RD or choroidals is suspected, 6-mm cannulas can be helpful in ensuring the proper entry of the distal tip into the vitreous cavity. These longer cannulas are easier to visualize behind the iris and the length also provides better stability to avoid migration of the cannula into the choroidal space intraop.
  - If possible, keep the superior cannulas sufficiently separated to allow for efficient bimanual surgical maneuvers.
  - In some cases, especially when a bullous and/or anterior RD is suspected, insert the trocars 2-3 mm from the limbus and parallel to the iris to avoid further damage to the detached retina upon entry.
- If you cannot see the tip of the infusion cannula in the vitreous, consider an AC maintainer (Fig. 62.2), a combined infusion/light pipe (20G), or a 6-mm infusion line tip if you do not have a 6-mm cannula in place. Place the AC maintainer in a location that avoids the open globe wound and minimizes interference with the vitrectomy instruments.
- Decide if the lens will need to be removed. In cases where the lens interferes with visualization, cyclitic membranes are present, and/or anterior hyaloid hemorrhage is present, consider removing the lens. If the anterior structures are mostly devoid of injury, a straight phacoemulsification through a clear corneal/scleral tunnel incision can be performed. Otherwise, a pars plana lensectomy can be performed utilizing the AC maintainer as the infusion source when needed. See chapter titled *Pars Plana Lensectomy*.
- In most cases, a PVD will be present by day 10 after the injury, but if not, induce a PVD at this stage. Creating a PVD in eyes that are inflamed and with an RD can be challenging. See chapter titled *PVD Induction*. Use the vitreous cutter in suction mode, and in many cases a membrane pick or forceps may also be needed, to separate the posterior hyaloid from the retina. In cases where the RD is long-standing and/or apposed choroidals are present, address the vitreous adhesion anterior to the equator (forceps, vitreous cutter).
- Identify and mark all retinal breaks with diathermy. See chapter titled *Retinal Break Localization*.
- Release all tangential and AP vitreous traction and remove membranes.
- Consider the need for a localized retinectomy circumscribing a retinal incarceration site, if present, with careful hemostasis using endodiathermy. If the incarceration site is in the inferior 180 degrees, consider a 180-degree relaxing retinectomy.
- Decide whether or not the retina is "relaxed" enough to reattach without a retinectomy. Instilling PFCL may help predict whether the retina will be relaxed or taut once flattened. If the retina is taut (especially inferiorly), an inferior 180-degree relaxing retinectomy may be needed. See chapter titled *Proliferative Vitreoretinopathy Surgery*.

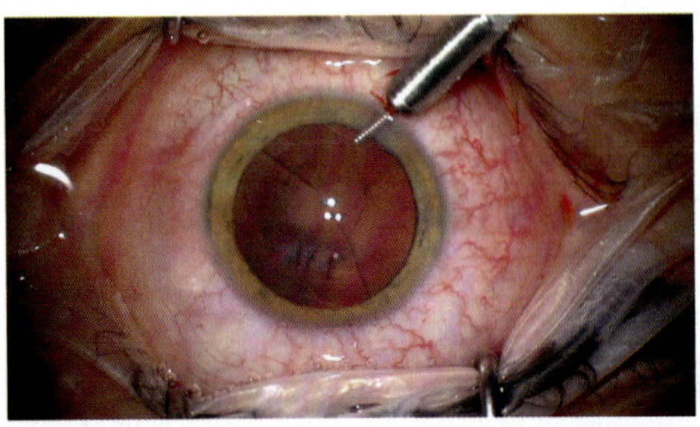

FIGURE 62.2. A straight, corrugated AC maintainer.

- Use PFCL to flatten the retina and drain anterior SRF.
- Apply endolaser to retinal breaks and retinectomy edges.
- In most cases, silicone oil is used as a tamponade. Silicone oil allows for good visualization during the initial healing period to monitor for occurrence of PVR and recurrent RD. Silicone oil is instilled following a PFCL air exchange or utilizing a direct PFCL silicone oil exchange. See chapter titled *Perfluorocarbon Liquid Silicone Oil Exchange*.
    - In eyes that are aphakic or if the lens (either crystalline or implant) is not stable, perform an inferior PI. The PI should be large enough to avoid the possibility of blockage of the opening due to fibrin or buildup of debris.

POSTOPERATIVE CONSIDERATIONS

- The risk of developing PVR and recurrent RD is high. The overall single surgery success rates for retinal reattachment are ~60%. Complications, such as endophthalmitis, are higher after open globe injury compared to standard RD repair.
- In eyes where there is no plan to remove silicone oil (due to the retinal reattachment status, hypotony, and poor prognosis), long-term complications of silicone oil must be monitored, including silicone oil emulsification, inflammation, and increased IOP. See chapter titled *Silicone Oil Tamponade*.
- The fellow eye should be monitored for any signs of sympathetic ophthalmia.
- Advise your patient to wear eye protection with 3 mm polycarbonate lenses.

CHAPTER 63

Macular Hole Retinal Detachment

Max Treacy, BA, BAI, MSc, FRCSI, FRCOphth, FEBO • Mark Cahill, MCh, MMedSci, FRCSI, FRCOphth, FEBO

A FTMH with RD usually occurs in highly myopic eyes. The pathogenesis is unclear, but VMT along with staphylomatous elongation of the eye are thought to contribute, and in these cases, the FTMH is the causative retinal break. The goals of treatment (in order of importance) are to

- Reattach the retina
- Close the FTMH

Macular hole RD is different than a rhegmatogenous RD with a coexisting FTMH, which occurs in 1%-4% of RRD.

PREOPERATIVE CONSIDERATIONS

Choice of Surgery

The main treatment options are scleral imbrication (macular buckle) or PPV or a combined procedure. Scleral imbrication may be especially difficult in myopic eyes with thin sclera. PPV with PVD induction, ILM peel with inverted ILM flap insertion may be more likely to reattach the retina and close the FTMH and that is the procedure described herein. If an inverted ILM flap is not technically possible, then peeling the ILM without a flap would be the next choice. If it is not possible to peel the ILM at all, then just a PPV with creation of a PVD and release of VMT may also work. See chapter titled *PVD Induction*.

Patient Assessment

- Is the eye myopic? Or, pseudophakic but previously myopic with a long axial length?
- Is the fundus anatomy normal? Are there staphylomas or areas of lattice degeneration?
- How extensive is the RD? Is it confined to the macular area or does it extend peripherally?
- Is there a PVD?
- Is the FTMH the causative retinal break or are there other breaks and the FTMH is incidental?
- Is there an ERM?

Patient Counselling

- The condition is neither a straightforward RD nor a straightforward FTMH and the prognosis for restoration of central vision is guarded.
- The retina is especially thin and fragile and the ILM is more difficult to peel safely.
- The published rates of reattachment of retina with and without FTMH closure are highly variable. The largest published retrospective series showed a retinal reattachment rate of 81%, and a FTMH closure with reattachment rate of 48% after one operation.

VIDEO SURGICAL PROCEDURE: PPV AND INVERTED ILM FLAP (VIDEO 63.1)

- Set up standard three-port 23G or 25G vitrectomy (triamcinolone is useful in these cases and the crystals do not flow through 27G instruments as well so a larger gauge is advised).
- In these highly myopic eyes, carefully control the IOP using plugs or valved trocars to avoid hypotony and reduce the risk of choroidal hemorrhage or effusion.
- Use triamcinolone to better visualize the vitreous and check for a PVD.
- If the posterior hyaloid is still attached to the optic disc, use the vitrector to induce a PVD in the standard fashion. See chapter titled *PVD Induction*.

> **Use a lighted pick when the hyaloid is particularly difficult to lift.**
> **Use a flat macular contact lens for enhanced visualization. See chapter titled *Lenses and Viewing Systems*.**

- Propagate the PVD carefully, remembering that a myopic eye may have coexisting peripheral retinal changes such as lattice degeneration that may make iatrogenic peripheral tears more likely.
- Inject ICG (see chapter titled *Intraoperative Visualization Agents*) or other dye such as Brilliant Blue G (if available) over the posterior pole.
  - Allow the ICG to sit and stain the ILM for 30 seconds and then aspirate it out.
  - Allow the Brilliant Blue G to sit on the posterior pole for 2 minutes, then aspirate it out.
- Use a Finesse Flex Loop (Alcon) or Tano Diamond Dusted Membrane Scraper (Synergetics) to carefully initiate a flap of lifted ILM. Avoid scratching the bare retinal surface.

> **In a right eye, start the flap close to the optic disc along the direction of the inferior arcade (assuming a right-handed surgeon). In the left eye, start the flap temporal to the fovea along the direction of the inferior arcade.**

- Use an end-gripping or ILM forceps to complete the ILM peel in a circular manner around the fovea to create a doughnut-shaped area of retina stripped of ILM with an island of attached ILM around the FTMH (Fig. 63.1). This island should be ~1.5 times the size of the optic disc.
- Extend the ILM that is still attached anterior to the circular peel at least as far as the arcades. Perform larger than normal ILM peels in eyes with a posterior staphyloma, RD due to FTMH, and large FTMH.
- Lift the circular island of attached ILM around the FTMH in a centripetal fashion toward the center of the FTMH so it is entirely reflected off the surface of the retina,

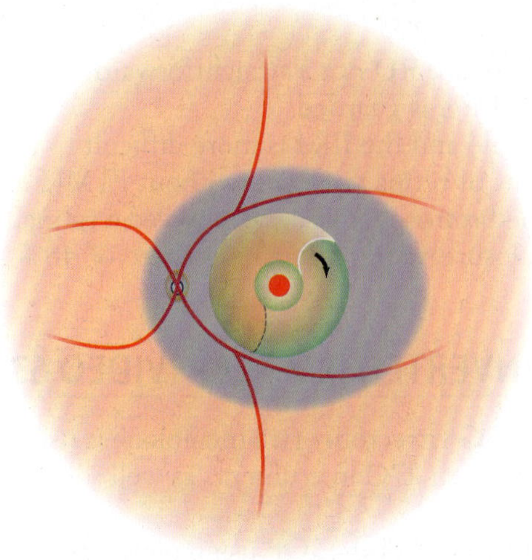

FIGURE 63.1. Use an end-gripping or ILM forceps to complete the ILM peel in a circular manner around the fovea such that there is a doughnut-shaped area of retina stripped of ILM with an island of attached ILM left around the FTMH.

except for a central cuff of attachment around the rim of the MH. Fold this frilled collar of ILM over the MH and this is the inverted ILM flap (Fig. 63.2). It can be difficult to get the inverted flap to stay in the FTMH, particularly in these cases where the retina is detached. A blob of viscoelastic can be placed over the MH and inverted flap to hold the flap in place. See chapters titled *Macular Hole* and *Advanced Vitrectomy Techniques for Macular Holes* for other methods of performing an ILM flap for FTMH.

- Perform 360-degree scleral depression and treat any peripheral pathology with endolaser or external cryotherapy.
- If the RD only extends to the arcades, do not drain SRF. However, if the SRF extends beyond the arcades, create a small drainage retinotomy. See chapter titled *Posterior SRF During Vitrectomy for RRD* for drainage retinotomy tips. Prior to the FAX, use diathermy to make the drainage retinotomy site. Then, using a soft-tip cannula, the SRF can be drained during the FAX. Maintain the pressure in the subretinal space relatively less than or equal to the vitreous cavity so that the inverted flap and viscoelastic blob is not blown upward out of the FTMH. During the FAX, the retinotomy should be the most dependent part of the posterior pole and the entire FAX should be completed with the soft-tip cannula held there, rather than over the optic disc.

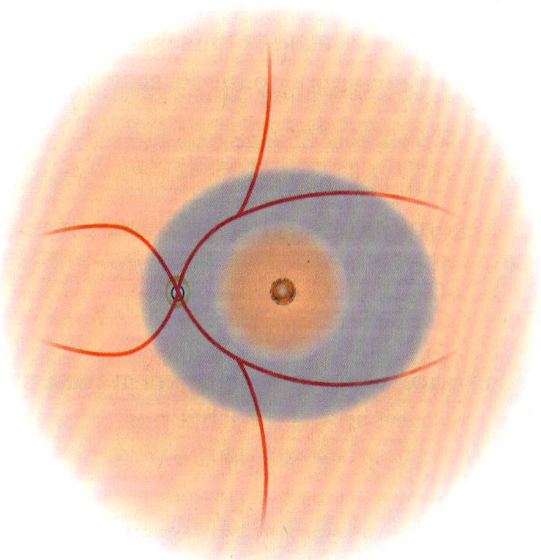

FIGURE 63.2. Inverted ILM flap. Carefully lift the circular island of attached ILM around the FTMH in a centripetal fashion toward the center of the FTMH so that it is entirely reflected off the surface of the retina except for a central cuff of attachment around the rim of the MH. Fold this frilled collar of ILM over the FTMH.

- When the FAX is complete, apply gentle laser retinopexy to the edge of the retinotomy.
- Perform an air gas exchange. Total of 14% C_3F_8 gas provides a longer tamponade in these more complicated cases. See chapter titled *Gas Tamponade.*

If it is not possible to fashion an inverted ILM flap, drain through the FTMH (rather than make a drainage retinotomy) but do this very slowly and carefully so as not to enlarge the FTMH or touch the underlying RPE. Leave a small amount of fluid behind rather than risk touching the subfoveal RPE.

POSTOPERATIVE CONSIDERATIONS

Instruct the patient to posture facedown postop: 45 minutes out of every hour while awake and to sleep on the right side for the left eye and on the left side for the right eye. See chapter titled *Postoperative Positioning.*

If the operation fails to reattach the retina, it may be necessary to reoperate to extend the ILM peel, make absolutely sure that there are no PVR or vitreoschitic membranes and to use silicone oil as a tamponade.

CHAPTER 64

Retinoschisis Retinal Detachment

Harsha A. Sen, MD

PREOPERATIVE CONSIDERATIONS

A RRD secondary to retinoschisis usually develops when there is a retinal break in both the inner and outer layers of the retinoschisis cavity, creating contiguous communication between the liquefied vitreous in the vitreous cavity and the subretinal space. However, fluid within the schisis cavity itself can migrate through an outer layer break and create a localized RD in association with the schisis cavity, even in the presence of an intact inner layer. Distinguishing between a simple schisis cavity and one with part or all of the outer layer elevated can be challenging, especially if the outer break is large, irregular, thin, or the rim of the break is contiguous with the margin of the schisis cavity. Schisis fluid is thick, so the inner surface of the schisis detachment may continue to resemble simple schisis, that is, be convex, smooth, and transparent, as opposed to corrugated, mobile, and more opaque as is typical of RRD. Careful clinical examination using indirect ophthalmoscopy with scleral depression is often needed to make an accurate assessment. Imaging the more posterior areas of retinal elevation with OCT can distinguish the various layers and be diagnostic. In eyes with RRD, OCT will show SRF under full-thickness retina. In eyes with retinoschisis, OCT will show splitting of the retina without SRF (Fig. 64.1A and B). See chapter titled *RRD vs Exudative RD vs Retinoschisis*.

Management Considerations

- Retinoschisis without inner or outer layer breaks
  - Observe, as this can remain stable for years.
- Retinoschisis with inner layer breaks
  - Inner retinal breaks may be round and atrophic or tractional (irregular, jagged, horseshoe) and may be associated with lattice degeneration.
  - As long as there are no outer layer breaks, the schisis cavity can remain stable for years, even with large or multiple inner breaks.
  - Periodic monitoring for the development of outer layer breaks is prudent, particularly if vitreoretinal traction is present or the outer layer is thin.

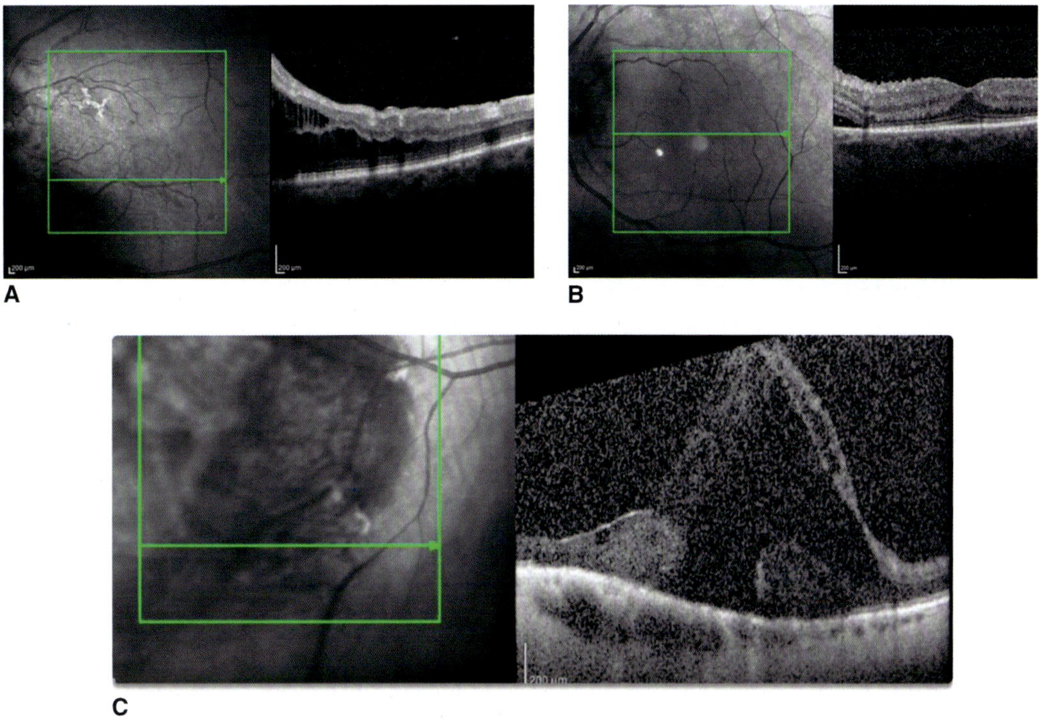

FIGURE 64.1. **A.** OCT of an eye with retinoschisis. Intraretinal fluid is present which by definition is within the neurosensory retina. There is no SRF. **B.** OCT of an eye with a rhegmatogenous RD. SRF is present which by definition is under full-thickness retina. Sometimes, there may also be intraretinal fluid (not pictured). **C.** OCT of an eye with retinoschisis and an outer layer break. Intraretinal fluid is evident in the inner layer of the schisis cavity. There is an outer layer break but no SRF and thus, no retinal detachment.

- Retinoschisis with outer layer breaks
  - If the area of schisis is small, this may be observed, particularly if located inferiorly, even if SRF is present.
  - Small retinoschisis RDs, especially in an inferior location, can remain stable for years.
  - Larger areas of retinoschisis may contain significant intraretinal fluid, which can migrate into the subretinal space and even detach the macula in the absence of a coexisting inner layer break. Consider barrier laser photocoagulation of all outer layer breaks prior to the development of SRF.
  - Consider barrier laser photocoagulation or surgical management (eg, primary SB) of localized retinoschisis-related RDs associated with moderate to large schisis cavities.
- Retinoschisis with both inner layer breaks and outer layer breaks
  - This is the highest risk condition, warranting management similar to RRD. Consider barrier laser photocoagulation for localized peripheral RD.
  - Larger RD, even if not involving the macula, may have better long-term results if managed surgically. A retinoschisis RD involving the macula requires surgical management.

SURGICAL PROCEDURE (VIDEO 64.1)

The principles of repair of retinoschisis RD are the same as for primary RRD. See chapters titled *Retinal Break Localization* and *Scleral Buckling Basics*.

- Find and treat all causative breaks, which in retinoschisis RDs are the outer layer breaks.

- Relieve vitreoretinal traction.
- Reappose the outer retina to the RPE.
- Maintain retina-RPE apposition during the postop period.

Many of these patients are younger and phakic. If the area of RD is localized and the outer layer breaks are small and peripheral, consider a primary SB with cryopexy of the outer layer breaks and external drainage of subretinal and schisis fluid using standard radial sclerotomy with choroidal puncture or transscleral needle drainage techniques. See chapters titled *External Subretinal Fluid Drainage* and *Posterior Subretinal Fluid During PPV for RRD*.

Remember, outer layer breaks may be quite posterior.

However, these are often complex cases that require PPV with internal drainage of fluid from multiple layers and gas or silicone oil tamponade. The causative outer layer breaks may be large, posterior, and multiple. Broad anteroposterior and tangential vitreous traction may be present, and multiple layers of the retina may be elevated, each with loculated fluid. In approaching these complex cases:

- Find and treat all the outer layer breaks, which are the causative breaks. The inner layer breaks do not necessarily require treatment. If the outer layer is very thin, an outer break may be obscured intraop by edema of the elevated inner layer, even after FAX. These may become evident postop and can be encircled with laser in the office.
- Relieve all vitreoretinal traction. Vitreous traction in retinoschisis RD can be significant and extensive. Consider an encircling buckle, such as a #240 band with a #220 strip or #286 tire element supporting the areas of pathology in eyes with significant peripheral traction, especially if phakic, as the posterior hyaloid may be so tightly adherent to the inner layer that the hyaloid cannot be peeled from the retina. See chapter titled *Scleral Buckling Basics*. Excise the inner and occasionally outer layers in the involved area(s) using relaxing retinectomy techniques. See chapter titled *Proliferative Vitreoretinopathy Surgery*.
- Reappose the outer retina to the RPE. Schisis fluid is thick and can take months to years to reabsorb, or may remain unabsorbed. Drain as much of the subretinal and intraretinal fluid as possible. Complete internal drainage may require one or, in the case of multiple noncontiguous areas of schisis detachment, multiple drainage retinotomies. Use existing outer layer break(s) to drain SRF if suitably located by creating a retinotomy in the overlying inner layer.
- Tamponade to maintain postop retinal apposition. Gas tamponade may be adequate for RD with superior and peripheral breaks, and for simpler cases. Complex cases, particularly those involving inferior pathology, multiple breaks, and/or collections of SRF in different quadrants, paramacular breaks, loculated intraretinal fluid, or cases requiring relaxing retinectomy carry significant risk of early redetachment due to insufficient duration of tamponade over the affected areas. For these cases, silicone oil tamponade allows consistent long-term tamponade over a large area of retina and allows the best postop visualization regardless of lens status. See chapter titled *Silicone Oil Tamponade*.

POSTOPERATIVE CONSIDERATIONS

If retinal breaks that were not evident intraop become evident once the retina is reattached and retinal edema has resolved, the visualization afforded by silicone oil facilitates postop laser treatment in the office.

CHAPTER 65

Postop Retinal Fold

Akshay S. Thomas, MD, MS • Avni P. Finn, MD, MBA

PREOPERATIVE CONSIDERATIONS

Risk Factors for Development of a Retinal Fold

- Superior bullous RD
- High circumferential SB creating redundant retina
- Gas tamponade
- Incomplete SRF drainage
- Poor postop positioning

To avoid the development of a retinal fold following RD surgery, see chapter titled *Postop Positioning*.

Surgery is Indicated for a Postop Retinal Fold if:

- The retinal fold involves the macula and is full thickness.
  - Full-thickness retinal folds are unlikely to resolve on their own, while partial-thickness folds, especially those not involving the fovea, may be observed.
- The patient is symptomatic with reduced vision, metamorphopsia, or diplopia.
  - If you decide to intervene surgically for a full-thickness macular fold, early intervention may be favorable as the retinal fold may flatten more easily.

SURGICAL PROCEDURE: MANAGEMENT OF POSTOP RETINAL FOLD

- Set up for a standard 3-port vitrectomy. See chapter titled *Vitrectomy Surgery Steps.*
- Remove any residual tamponade agent leftover from the previous surgery.
- Using a 41G subretinal cannula, induce a paramacular RD with BSS.
  - Create SRF blebs at one or more locations (Fig. 65.1).
  - Try not to detach the fovea even if the retinal fold involves the fovea during this step to avoid creating a FTMH.
- Perform a FAX. See chapter titled *Fluid Air Exchange.*
  - This forces the SRF posteriorly, which helps coalesce the SRF blebs and detaches the fovea in a more controlled fashion.

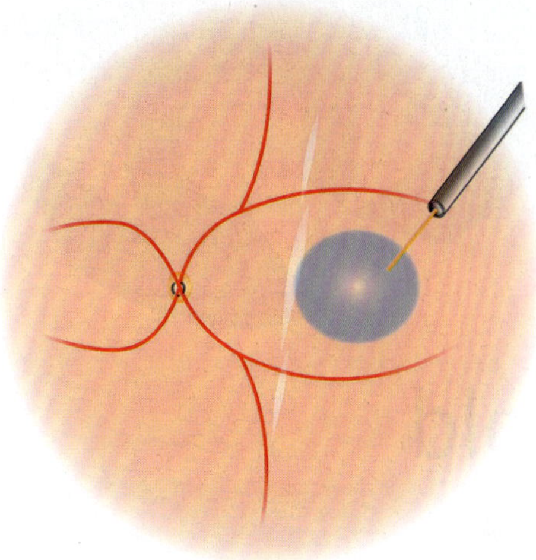

FIGURE 65.1. Using a 41G subretinal cannula, induce a paramacular RD with BSS. Create SRF blebs at one or more locations.

- Perform an air fluid exchange.
  - Perform this step by either venting air out of a cannula or passively aspirating air with a backflush cannula. Active aspiration of air can collapse the eye as the infusion may not be able to keep up with active aspiration of air.
- Massage the retinal fold gently with a Tano Diamond Dusted Membrane scraper (Synergetics) or Finesse Flex Loop (Alcon).
- Flatten the macula with PFCL.
  - You could consider skipping the air fluid exchange and attempt to flatten the retina under air. However, visualization may be suboptimal and there is a greater chance of creating a new retinal fold if retina is flattened with PFCL under air.
  - Confirm that the retinal fold has flattened under PFCL.
    - If it has not, massage the fold further.
  - Continue to inject PFCL until the SRF has been pushed peripherally.
- Create a small drainage retinotomy peripherally using diathermy.
  - In the case of a giant retinal fold following surgery for a GRT or following a case in which a retinectomy was created, a drainage retinotomy may not be adequate. In such cases, the lasered retinectomy or GRT edge may need to be elevated with forceps, flattened with PFCL, and then lasered.
- Drain SRF through the drainage retinotomy and then remove all PFCL.
- Confirm once again that the retinal fold has not recurred.
- Laser the drainage retinotomy.
- Perform an air gas or air silicone oil exchange and position the patient facedown for the first 48-72 hours. See chapters titled *Air Gas Exchange* and *Air Silicone Oil Exchange.*

CHAPTER 66

Vitrectomy With the Endoscope

Brendan Seto, BA • Jorge Arroyo, MD, MPH

PREOPERATIVE CONSIDERATIONS

- **Bypassing anterior segment opacities**
  Sometimes, anterior segment opacities do not allow a view of the fundus, yet vitreoretinal surgery is needed. Such scenarios may include eyes with an IOFB, endophthalmitis, corneal scarring, or open globe injury, particularly ascertaining viability of optic nerve and retina after open globe injury with no view. In these scenarios, use of an endoscope may be considered.
  Considerations
  - Timing of vitreoretinal surgery
    - How urgent is it?
    - Can it wait until the media opacity or other anterior segment condition is resolved?
  - Endoscopy vs keratoplasty? Specific contraindications for keratoplasty that do not impede endoscopy use include:
    - Grossly deformed anterior segment structures
    - Severe autoimmune ocular surface diseases
    - Consideration of silicone oil use in eyes with no iris diaphragm and poor anatomy for iris retention sutures
- **Unique viewing plane**
  In some clinical situations, a particular viewing plane may be needed. Some examples include endocyclophotocoagulation for glaucoma, trauma (sutured IOLs, sub-iris and ciliary body abscesses, and anterior PVR), when aggressive scleral depression is contraindicated (open globe injury, unstable IOL, and filtering blebs), visualization of anterior structures or subretinal space, visualization of vitreous in ROP detachments.
- **Limitations of the endoscope**
  - No stereopsis
  - No shadowing
  - Narrow field of view with "first person shooter" view, rather than "bird's-eye"
  - No bimanual techniques

Even if the endoscope allows for bypass of anterior opacification, the postop exam is still limited. Diligent ultrasonography or further procedures may be required.

SURGICAL PROCEDURE

- The modern endoscope comes in a 23G system, which fits through 23G trocars, or a 19G system placed through a sclerotomy.
- The endoscope is primarily composed of three parts:
  - Camera
  - Light source (300 W)
    - Camera and light source are housed by a base unit, which transmits images through fiber optics to the handpiece and connects to a monitor and image capture unit.
    - The video feed can be viewed simultaneously on a 3D heads up display.
  - Laser unit (810 nm diode laser with pulses of 50-2000 ms and power of 0-1200 mW)
    - Can also be incorporated into base unit or attached as a separate component with a footswitch control.
- Set-up (Video 66.1)
    - Power on endoscope.
    - Choose tip: straight for PPV, curved for anterior dissection.
    - Connect 23G or 19G endoscope probe to illumination and laser ports on machine.
    - Focus endoscope by aiming at text on paper and then rotating knob at the endoscope port (Fig. 66.1).
    - Orient endoscope by rotating endoscope port attachment.
    - Set laser power to 0.5-1.2 W depending on level of tissue pigmentation.
    - Set duration to continuous laser. See chapter titled *Endolaser Types and Settings.*
    - Set illumination to highest level possible.
    - Turn laser from standby to active.
    - Set aiming beam intensity to 30.

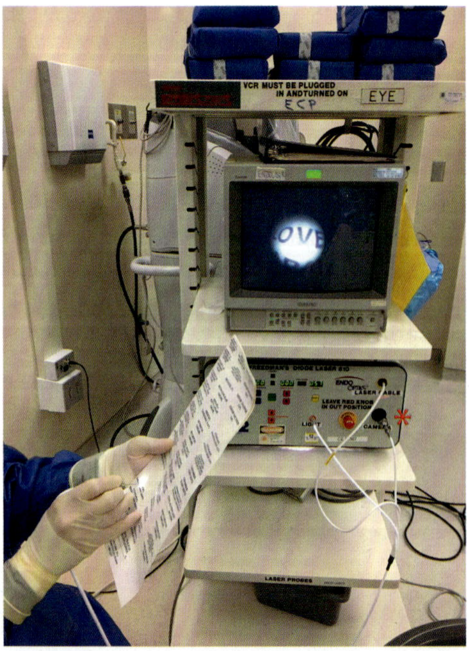

FIGURE 66.1. Focus endoscope by aiming at text on paper and then rotating knob at the endoscope port.

- Foot pedal
  - Depress for laser.
  - Right to increase illumination.
  - Left to decrease illumination.
- Use of endoscope
  - Orient endoscope image outside of the eye (Fig. 66.1).
  - Enter eye through 23G cannula or 19G sclerotomy.
    - For 19G sclerotomy, approach sclerotomy at a 45-degree angle and twist probe to facilitate entry into vitreous cavity.
  - Begin by using endoscope probe only as a light pipe during case.
  - Alternate views inside eye between microscope view and endoscope view.
  - As your comfort increases, begin utilizing the endoscopic view for peripheral vitreous base dissections.
- Use of endoscopic laser
  - Set laser intensity to 0.8-1.2 W for retinal laser photocoagulation depending on level of RPE pigmentation.
  - Set laser intensity to 0.3-0.5 W for endoscopic cyclophotocoagulation.
  - Utilize distance of probe tip to retinal structures to modulate laser power absorption.
  - Be careful with retinal laser close to the macula, given narrower field of view. Pull probe back regularly to re-orient location of nerve and macula.
  - During PRP, initially and carefully place laser spots to demarcate the posterior extent of laser.

With repeated use of the probe, black spots may appear in the image, signifying broken fibers in the fiberoptic bundle. Never kink the fiberoptic bundle. Replace endoscope probe as needed.

If tip of endoscope fogs up during FAX, use soft-tip cannula to wipe tip of probe when inside the eye. See chapter titled *Fluid Air Exchange*.

CHAPTER 67

Optic Pit Maculopathy

Wenlan Zhang, MD • Eric Postel, MD

There are no fixed guidelines for treatment, although a number of techniques have been described, including observation, laser adjacent to the pit at the temporal disc margin, intravitreal gas, macular buckling, and PPV with/without adjuvant techniques such as PVD induction, peripapillary laser (as above), ILM peeling, ILM flap, ILM plug, placement of platelet rich plasma, gas tamponade, etc. These techniques are guided by case reports/case series without the availability of comparative studies.

This rare congenital optic disc anomaly is unilateral, sporadic, and associated with intraretinal fluid and/or SRF in the macula with progressive vision loss. The source of the fluid is unclear and theories abound (vitreous fluid, CF, leakage from blood vessels at pit base, choroidal leakage). Rates of optic disc maculopathy in those with pits vary from 25% to 75%.

PREOPERATIVE CONSIDERATIONS

- Is there another explanation for macular intraretinal fluid and SRF?
- Consider initial monitoring (at least 3 months) as spontaneous resolution with VA improvement has been reported in up to 25% of cases. However, recurrences may be common and persistent fluid may result in RPE atrophy and subsequent VA deterioration.
  - Use this monitoring period to educate patient about clinical and surgical options.
- Is there any vitreous traction that might be contributing to optic pit maculopathy?
  - If there is evidence of partial vitreous separation, consider monitoring through completion of PVD to see if this leads to spontaneous resolution.
- Careful discussion of risks of intervention.
  - Laser: possible visual field defects, may take time for effects to manifest.
  - Intraocular gas: positioning issues, gas precautions.
  - PPV: infection, bleeding, MH, RD, IOP issues, positioning, etc.
  - Macular buckling: technically challenging, special equipment, few have expertise.
- If plan is proceeding with PPV, weigh risks and benefits of additional adjuvant steps.

- If platelet rich plasma is planned,
  - Make sure all equipment is in the room and OR staff knows how to set up for platelet rich plasma.
  - Ensure second IV is placed for ease of drawing blood when ready for sample *prior* to prep and drape.
  - Make sure the centrifuge is in the room, including the balance for centrifuge.
  - Review with OR scrub and circulator how to draw platelet rich plasma from spun-down sample.

SURGICAL PROCEDURE (VIDEO 67.1)

- Set up for a standard three-port PPV. See chapter titled *Vitrectomy Surgery Steps.*
- Induce a PVD. See chapter titled *PVD Induction.*
- If ERM/ILM peeling planned, perform this in the standard fashion, though some will hinge the ILM flap at the temporal edge of the disc to essentially create an inverted ILM flap over the optic pit (Fig. 67.1; Video 67.1). See chapter titled *Macular Hole* for tips.
- If you plan to use platelet-rich plasma, perform FAX first before adding 1-2 drops over pit and/or flap.

Platelet-rich plasma preparation. See chapter titled *Advanced Vitrectomy Techniques for Macular Holes.*

Collect autologous whole blood from the peripheral IV (2nd IV placed preop).
Centrifuge in tabletop centrifuge to fractionate platelet-rich plasma (Fig. 67.2).
Collect fractionate in a 5-mL syringe.
Connect syringe to a 25G dual-bore cannula.
Use within 20 minutes.

- Endolaser or not to area just temporal to pit. See chapter titled *Endolaser Types and Settings.*
  - Keep in mind that if there is significant SRF, laser uptake may be limited.
  - Only a light laser treatment should be done, if performed.

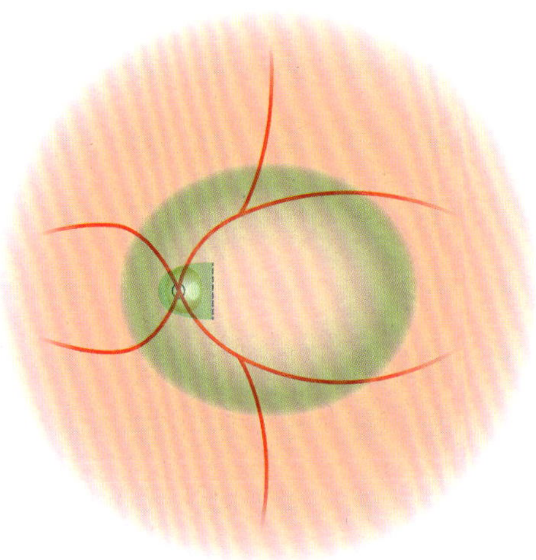

FIGURE 67.1. If ERM/ILM peeling planned, perform this in a standard fashion, though some will hinge the ILM flap at the temporal edge of the disc to essentially create an inverted ILM flap over the optic pit.

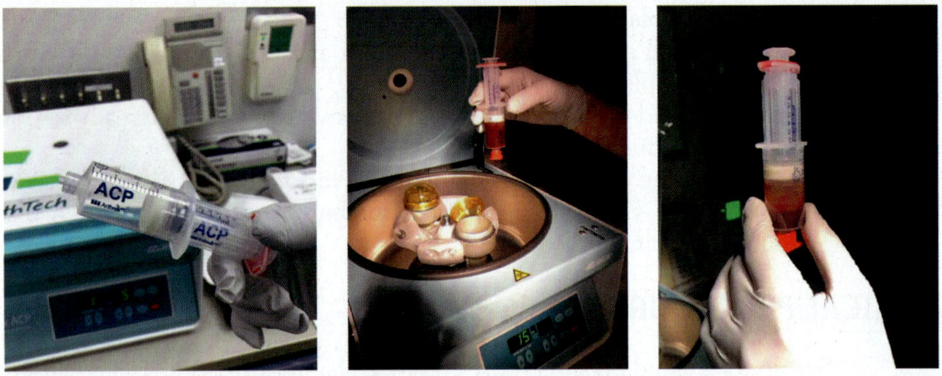

FIGURE 67.2. Centrifuge the whole blood in Arthrex Rotofix tabletop centrifuge to fractionate the plasma from the cellular components at 1500 rpm for 5 minutes. This will separate the whole blood into red blood cells and white blood cells at the bottom and a supernatant containing platelets in the bottom one-third and platelet poor plasma on the top two-thirds.

- Gas tamponade or not. Gas selection is surgeon preference. See chapter titled *Gas Tamponade.*
- Consider use of intraop OCT (if available).

Be careful with possibility of subretinal migration of tamponade, particularly PFCL and silicone oil, although air and gas can also migrate through the optic pit. Care in postop positioning has been suggested to minimize this risk.

POSTOPERATIVE CONSIDERATIONS

The time required for anatomic and visual improvement is variable and can be lengthy (months).

CHAPTER 68

Argus II Retinal Prosthesis

Paul Hahn, MD, PhD

The Argus II retinal prosthesis (Second Sight Medical Products, Inc., Sylmar, CA) was FDA approved in 2013 (and obtained the European CE mark in 2011) for patients with end-stage RP. The device consists of a surgically implanted array that communicates wirelessly with a camera-embedded pair of custom glasses.

PATIENT ELIGIBILITY

- FDA approval is currently only for adults with RP and bare or no light perception vision in both eyes.
- Conditions that may prevent adequate implantation of the Argus II:
  - Conjunctival thinning
  - Axial length <20.5 mm or >26 mm (given the fixed intraocular cable length)
  - Conditions that prevent implant visualization such as corneal opacities or other media opacity
  - Phakic patients will require removal of the lens prior to or during Argus II implantation.
- The device cannot be implanted in patients with a cochlear implant or other metallic/active implantable device in the head.

PREOPERATIVE CONSIDERATIONS

- Ideal patients will have appropriate expectations and dedication to visual rehabilitation.
- Make sure that you have several specialized instruments:
  - Angled forceps with silicone sleeves (to safely handle cable and array)
  - 20G Eckhardt end-gripping forceps (for insertion/positioning of array)
  - 19G Tack forceps
  - Second Sight laptop and probe (to test device; operated by Second Sight field engineer in OR)
- Surgery is performed under general anesthesia.

Special Considerations

- Implant (coil, cable, and array) must be handled carefully with silicone-tipped forceps, avoiding any sharp or toothed instruments, which can damage the delicate electronics.
- The array will be tested intraop before, during, and after surgery with a diagnostic laptop computer and probe operated by a Second Sight field engineer present during the case.

SURGICAL PROCEDURE: ARGUS II IMPLANTATION (VIDEO 68.1)

- Perform 360-degree conjunctival peritomy. Avoid radial incisions supero- and inferotemporally where the bulk of the implanted device lies.
- Isolate each of the four rectus muscles with a silk traction suture.
- Carefully remove the implant from its packaging.
- Pass the implant and straps under the isolated rectus muscles such that the electronics case is in the superotemporal quadrant and the coil is in the inferotemporal quadrant. A Watzke sleeve is used to secure the straps to each other, avoiding tension that will elongate the axial length.

The array can be optionally protected with a cover (eg, a phaco tip cover or the tip of a sterile glove loosely tied around the cable).

- Secure the electronics case to the underlying sclera first then the coil (followed by the implant straps) with 5-0 Mersilene (Dacron) suture at distances prespecified by a nomogram based on axial length provided by Second Sight. The suture knots should be positioned to minimize risk of conjunctival erosion.

The placement of securing sutures to the electronics case is critical to properly orient the implant. The final position of the intraocular cable and array will be predetermined in a large part by the accurate placement of these extraocular sutures.

TIP: The cable should be centered when reflected over the cornea (Fig. 68.1). If not, the securing sutures should be carefully inspected and repositioned if needed.

- Perform vitrectomy with vitreous base shaving, particularly superotemporally where the array is inserted and nasally where the Tack forceps are inserted.

TIP: The temporal and nasal ports should be placed at 3:00 and 9:00 to avoid the insertion site of the cable superotemporally and facilitate tack placement nasally.

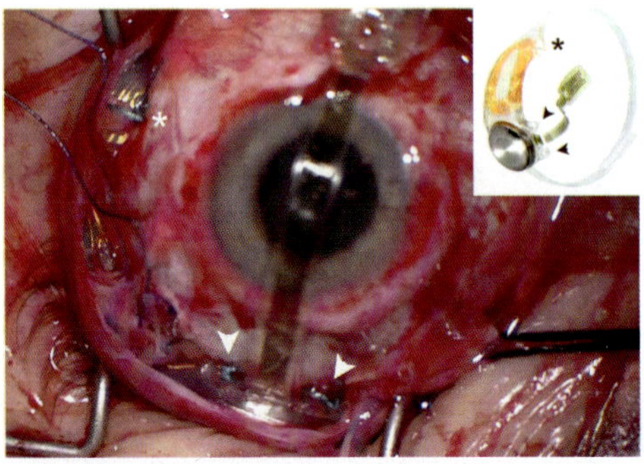

FIGURE 68.1. Suture the electronics case (metallic disc) in the superotemporal quadrant (*arrowheads*). Use silicone-tipped forceps to carefully reflect the cable and array over the cornea. A centered position confirms appropriate extraocular placement. Position the racetrack-appearing receiving coil under the lateral rectus muscle, also with a securing suture inferotemporally (*asterisk*).

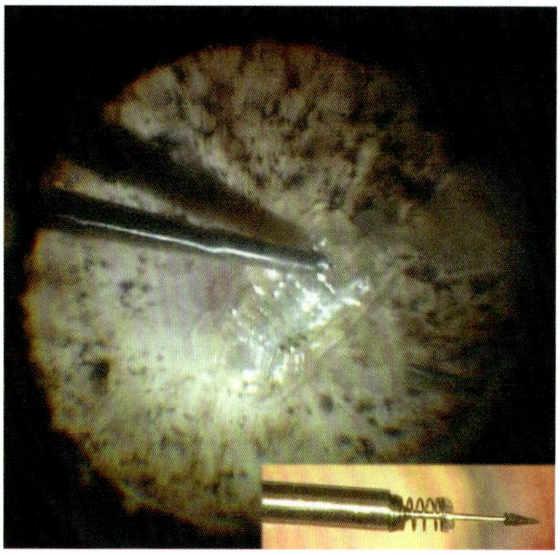

FIGURE 68.2. Use a retinal tack on specialized 19G Tack forceps to fixate the array to the retina/choroid/sclera centered over the fovea.

- Create a <5.5-mm sclerotomy in the superotemporal quadrant. This sclerotomy should be a clean linear cut centered over the cable.
- Use 20G Eckhardt forceps to engage the array handle and insert the array into the vitreous cavity.
- Close the <5.5-mm sclerotomy with multiple 6-0 Vicryl sutures with long passes to help with complete closure. An optional purse-string suture around the cable may also be helpful. Ensure that this sclerotomy is watertight.
- Remove the nasal vitrectomy cannula and enlarge the sclerotomy to >19G for insertion of the Tack forceps.
- Use the Tack forceps to place a tack through a securing ring on the array and through the retina/choroid/sclera to center the array over the fovea (Fig. 68.2). Various unimanual or bimanual techniques for this step have been described.
- Remove the vitrectomy cannulas and close the sclerotomies (sutured as needed).
- Place a 9-0 Prolene mattress suture to flatten the short extraocular course of array cable.
- Cover the electronics case and coil suture tabs with Tutoplast (RTI Surgical Inc) or corneal graft sutured to the surrounding sclera.
- Close conjunctiva and Tenon's with particular attention over the electronics to ensure complete coverage.

POSTOPERATIVE CONSIDERATIONS

- Patient recovery is similar to a SB procedure.
- A few weeks following recovery, the device is programmed and turned on for the first time, followed by visual rehabilitation.
- Postop complications include hypotony, usually due to leakage from the superotemporal cable sclerotomy, conjunctival erosion, and rarely retinal detachment and endophthalmitis.

CHAPTER 69

Physiology of Vitreous Surgery

Jóhann Ragnar Guðmundsson, MD • Einar Stefánsson, MD, PhD

The idea behind vitreous surgery was entirely mechanical in the beginning. The notion that vitreous surgery would have physiological or biochemical consequences was not considered at all. However, the delayed clinical effects of vitreous surgery soon became apparent.

THE LONG-TERM CLINICAL EFFECTS OF VITRECTOMY

In the early 1980s, George Blankenship and Robert Machemer noticed that NVE did not recur following PPV in eyes with PDR. The mechanical way of thinking was so strong that most surgeons sought mechanical explanations for the disappearance of NV. The most popular explanation was that the vitreous gel provided a mechanical scaffold for new vessel formation, and without this scaffold, the new vessel growth would not take place. The exception that proved the rule was the observation was that in areas still covered by vitreous gel, new vessels may still grow. Blankenship and Machemer also documented that while NVE stopped after PPV, there was an increased risk of NVI and NVG.

It was a decade later that Hilel Lewis (1992) pointed out that not only does NVE stop in diabetic eyes after PPV but diabetic macular edema (DME) also improves following PPV. Lewis did maintain the mechanical school of thought and focused on vitreoretinal traction and DME. It has since become apparent that PPV reduces DME, even if traction is not present.

The long-term consequences of vitreous surgery were not entirely beneficial. The vitreoretinal surgeons at the Wilmer Eye Institute under the leadership of Ronald G. Michels reported that the risk of cataract is substantially increased following PPV. Later, Stanley Chang (2006) proposed that PPV also influenced IOP and might increase the risk for glaucoma.

None of these clinical consequences was expected by the early vitreous surgeons and no realistic explanation was being offered. However, while these clinical phenomena were being documented by Robert Machemer, Brooks McCuen, and their fellows on the main floor of the Duke Eye Center, the physiological mechanisms were already being studied in the basement.

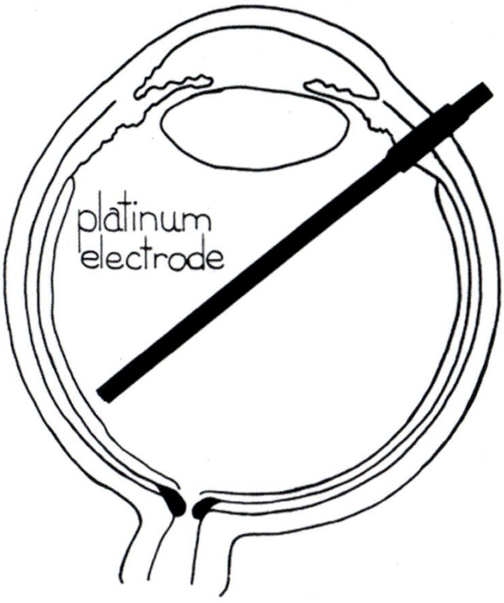

FIGURE 69.1. A polarographic oxygen sensor placed into the eye through the pars plana across the vitreous cavity to measure oxygen tension at the retinal surface. (From Stefánsson et al. (1981) with permission from the American Ophthalmological Society.)

PHYSIOLOGICAL MECHANISMS OF VITREOUS SURGERY

Following Robert Machemer's arrival at the Duke Eye Center in 1978, it quickly became the premier vitreous surgery center in the world. The following year, in the basement of the Duke Eye Center, Reece Landers and Mike Wolbarsht recruited an Icelandic graduate student to study the oxygen physiology of the eye, and this quickly developed into research on the physiology of vitreous surgery. They vitrectomized cats and used polarographic electrodes to measure oxygen level in the eye (Fig. 69.1).

In 1981, the first publication by Stefánsson et al demonstrated that vitreous surgery in cats influences the oxygen distribution and levels within the eye (Fig. 69.2).

Later in the same decade and still working in the basement of the Duke Eye Center, Stefánsson, Roger Novack, and Dianne Hatchell demonstrated that PPV prevents retinal hypoxia as a consequence of BRVO in cats (Fig. 69.3) (1990). At the time, the most credible explanation for this effect on oxygen distribution and metabolism was found in the fluid currents in the vitreous cavity (Fig. 69.4). The vitreous gel is viscous and fluid currents are therefore very slow. When the viscous gel is removed and

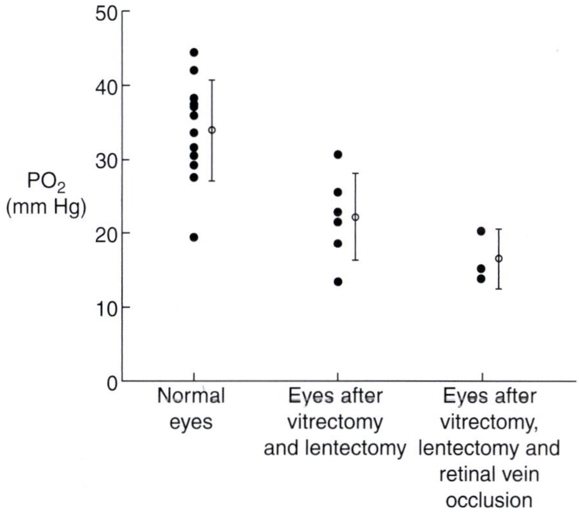

FIGURE 69.2. Oxygen tension in the aqueous humor in cats following vitrectomy and lens extraction. (From Stefánsson et al. (1981) with permission from the American Ophthalmological Society.)

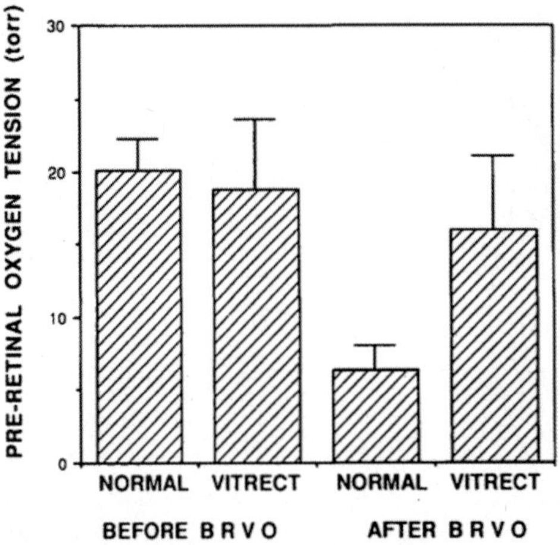

FIGURE 69.3. Retinal oxygen tension at the retinal surface in normal and vitrectomized cat eyes with and without BRVO. (From Stefánsson et al. (1990) with permission from Investigative Ophthalmology and Visual Science.)

replaced with saline and ultimately aqueous humor, the viscosity is much less and fluid currents are free to flow. Indeed, Robert Machemer confirmed at the time that such fluid currents are clinically visible in vitrectomized eyes.

Twenty years later, Svandis Gisladottir, Thorsteinn Loftsson, and Stefansson, now working in Iceland, pointed out that these phenomena were entirely predictable using the axioms of classical physics. The critical fact is that the vitreous gel is viscous and this regulates the transport of molecules within the vitreous cavity. When the gel is removed and replaced with water, the viscosity is reduced from 5 to 200 centipoise (cp) in vitreous gel to 1 cp in water and transport of molecules becomes at least 5 times faster.

The Hagen-Poiseuille equation stipulates that fluid currents are inversely related to the viscosity of the medium. Similarly, Fick's law and the Stokes-Einstein equation propose that rate of diffusion is also inversely related to the viscosity of the medium. What this means is that all transport of molecules is slow in the vitreous gel but is greatly increased when the vitreous gel has been replaced with water. This influence on molecular transport within the eye is not limited to oxygen but includes all molecules that are transported, such as drug molecules, VEGF, and others.

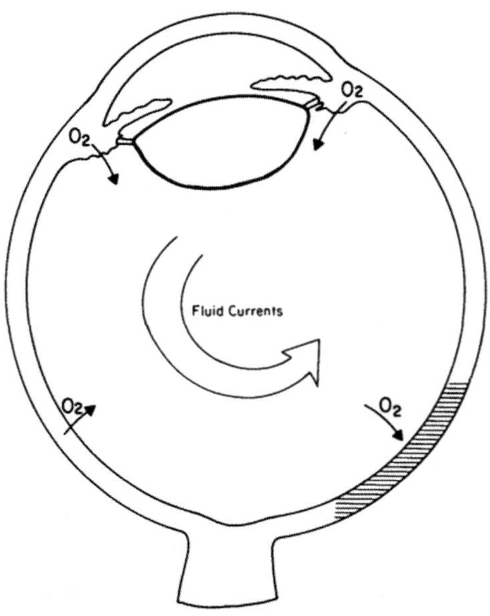

FIGURE 69.4. A schematic drawing explaining how fluid currents in the vitrectomized vitreous cavity transport oxygen from well-perfused areas of the retina to the nonperfused and hypoxic areas. (From Stefánsson et al. (1990) with permission from Investigative Ophthalmology and Visual Science.)

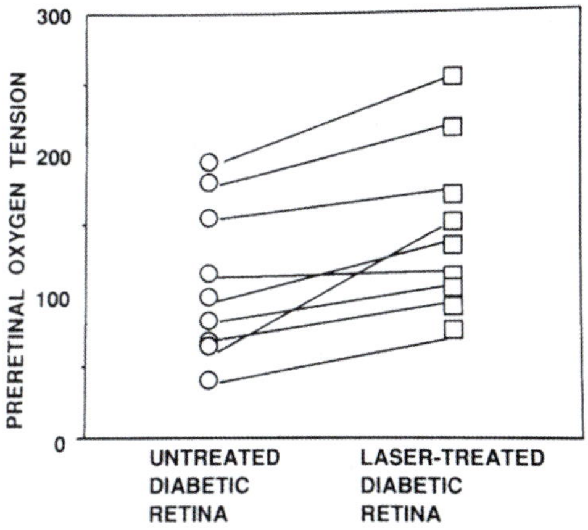

FIGURE 69.5. Oxygen tension in human diabetic eyes in the vitreous cavity over untreated and laser-treated areas of the same eye. The probes were placed by Robert Machemer, Brooks McCuen, and Eugene de Juan, Jr. (From Stefánsson et al. (1992), with permission from the American Journal of Ophthalmology.)

All of these studies were conducted in animals. The Duke group did take some of the first steps to develop oxygen sensors suitable for human studies. A fiberoptic sensor was first tested in diabetic dogs (1989) and then a major study of retinal oxygenation in human eyes was conducted in Duke Eye Center operating rooms by the vitreoretinal team at the time, Robert Machemer, Brooks McCuen, Eugene de Juan, Jr., and Einar Stefánsson using pars plana transvitreal fiberoptic probes to measure oxygen tension (Fig. 69.5).

A decade later, Nancy Holekamp and DC Beebe used similar oxygen sensitive optical fibers to advance this field in the human eye. Holekamp and Beebe demonstrated that after PPV, oxygen levels in the eye are indeed altered (Fig. 69.6) and oxygen

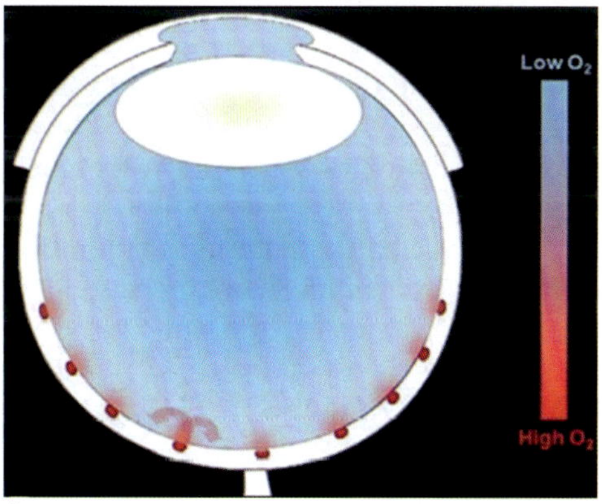

A

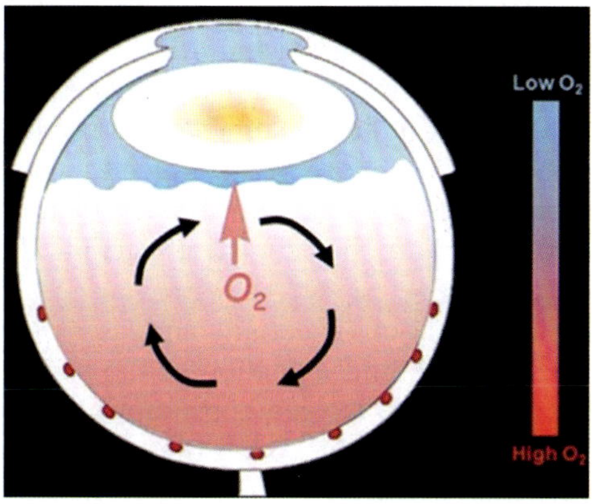

B

FIGURE 69.6. A, B. A schematic drawing showing the change in oxygen transport following vitrectomy. (From Beebe et al. (2010) with permission from Ophthalmic Research.)

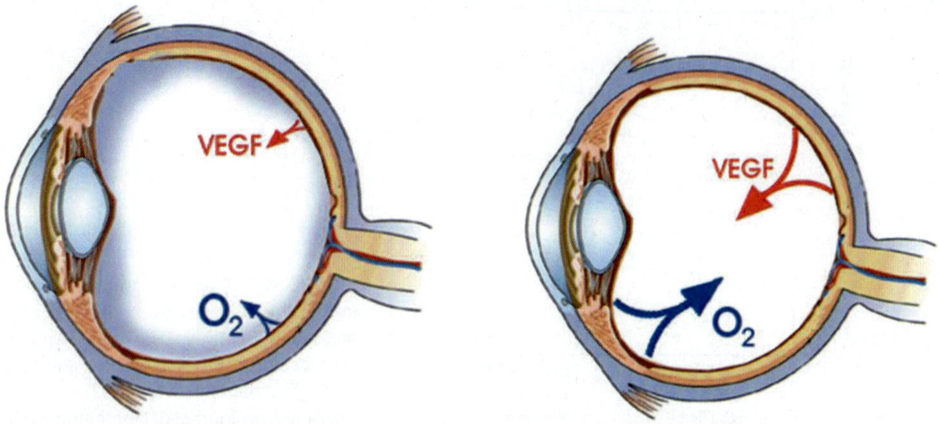

FIGURE 69.7. The *left image* depicts the slow transport of oxygen and VEGF (and other molecules) in an eye with intact vitreous humor. The *right image* shows the relatively fast transport of molecules following PPV.

gradients flatten; they confirmed the basic principles previously demonstrated in the cats in the basement of the Duke Eye Center. They acknowledged the fluid currents and also pointed out the influence of ascorbate working as an antioxidant in the vitreous gel.

The physiological changes following vitreous surgery are shown schematically in Figure 69.7. Following PPV, the transport of oxygen and all other molecules is at least five times faster than in the nonvitrectomized eye. This has several consequences:

- Oxygen can diffuse from well-perfused areas of the retina to those areas that are nonperfused and hypoxic and thereby reduce hypoxia and the production of hypoxia induced growth factors, that is, VEGF.
- Hypoxia-induced growth factors such as VEGF that are produced in the retina can easily diffuse into the fluid in the vitreous cavity and be transported away through fluid currents and/or diffusion. The accumulation of VEGF in the retina is thereby reduced.
- Oxygen diffuses more readily from the retina to the anterior portion of the vitreous cavity and to the crystalline lens where oxygen levels are increased and cataract formation stimulated.

VITRECTOMY AND LASER TREATMENT HAVE SOME OF THE SAME CONSEQUENCES

In the early days of vitreous surgery and retinal laser photocoagulation, the empirical effects of these treatment modalities on NV were well documented. However, the popular physiological explanations at the time were primitive and mostly mechanical. We previously mentioned the obsolete thesis of the vitreous gel being a necessary scaffold for vascular growth. The most popular explanation for the effect for laser photocoagulation was that it destroyed hypoxic retinal tissue and thereby reduced the production of vascular growth factors. Both of these theses had many obvious problems and they certainly did not explain why laser and vitrectomy had similar effects on NV as well as DME.

The unifying principle for the clinical effect of vitrectomy and laser photocoagulation was proposed in the 1980s. Panretinal photocoagulation of the retina destroys 20%-30% of the photoreceptors. This reduces the oxygen consumption of the outer retina and allows oxygen to diffuse from the choroid through the laser scars into the inner retina where it reduces retinal hypoxia. Reduced hypoxia results in reduced production of hypoxia-induced growth factors, such as VEGF.

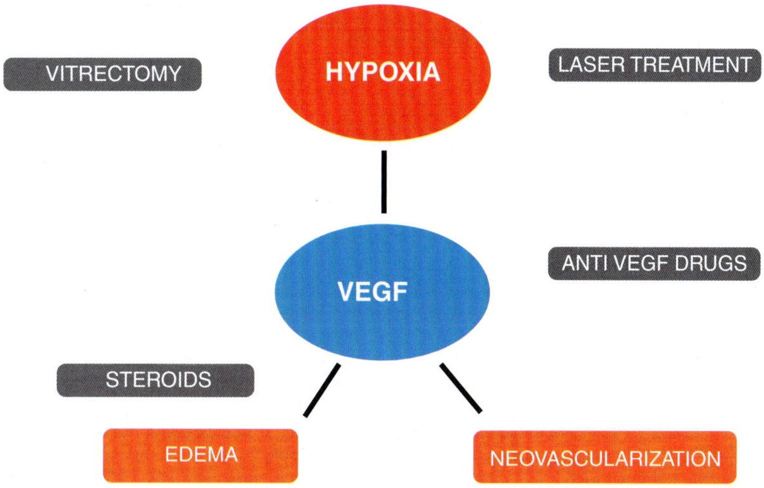

FIGURE 69.8. Retinal ischemia (nonperfusion) causes hypoxia, which stimulates production of VEGF, resulting in edema and new vessel formation. Retinal hypoxia is mitigated by either PPV and/or laser photocoagulation of the retina. Both vitrectomy and anti-VEGF drugs reduce VEGF levels in the retina. Steroids do that also to some degree and reduce vascular permeability.

From the other side of the retina, the removal of the vitreous gel allows oxygen to diffuse to the hypoxic inner retina from well-perfused areas of the same retina and thereby reduces VEGF formation. At the same time, VEGF that is produced can escape into the vitreous cavity and be transported away through the fluid currents and diffusion.

Both vitrectomy and laser photocoagulation thereby reduce retinal hypoxia, reduce VEGF concentration in the retina, and thereby reduce both new vessel formation and edema formation. This way, one physiological principle explains both clinical phenomena and multiple explanations may not be needed (Fig. 69.8).

The interplay of laser and vitrectomy is demonstrated in Figure 69.8. This thesis also explains why panretinal photocoagulation and vitrectomy can be complementary in treating PDR. For example, eyes that have recurrent VH following panretinal photocoagulation can be treated with PPV, which not only removes the VH but also reduces the risk of further neovascularization and recurrent hemorrhage.

HOW VITRECTOMY INTERACTS WITH INTRAVITREAL ANTI-VEGF INJECTIONS

Injecting antibodies against VEGF into the vitreous gel has a similar effect on intraocular VEGF levels as does vitrectomy. In a normal eye, the presence of anti-VEGF antibodies in the vitreous gel creates a gradient where VEGF diffuses from the retina into the vitreous gel where it is neutralized by the antibodies. Following vitreous surgery, the VEGF molecules diffuse from the retina into the fluid in the vitreous cavity and are transported away with fluid currents and/or diffusion. This way, the removal of VEGF from the retinal tissue can continue and the VEGF molecules disappear into the vitreous cavity. From the standpoint of the retina, it makes no difference whether the VEGF disappears into the mouth of an antibody or is transported away with fluid currents in the vitreous cavity. In both cases, the VEGF leaves the retina and does not accumulate as it otherwise would have. In this way we can understand why PPV, laser treatment of the retina, and injection of antibodies into the vitreous cavity have some of the same effects on DME, PDR, and other ischemic retinopathies. This is shown schematically in Figure 69.7.

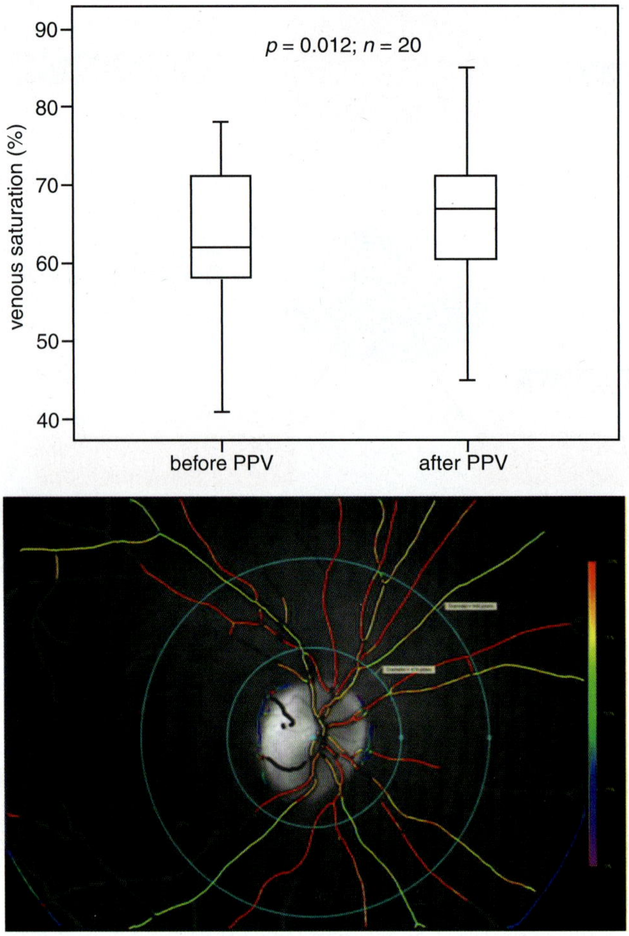

FIGURE 69.9. Top: Retinal venous oxygen saturation before and after PPV. **Bottom:** Retinal oximetry image. (With permission from Sin et al. (2014, 2016) Acta Ophthalmologica.)

RETINAL OXIMETRY AND VITRECTOMY

The physiological studies reviewed above all rely on invasive technologies and oxygen-sensitive probes that were inserted into eyes of animals or patients undergoing vitreous surgery. Over the last two decades, a noninvasive retinal oximeter has been developed that is used in noninvasive clinical studies to better understand the physiology of the vitreous (Fig. 69.9) and the sequelae following its absence (Sin et al. 2014, 2016 and Stefánsson et al. 2019).

CONCLUSION

The Duke Eye Center was pivotal in the rise of vitreous surgery and its application in ophthalmology. At the same time, the Duke Eye Center vitreoretinal group played a crucial role in understanding the physiological mechanisms that explain the clinical consequences of vitreous surgery.

Index

Note: Page numbers followed by "*b*", "*f*", and "*t*" indicate boxes, figures and tables, respectively.

C

D

E

R